Behavioral Concepts and Nursing Throughout the Life Span

Sharon L. Roberts
Associate Professor
California State University, Long Beach

Prentice-Hall, Inc., Englewood Cliffs, N.J. 07632

Library of Congress Cataloging in Publication Data

ROBERTS, SHARON L (date)
 Behavioral concepts and nursing throughout the life span.

 Bibliography: p.
 Includes index.
 1. Nursing—Psychological aspects. 2. Hospital
patients—Psychology. I. Title.
RT86.R56   610.73'01'9   77-10970
ISBN 0-13-074559-6
ISBN 0-13-074567-7 pbk.

10   9   8   7   6   5

Printed in the United States of America

PRENTICE-HALL INTERNATIONAL, INC., *London*
PRENTICE-HALL OF AUSTRALIA PTY. LIMITED, *Sydney*
PRENTICE-HALL OF CANADA, LTD., *Toronto*
PRENTICE-HALL OF INDIA PRIVATE LIMITED, *New Delhi*
PRENTICE-HALL OF JAPAN, INC., *Tokyo*
PRENTICE-HALL OF SOUTHEAST ASIA PTE. LTD., *Singapore*
WHITEHALL BOOKS LIMITED, *Wellington, New Zealand*

To

*My parents who by their own example have taught me
the importance of caring*

*My students who throughout the years have taught me
the art of patience*

*My friend Geron who has taught me
the joy of creativity*

Contents

Foreword

The nursing profession's very special contribution to the health of people lies in its ability to provide holistic, continuous, and integrated care. Nurses who are well-grounded in theories from the biological, psychological, and social sciences from which nursing derives its theoretical base, and who can synthesize this knowledge in order to apply it, are able to provide high-quality nursing care to their patients. Today, due to technological advances in hospital monitoring-mechanisms and life-sustaining devices, there is a tendency toward care that is fractionated, depersonalized, and isolated. It is now absolutely essential that nurses understand and foster the relationshipa that help a patient regain or retain behavioral integrity.

Through the integrating mechanism of the systems model, Sharon Roberts skillfully focuses on each of the eleven major behaviors common to all hospitalized patients while not losing sight of the total human being. In addition, she describes and analyzes the balance of relationships among patients, family, and health providers, their critical interactions, and the influencing factors such as economic, educational, health, social, and those involving roles, expectations, and power relationships. Sharon Roberts stresses many times and in different ways that nurses must acknowledge, accept, and understand behavioral phenomena.

By her use of carefully selected examples, the author assists the student in gaining an understanding of the open systems theory as a model for the interaction of the patient with his or her environment. As a result, the student will be closer to attaining the goal of providing holistic care and maintaining the delicate balance of all interrelated systems.

Through a unique presentation of the major behaviors present in hospitalized persons, the systems theory, and its application to nursing practice, Sharon Roberts has given the nursing profession and its many practitioners and students a valuable and needed reference. I believe this volume will make a significant advance toward our goal of providing high-quality nursing care.

School of Nursing   *Rheba de Tornyay, R.N., Ed.D.*
University of Washington   *Dean and Professor*
Seattle, Washington

Preface

Nursing has steadily evolved into an independent discipline. As this development has continued, educators and practitioners have explored new areas in which the nurse can initiate and implement health care programs independent of the physician. It is exciting to note that one such area is the behavioral domain. Behavioral concepts have been discussed by educators, integrated into school curricula, and applied to one age group or another at various times.

This book covers the most frequently utilized behavioral concepts as applied to all age groups. Because the child, adult, and aged patient is dealt with comprehensively, this book is unique. In this respect, it has significance for undergraduate and graduate students, as well as practitioners.

Incorporated into the discussion of each behavior is the author's belief in the humanistic approach to health care. For it is the nurse who can assess a patient's loneliness, powerlessness, body image disturbance, or pain. It is the nurse who can formulate and carry out a plan to alleviate these feelings and to help a patient keep a sense of dignity, worth, and positive self-concept. The author hopes that this book will inspire its readers to research the behavioral aspect of nursing, to develop the ability to detect potentially harmful behavior, and to apply the behavioral concepts to help the patient as a human being.

I wish to express my gratitude to the people who have encouraged me in this endeavor and to those who have taught me the joy of caring for the well-being of others.

Sharon L. Roberts

Behavioral Concepts
and
Nursing
Throughout
the Life Span

1
Open System

Man, as a living open system, is subject to the universal laws of nature, allowing us to use the principles and concepts of systems theory in the field of human biology. Buckley has said that "we cannot make a neat division of those things that are and those that are not systems; rather, we shall have to recognize varying degrees of systemness. And if we also recognize that the substances or entities that the various scientific disciplines study—nuclear particles, atoms, molecules, solar systems, cells, organs, organisms, ecological communities, societies—are all subsumable under a definition of system, then we seem forced to accept the notion of varying degrees of 'entity.' "[1] The systems model provides an overall conceptual framework by which otherwise unconnected parts may be integrated. The individual is composed of a well organized system of molecules, cells, organs, and a system of organs. The individual is a unique whole because of this highly integrated system. When interacting with the environment, however, the individual becomes aware that he or she is simply one of many within the social hierarchy.

Therefore, as a concept applied to care of the hospitalized patient, the systems theory is concerned with the total system; namely, the whole individual, not simply the subsystems or parts. An open system interacts with its environment and with other systems such as the health team, family, or friends. The patient interacts with the environment, the setting in which care is received. This setting varies according to a particular patient's age and biological or emotional problem. Interaction with the environment takes any one of several forms. The individual may interact verbally, behaviorally, socially, or physically with the environment. However, there are times when an individual finds the immediate environment too threatening for meaningful interaction. Take, for example, a newly admitted patient experiencing biological or emotional crisis. The

[1]Walter Buckley, *Sociology and Modern Systems Theory*, (New Jersey: Prentice-Hall, Inc., 1967), p. 42.

patient may be too involved with biological crisis, anxieties, and fears to interact with the environment or the people therein. To members of the health team, the behavioral response is understood in light of the presenting problems.

A system refers to a set of parts or components with a relationship between the parts and between the property of the parts. In the hospital, the system consists of three subsystems; the patient, the family and the health team. The patient's physical state can improve or decline; the family's anxiety can increase or decrease; and, the health team's involvement can intensify or subside. Therefore, "A system model assumes that organization, interdependency, and integration exists among its parts and that change is a derived consequence of how well the parts of the system fit together, or how well the system fits in with other surrounding and interacting systems."[2]

SYSTEMS THEORY COMPONENTS DEFINED

Living Organisms

A living organism, as an open system, is continually exchanging matter with the outer world, while maintaining or approaching a variation of a steady-state. Therefore, the living organism contains many interrelated elements. As a system it is capable of developing as states of order, organization, differentiation, or disintegration. Wholeness, growth, differentiation, hierarchial order, dominance, control, and competition are characteristics of organization for both living organisms and societies. According to the law of instability, many organizations do not exist as a stable equilibrium but show cyclic fluctuations resulting from the interaction of subsystems.[3] Interaction among the patient, the environment, and the health team can result in instability or stability of the behavioral system.

The hospitalized patient regardless of age or problem represents a living system. The living system consists of both matter and energy, which is organized by an information system. The living system is able to exchange content with the outside environment through the information system. This process of exchange is possible through communication. For

[2]Robert Chin, "The Utility of System Models and Developmental Models For Practitioner," *Conceptual Models for Nursing Practice*, (Ed: Callista Roy and Joan Riehl), (New York: Appleton-Century Crofts, 1974), p. 60.

[3]Ludwig von Bertalanffy, *General Systems Theory*, (New York: George Brazillen Inc., 1968), p. 27.

the living human system to survive, it must have adequate information and the ability to process the information as it relates to previous or current experiences. Thus, communication is an important aspect of the interaction process between the patient and the significant people in the patient's environment.

Matter and Energy

Matter and energy are both integral parts of the system and its environment. Matter is anything that has mass and occupies space, whereas energy is the ability to do work. There are two types of energy: kinetic and potential. Kinetic energy is energy of movement, and movement is work. Anything capable of doing work has potential or stored energy. Patients may have an excess or deficiency of stored energy. Just as the patient represents an energy system, the family and health team symbolize social energy systems. Anderson states "The energy derives from a complex of sources including the physical capacities of its members; social resources such as loyalties, shared sentiments, and common values; and resources from its environment."[4] In other words, the system is capable of actions and has power to bring about change or it can simply maintain itself in its existing state.

Open System Versus Closed System

There are basically two types of systems within the framework of systems theory. The first type is a closed system. By definition, a closed system is one in which matter and energy are not exchanged with environment. Mathematics and physics are common examples of this. People can have a tendency toward closure. In behavioral terms, both the nurse and patient can become closed systems. The patient may refuse to take medication, limit fluid intake, exercise an arthritic arm, limit activity, or participate in group therapy. Likewise members of the health team may unintentionally or unknowingly become closed to input from the patient. The child may want to watch a favorite program instead of having treatment that could be given at anytime. A schizophrenic patient may desire to interact with one individual rather than a group. Likewise a geriatric patient may want to sleep rather than be bathed. Regardless of each patient, the nurse's goal becomes focused on the patient's treatment, group involvement, or bath. Thus the nurse and patient each share

[4]Ralph Anderson, *Human Behavior and Social Environment: A Social System Approach,* (Chicago: Aldine Publishing Company, 1974), p. 11.

different goals. The nurse's tendency to closure may stem from environmental pressures such as the need to complete certain time-oriented tasks. Such closure can result in depersonalization. In addition, closed systems lose their sense of organization because both individuals view the other's goal as intrusive. Buckley has stated that "The typical response of natural, closed systems to an intrusion of environmental events is a loss of organization, or a change in the direction of dissolution of the system."[5] To avoid depersonalization and disorganization, the nurse should assess the personal meaning of the patient's goal.

The second type of system is an open system. An open system is one that exchanges matter with its environment, building up and breaking down its material components, presenting intake and output. Under certain conditions, open systems approach a time-independent state, called a steady-state. Man represents an open system. The open system responds to external stimuli in its environment. Unlike the closed system, the open system responds to environmental intrusion with organization and change.

Buckley and others have made various distinctions between open and closed systems. "The important distinction between open and closed systems has often been expressed in terms of entropy: closed systems tend to increase in entropy—to run down; open systems are negentropic—tending to decrease in entropy or to elaborate structure."[6]

Entropy, Negentropy, and Equifinality

Entropy has been defined as that quantity of energy within a system that is not capable of conversion into work. The second principle of thermodynamics states that, "in a closed system, a certain quantity, called entropy, must increase to a maximum, and eventually the process comes to a stop at a state of equilibrium."[7] The changes of entropy in a closed system are always positive; order is continually destroyed. Open systems exhibit both increased and decreased entropy, because of their reversible and irreversible processes. Thus, living systems, maintaining themselves in a steady-state, can avoid the increase of entropy and may even develop toward a state of increased order and organization.

Negentropy is a measure of the order of the system and may be referred to as energy that is available to do work. Therefore negentropy is

[5]Buckley, *Sociology and Modern Systems Theory*, p. 50.

[6]Leon Brillovin, "Life Thermodynamics and Cybernetics," *American Scientist*, Volume 37, 1949, pp. 554–568.

[7]Bertalanffy, *General System Theory*, p. 39.

the tendency toward order and organization. Equifinality involves moving toward a final state and is based upon dynamic interaction in an open system attaining a steady-state. In other words, the open system may attain a time-independent state.

Feedback

Applied to the living organism, the feedback scheme is called homeostasis. Homeostasis is the ensemble of regulations that maintain constant variables and direct the organism toward a goal. These regulations are performed by feedback mechanisms; that is, the result of the reaction is monitored back to the "receptor" side so that the system is held stable or led to a target or goal.

The living organism is an open system, maintaining itself in, or approaching, a steady-state. Superposed are those regulations that are controlled by fixed arrangements, especially of the feedback type. This evolves from a general principle of organization known as progressive mechanization. Initially, it is the dynamic interaction of their components that governs biological, neurological, psychological, or social systems. Then fixed arrangements and conditions or constraints take shape. They render the system and its parts more efficient but also gradually diminish and eventually abolish its equipotentiality.[8]

Self Regulation

A characteristic of living open systems is that they are capable of self-regulation, or steady-state. Input in the form of matter, energy, and information taken into the system is subsequently released to the environment. It represents a balanced relationship between parts that is not necessarily dependent upon a fixed equilibrium. There are times, as shall be discussed later, when the hospitalized patient reaches a premature steady-state or fixed balance. For the most part, the living organism is able to advance to a higher order of organization. "When self-regulatory processes fail, the system may be referred to as diseased and may be so altered as not to survive. Disease is the process whereby the living system attempts to return within the predetermined variable limits after some disturbance has shifted these. This is an expression of the dynamic tendency of living systems to maintain and reestablish as far as possible the steady-state."[9]

[8]*Ibid.*, p. 44.

[9]Mary Hazard, "Overview of Systems Theory," *Nursing Clinics of North America,* Volume 6, September 1971, p. 390.

THE PURPOSE OF THE SYSTEMS
APPROACH

Systems approach can be a helpful tool for the health team, particularly the nurse. It helps the nurse to understand the relationships that link the elements of systems in a significant way. The hospitalized patient appears as a complex of unrelated parts. Various specialists examine pulmonary, cardiovascular, neurological, renal, and psychological systems. Nurses and other members of the health team must be concerned with the patient's totality, not just elements or parts. The nurse attempts to integrate all elements or parts, realizing that behavioral disturbances are a system of disturbances, rather than a single malfunction.

Systems approach helps the nurse remember that each patient system interrelates with others. Therefore, while directly caring for one system, the nurse is indirectly caring for all patient systems. Each system, whether behavioral, physiological, environmental, or social, should be open and in communication with the others. The patient's behavioral system affects and is affected by physiological, environmental, social, or family systems. These systems together with demographic variables become the praxis around which the health team functions. For example, the patient may be anxious about an illness and may react to the environment through anger or negativism. The significant people in the immediate environment may consist of the nurse and family. These people, as receivers of the patient's feelings of anger, experience temporary alteration. They may feel hurt by the patient's sudden behavioral display, and may alter their approach to the patient. They may choose to rationalize, avoid, or handle the patient's feelings as well as their own. The nurse realizes a dynamic relationship among the nurse-patient-family system that causes the parts to behave differently. The family system may not understand the emotional outburst of a wife, husband, mother, or father, failing to realize that the patient is coping on a different level. The family member may have accepted the crisis, which might anger the patient who still denies that a crisis exists. Therefore, it is important to understand not only the elements of a system but also their overall organization, which may control behavior resulting from internal tension. According to Buckley, "tension, in the broad sense, of which 'stress' and 'strain' are manifestations under conditions of felt blockage, is ever present in one form or another throughout the sociocultural system."[10]

Illness can be the origin of a patient's tension. If illness or admission

[10]Buckley, *Sociology and Modern Systems Theory*, p. 51.

into unfamiliar territory are new experiences for the patient, coping abilities may be limited. Thelen believes that "man is continually meeting situations with which he cannot quite cope. In stress situations, energy is mobilized and a state of tension is produced. The state of tension tends to be disturbing, and man seeks to reduce the tension."[11] In this respect, a patient's anger becomes a way of reducing tension.

The open system model provides an organizational framework for the holistic assessment of individuals. The overall purpose of an open system model is to integrate otherwise unconnected parts.

APPLICATION OF OPEN SYSTEM
MODEL TO PATIENT CARE

There are four elements of an open system, as indicated by the following flow chart, that have significant application to the hospitalized patient.

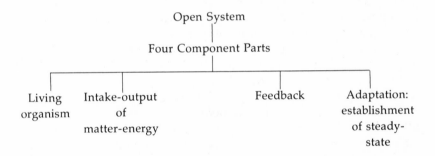

The open system model is a living organism which is continually exchanging matter with the outer world. It seeks to maintain this continuous exchange in a steady-state, or to approach such a steady-state in its variation.

The Living Organism

All living organisms are open systems. As open systems, they are in contact with their environment by means of input and output across system boundaries. Normally the open system is responsible for choosing and deciding those things that alter one's life. In health, the individual

---

[11]Herbert Thelen, "Emotionality and Work in Groups," *The State of Social Science*, (Ed: Leonard White), (Chicago: University of Chicago Press, 1956), pp. 184–186.

has selective control over life. However during illness control is reduced or altered. The hospitalized patient, regardless of the biological crisis, loses freedom of choice and decision-making ability. Of course the loss is dependent upon the severity of the biological or emotional crisis. One must also recognize that what appears to be an insignificant curtailment of decision-making activities for the health team can be interpreted as significant losses to the patient. What is defined as reality by one open system may not be similarly defined by the other interacting open system.

While in the hospital, the patient comes in contact with other systems: nurses, family, friends, doctors, technicians, and the environment. Of all systems with which the patient interacts, it is probably the nurse who is most influential. Doctors enter and leave the patient's intimate territory, but the nurse remains to explain and interpret the confusion created by meaningless technical jargon. The nurse sometimes curtails activities within the patient's environment in order to protect him. Take for example the newly admitted critically ill patient. When the patient arrives in a critical care unit, a nurse makes the decisions involving connection to various monitoring devices that restrict his activity. The patient may feel that partial control over intake and output of matter and energy has been lost, and this loss of control to machines and strangers becomes a threat to the critically ill patient.

Furthermore, the patient loses temporary control over his biological well-being. Prior to hospitalization, the individual's biologically healthy state permitted movement through his or her environment and the ability to make beneficial decisions. Suddenly a biological crisis occurs and the individual is in a strange environment while he or she is dependent upon others. This in itself can be a threatening experience. Whatever the biological crisis, the injured or diseased system now assumes control over the individual. It gains controls through pain, temporary immobility, complications, or the fear of death. Hopefully, in time, the living organism's biological crisis reaches a level of stability. The patient hopes that the losses associated with the disease will not constitute either continuous dependency on others or further physical immobility. As the body regains biological control, the patient can begin to think about the future.

The hospitalized patient is thrust into a future created by others. Keeping this in mind, the health team must include the patient and family in the planning of that future. Each system has the potential for dynamic interaction with the other. Such interaction helps the patient and family transcend the immediate situation, since each has the ability to take in and give out matter and energy to the environment.

Intake and Output of Matter and Energy

The intake system Matter and energy are an integral part of a system and its environment. In an open system, input and output are continuous and cyclic. The system receives energy from the environment, uses it, transforms it as needed, and then loses it in output to the environment where it is changed again. The intake system involves two components. First, there are internal and external patient variables. Second, there are boundaries that exist between the individual and the environment. Each component can directly and/or indirectly alter the amount of input received by the patient.

Variables as applied within the open system model are twofold. First, there are variables referred to as influencing systems. These include economic, educational, health, and social systems. The exorbitant cost of hospitalization is a major concern to most patients, especially the young male with an expanding family; the critically ill patient who conceivably can spend a month in critical care; and the aged patient on a fixed income whose insurance fails to cover the cost of all expenditures. In addition to the cost of the hospital room, the individual is subjected to various chargeable items such as diagnostic studies or treatment procedures. They are presented to the patient as necessary for confirming his diagnosis or treating his illness. Nothing is said of the validity of numerous unrelated diagnostic studies which serve to confirm one centralized problem, (e.g., myocardial infarction). In other words, the quantity of these studies does not insure the quality of diagnostic interpretation. It implies that the diagnostician is uncertain of the patient's biological problem. If one study is helpful, then several additional related studies will be even more helpful. Thus technology becomes diagnostic rather than clinical. As a result, patients are questioning the validity of these various diagnostic studies based on cost instead of diagnostic confirmation. The economic system can alter the patient's intake system. The patient's goal direction is to attain biological stability and then be home in the shortest period of time.

Education is another influencing system. Patients enter the hospital with varying educational backgrounds. Age is coupled with education. Needless to say, the small child has less experiential knowledge than the older patient. Since the patient is relating to a professional with years of formal and experiential knowledge, one may feel threatened to admit not understanding the technical jargon. In doing so one actually relinquishes power to professionals over one's being. In other words, one may agree to a diagnostic procedure or therapy due to a lack of understanding its implications or consequences. Nurses have a significant role to assess the patient's knowledge level and provide educational input that will enhance or reinforce the knowledge base to aid decision making. The nurse realizes that during the initial biological or emotional crisis the patient's intake system is limited, and besides assessing the knowledge level, must also assess the patient's readiness for such input.

Health is also an influencing system. Restoration to good health is the patient's primary goal. After the illness has been legitimized by a professional, the patient seeks ways to achieve wellness and thus return to all previous roles and obligations. How quickly these goals are accomplished depends upon the severity of and one's previous experience with illness. Naturally, more serious biological or emotional illness requires more time before one can return to a level of wellness. In addition, more serious biological losses imply that one may never completely achieve a total recovery. Previous experiential knowledge of illness can enhance or diminish the patient's intake system. For example, a patient hospitalized for the second time with bronchitis is hopeful that the biological problem can be stabilized. Finding success in previous treatments there is anticipation of the same success with the present therapy. On the other hand another respiratory patient hospitalized for the third time in one year because his biological problem is more complicated and serious, begins to have less hope in current therapeutic procedures resulting in a greatly diminished intake system.

The last major variable is the social system. The social system includes both the social unit or environment in which a patient is hospitalized and the various supportive subsystems including family, friends, and the health team. The social unit or environment has been defined as follows: "For a given system, the environment is the set of all objects a change in whose attributes affects the system, and also those objects whose attributes are changed by the behavior of the system."[12] The environment is the patterned wholeness of all that is external to a given individual. The constant interchange of matter and energy between man and environment is the basis of the patient's becoming and achieving being. Ideally the patient and social unit exchange matter and energy continually with one another, implying a transactional relationship between parts of the whole individual and the immediate environment.

The transactional relationship is not possible in a crisis. The adult or aged patient with acute myocardial infarction, respiratory failure, chronic renal failure, acute schizophrenia, or serious burns is an open system, but

[12]Martha Rogers, "Man An Open System" *Theoretical Basis of Nursing,* (Philadelphia: F. E. Davis Company, 1970), p. 52.

at times assumes some of the characteristics of a closed system. Anxiety related to the nature of the illness and the limitations it imposes can delay the patient's receptiveness to environmental stimuli. The nurse's goal is to alleviate anxiety, leaving the individual free to perceive both oneself and the surrounding world. For example, the young male patient who experiences his first massive myocardial infarction may be so anxious about his condition that he becomes closed to his environment. The anxious schizophrenic patient can also become closed to input from the immediate environment. Each individual's anxiety state only serves to reduce one's ability to interact with those people in the environment who could both explain uncertain events and reduce fears. The crisis state causes the patient to become a constricted being. The patient "curls up," reducing the input from his environment. The constricted patient can focus only upon the surgery, pain, or injury and may withdraw into sleep and lose all track of time. In this respect, the patient reaches a time-independent steady-state.

According to Combs, any physical disturbance that seriously reduces the energy reserves of the organism affects the scope of perception. When an individual is sick enough to be confined to a bed, alertness may be restricted by an inability to get around. Whatever decreases alertness has inevitable effects upon perceptive efficiency.[13] As a result, the individual may not perceive any supportive subsystems. The child views the parents as abandoning him or her when the need for their support is strongest. Adult or aged patients sometimes perceive professionals as being more interested in their pathology than in the factors which contribute to it. Patients experiencing acute biological or emotional crisis may not be permitted to visit with friends and may falsely see their friends as deserting them at a time when they need support. It must be remembered that what seems supportive to one individual can be perceived as threatening to another. The nurse may feel that he or she is offering supportive care in terms of treatments and emotional input, while the patient's integrity and sense of dignity is being threatened.

The second set of variables or influencing factors are less specific involving roles, expectations, and power relationships. As the individual's illness is legitimized by a diagnosis, he or she is forced to assume the sick role, which may be a new experience for the individual. Consequently, the patient is unaware of what is expected. Both these factors can contribute to an existing anxiety state which further reduces the environmental intake. In addition to role changes and expectations, the individual can become involved in power relationships. The power is usually maintained by the professionals providing the care. They main-

---

[13]Arthur Combs and Donald Snygg, *Individual Behavior*, (New York: Harper and Row, 1959), p. 72.

tain power by restricting the individual's activity, choices, and decision-making ability. Occasionally patients react to their loss of power and demonstrate behavior designed to gain control of their environment. This will be discussed as output system.

The second component of the intake system is boundaries, which can be related to variables influencing the individual. According to Chin, "We can delimit the system . . ., by placing our boundary according to what variables are being focused upon. We can construct a system consisting of the multiple roles of a person; or a system composed of varied roles among members in a small work group, or a system interrelating roles in a family."[14] A boundary can become a line forming a closed circle around certain variables, causing a reduction in exchange of energy across the line. Hopefully the boundary will remain open to energy exchange. The self has to have boundaries as the body has to have a skin. Just as there is a semipermeable membrane, or boundary, between the capillary and alveolar sac, there is a boundary between the patient and the environment. We can view the energy field of man as a whole encased in a permeable boundary contiguous with the permeable boundary of the environment. At the capillary-aveolar level, there is an exchange of oxygen and carbon dioxide. The diffusion of both gases depends on compliant lungs, adequate muscles, and alveoli that can be aerated. There are times when the membrane between the capillary and alveolar sac becomes altered due to fibrosis. The patient in biological or emotional crisis uses the "protective membrane" selectively to allow certain aspects of the environment in and to keep other aspects out. During the initial crisis, the patient maintains some kind of boundary, or selective screening, which is essential to the maintenance of the self. It follows that the nature of the hospital environment, whether it is seen by the patient to be facilitating or endangering, will determine the permeability or intake through this screen. The more facilitating a nurse can make the environment, the less need the patient will exhibit for protection. The more endangering or crisis-oriented the environment, the greater the need for protection, demonstrated by a decrease in the intake system.

Boundaries become definable only when the interaction between the system and the environment can be seen. "Some boundaries are visible because of their impenetrability, for example, the rigid personality that permits little interchange with the environment."[15] The schizophrenic patient's boundary becomes impermeable as a defense against external threats, such as the patient's family. Since not all family systems are supportive, the close interaction between family members can contribute to schizophrenic behavior. Anderson points out that, "The

[14]Chin, *Conceptual Models for Nursing Practice,* p. 49.
[15]Anderson, *Human Behavior and Social Environment,* p. 21.

boundary of a family is behavioral and is evidenced by the intensity and frequency of interaction among its components. . . . It is within the interactional boundaries of the family that the member participates in a particularly close network of feelings, both positive and negative, with a minimal sense of needing to put up a front."[16] The patient attempts to maintain a positive self-concept by limiting communicational exchange with others outside the family subsystem.

Regardless of the individual's biological or emotional problem, the nurse as one energy system attempts to exchange energy with the patient. Both open systems are linked with each other since the open system can never be totally passive. As the anxiety decreases, it receives less selected matter and energy from the environment, as energy transformation takes place within the intake and output system. The body as a system continually utilizes psychological, behavioral, and emotional energy as it strives toward behavioral equilibrium. Such energy should flow between the nurse and patient in the form of communication. The nurse and patient, as open systems, must have open communication. An important function of open communication is the presentation of information. The nurse's explanations become one way in which the patient picks up cues regarding any progress. This is possible because, "a solitary organism keeps its orienting system up to date in response to physical signs of the state of the environment, received by the sense organ. Communication is an extension of this process whereby some of the organizing work in one organism (patient) is attempted by another organism (nurse)."[17] As the patient becomes more active in seeking input from the environment, the output to the environment will be expanded.

The output system   Output is viewed as both physiological and emotional. Physiological output is measured through various diagnostic tests or procedures. The patient becomes frustrated because with each laboratory test or diagnostic procedure, a failing report card is received. Serum enzymes are elevated reflecting myocardial infarction; blood-gas changes reflect respiratory failure; or, personality studies reveal schizophrenia.

Emotionally the patient may manifest behavior associated with either reduced or excessive output. The patient who is constricted due to anxiety or immobility experiences reduced emotional output. Physical weakness and limited mobility often contribute to an emotional intolerance that complicates the process of recovery. Reduced emotional output

---

[16]*Ibid.*, pp. 107–108.

[17]David McKay, "The Informational Analysis of Questions and Commands," *Information Theory: Fourth London Symposium*, (Ed: Colin Cherry) (London: Butterworth, 1961), pp. 470–471.

can also occur because the patient loses autonomy over his or her body. In losing autonomy, one must "permit it to be handled and manipulated by those who purport to nurse him back to health. He is dressed and undressed; he is washed like an infant; while his bed is made he is pulled and pushed from one side to the other; the process of urination and defecation are suddenly no longer private; and he is subjected to the final indignity of having his nakedness exposed to the hospital personnel regardless of their sex."[18]

The hospitalized patient has been forced to absorb a variety of external environmental stimuli. People who profess to be supportive subsystems carry out diagnostic procedures on the patient. The patient's permeable membrane may have allowed relatively unimportant stimuli to pass by while blocking significant stimuli such as family visits. When the patient becomes less constricted as a system, there may be a feeling of lack of support from the family, even though their input was always present. As a result of reduced emotional output, the patient reacts behaviorally by becoming depressed, withdrawing, freezing, sleeping, or avoiding interaction with others. This behavior is normal when assessed in light of the praxis or influencing factors. To the patient the behavior is goal directed, conserving an already depleted emotional energy system. Depression, withdrawal, and avoidance behavior permits a temporary introspective retreat. The behavior is a protective defense understood only by the patient. For example, the patient with chronic respiratory failure focuses all energies toward the exhausting task of breathing. Likewise, the chronic schizophrenic or aged individual's energy may be invested in coping with a mobile and highly transitory environment. As the factors influencing behavior stabilize, the energies are directed outward, preparing the patient to interact with others. Buckley believes that, "The behaving individual—the psychological person—is essentially an organization that is developed and maintained only in and through a continually on going symbolic interchange with other persons."[19]

Depending upon the severity of the illness, the patient may not be able to care for oneself and may lack a vehicle for physical energy output. Nevertheless, input from the environment continue beyond control. Needs for protection prevent interaction with the environment as an open system. Such interaction, in the form of decision making and increased activity, dissipates energy. The health team either performs certain activities or assists in their accomplishment. As a result, the open patient's input of energy finally reaches the saturation point. Consequently, the patient is no longer able to receive additional input from the environment without some compensating output, which may be man-

[18]Sidney Smith, "The Psychology of Illness," *Nursing Forum*, Volume 3, 1964, p. 39.

[19]Buckley, *Sociology and Modern Systems Theory*, p. 44.

ifested in the form of overt and perhaps inappropriate behavior. Again it cannot be overly stressed that what seems to be inappropriate behavior to the health team, is perfectly rational and appropriate to the patient. Therefore, the patient's emotional output, in terms of behavior, must be assessed for its normalcy in view of the variables or influencing systems already discussed.

As the patient becomes less constricted, there are experiences of excessive emotional output. Behaviorally the emotional output is manifested as anger, hostility, or joviality. The patient's nonconstricted state heightens awareness of other feelings such as loneliness, hopelessness, or powerlessness. These behaviors can be physically or verbally expressed. A patient may verbally act out by yelling at a nurse or family member. If yelling doesn't facilitate emotional release, the same individual may act out by throwing an object or by physically striking anyone in the immediate environment. This could stem from an inability to express feelings of anger or frustration at having become ill. Once output as a behavioral response has occurred, the patient may experience guilt. The nurse must recognize that his behavior is an energy output mechanism. Furthermore, the nurse should understand that the patient almost involuntarily finds all concentration focused upon the individual misery, to the exclusion of whatever is happening in the surrounding environment. This causes the patient's system to become closed.

If the nurse acknowledges that the patient's behavior is an energy output system, permission will be given to express feelings verbally rather than physically. Once the significance of this behavior is realized, the nurse, with other members of the health team facilitate the achievement of a steady-state. This involves a feedback system between two open interacting systems.

Feedback

The concept of feedback is often represented by the example of homeostasis. A system may have both feedback within the system (internal feedback) and feedback that moves outside the system's boundary to the environment (external feedback). Input and output across the boundary implicates feedback as change. "While affecting the environment, a process we call output, systems gather information about how they are doing. Such information is then fed back into the system as input to guide and steer its operation."[20] Therefore the patient as an open system reacts only to the input received through its feedback system. Powers believes that, "Even when we speak of systems which deal in human interrela-

[20]Chin, *Conceptual Models for Nursing Practice*, p. 52.

tionships, these complex systems not only do not "care" about what is actually going on in the 'real' environment, they cannot even know what is going on 'out there.' They perform the sole function of bringing their feedback signals, the only reality they can perceive, to some reference-level, the only goal they know."[21]

The nurse, as an active member of the health team, receives feedback from a patient's internal environment. Such feedback consists of two types: internal biological and internal psychological feedback. Briefly stated, feedback from the patient's internal biological systems can be obtained through various diagnostic tests. The results of tests, whether negative or positive, reflect changes in the patient's internal biological being.

Internal psychological feedback is manifested through patient behaviors. The angry or hostile individual may be giving the nurse feedback regarding internal fears, frustrations, and stresses. Many patients do not know how to communicate these feelings to their nurse in a normal face-to-face dialogue. The admission of fears and anxieties for the male patient implies a loss of his masculinity. Consequently, such patients display their masculinity or self-assertiveness through more aggressive angry or hostile verbal feedback. Likewise the nurse needs to offer feedback on the normality of fears, frustrations, and anxieties, and their part in the illness experience. The patient's feelings may revolve around the forced dependency that illness creates. In addition there are feelings of guilt for leaving the family and work obligations. Each behavior whether it is actively or passively expressed requires energy that the patient needs for getting well.

The nurse should acknowledge, accept, and understand the patient's behavior. When necessary and realistic, permission is given to behave in a manner that seems appropriate (e.g., anger). Recognizing that a patient, as an open system, has vast potentialities and extensive strengths, the nurse should help that patient move beyond inappropriate behavioral outputs toward a positive and more beneficial steady-state. Achievement of a steady-state can be facilitated by offering positive feedback regarding learning and progress. The entire health team should help the living system use illness and crisis as a learning experience.

Adaptation: Establishment of Steady-State

An open system may attain a time-independent state, in which the system remains constant as a whole and in its phases, although there is a continuous flow of the component materials. This is called a

---

[21]W. T. Powers, "A General Feedback Theory of Human Behavior: Part I," *Perceptual and Motor Skills*, Volume 11, 1960, pp. 78–79.

steady-state.[22] The steady-state can also be referred to as self-regulation. Changes such as disease or illness can occur in an open system, causing an unsteady state. Normally the system attempts to achieve some balance among the internal and external influencing factors. This implies change and the understanding that, as an open system, the individual has the potential to change. Adaptation becomes the process of change, "whereby the individual retains his identity—his wholeness—within the reaction of his environment. A truly integrating system within the organism must be one that responds to environmental change, yet in the process defends the wholeness of the individual."[23] The individual moves toward a balance through adaptation and achievement of a steady-state.

After an emotional or biological crisis has occurred, the hospitalized patient can achieve one of two balances. First, one can adapt by reaching a fixed balance, a dependent steady-state in which the individual never moves beyond the limits of immediate illness. The individual behaviorally reaches a psychological fixed balance, becoming a psychological cripple and/or dependent upon supportive subsystems as the health team, the family, or technological equipment. The patient may fear the threat of another emotional or biological crisis, choosing to become an invalid or emotional cripple, failing to realize that although certain changes are necessary, one can continue with many aspects of the previous life style. To the professional team, the patient's psychologically fixed balance is not realistic in light of its knowledge and experience. However, to the patient the threat of additional illness becomes a reality. In a sense, the input boundary for changing to a higher level of wellness has become partially closed. A choice is made to become a cardiac, pulmonary, or emotional cripple dependent upon supportive subsystems.

Dependency, within the framework of fixed balance, can occur on three levels. First, the individual can become dependent upon the health team. This notion has particular significance for patients in psychiatric settings. It is here that patients have a greater potential to become emotionally dependent upon the staff's feedback for direction. Their feedback helps the patient stabilize and perceive the reality of the illness while gaining input as regards progress. If the staff fails to clarify information concerning the illness or progress, the patient interprets this as negative feedback. The patient feels that their uncertainty has negative connotations and therefore something must be terribly wrong. In reality the staff may simply be unable to stabilize the illness with a diagnosis or effective treatment plan. By not being open with the living system, the staff is

[22]Ludwig von Bertalanffy, "The Theory of Open Systems in Physics and Biology," *Science,* Volume III, January 13, 1950, p. 23.

[23]Myra Levine, "The Pursuit of Wholeness," *American Journal of Nursing,* 69, January 1969, p. 94.

simply contributing to the mystique and dependency surrounding illness.

Second, the individual can become dependent upon the family subsystem, transferring dependency behavior from the professional staff to the family. The patient wants to continue his dependency upon others for need fulfillment, and may feel safe in relinquishing roles and decision-making powers to family members. And the patient's biological problem may not warrant such behavior; however, the patient becomes psychologically dependent out of anticipatory fear.

Finally, a patient can reach a fixed balance by becoming machine dependent. A patient can become dependent upon a volume respirator, hemodialysis machine, temporary pacemaker, or cardioscope. This is a realistic problem in critical care units. Out of necessity a patient on long-term hemodialysis must become technologically dependent. With other patients the dependency should be only temporary. Take, for example, the respiratory care patient who can become too dependent upon the ventilator. Becoming too psychologically dependent makes the weaning phase more difficult due to the anxiety level. Therefore, the professional team, primarily his nurse, needs to foster security and the ability to maintain biological stability. This principle applies to all patients regardless of their problems. By transferring energies back into the patient, there will be less dependence upon supportive subsystems and more dependence upon oneself. Thus, the nurse helps the patient avoid negative adaptation.

The second balance to be achieved by the patient is a positive one. It implies the notion of achievement of new balance or new structure, signifying an increase in order and organization. The increase in order and organization takes place on two levels. Biologically the individual reaches a level of stability, as diagnostic studies reveal a reversal in the pathophysiological process which originally brought the patient into the hospital. On the psychological level, the individual learns from the biological or emotional crisis. A significant factor in the learning process is that the patient adapts psychologically to physical changes and/or limits. To accomplish the goal, continual positive reinforcement is needed. There must be a realization that regardless of what brought the patient into the hospital, the individual does have future value. By becoming aware of this value to others, the future becomes more hopeful.

THE ROLE OF THE OPEN HEALTH TEAM

All members of the health team, regardless of their roles, have the responsibility to help their patient achieve a steady-state of wellness.

Each professional assesses, intervenes, and evaluates those actions according to his or her own knowledge and skills.

The Living Organism

Members of the health team realize that illness in the human organism creates instability. They often witness situations in which some degree of disability has created imperfection in the patient's intake system, affecting the ability to gain, transmit, or utilize environmental information. Lack of information, or a failure anywhere in the circuit, changes the individual's response to the environment; this alteration frequently requires attention.[24]

The health team assesses when the living organism is able to participate in his or her own care. This includes making decisions about current and long term care. In many instances, the patient is in a better position to make decisions if there is knowledge regarding the environment and the illness. The nurse has a tremendous opportunity to facilitate the patient's understanding of the meaning of the environment. The nurse is in a position to facilitate educational intake regarding the biological and emotional status. Facilitation of educational input can only occur after the individual's readiness for input has been assessed. The child, adult, or aged patient due to their own anxiety states are not always ready for teaching input. Instead, their energies are focused on coping with the crisis, loss, or separation from significant others. In time as the nurse interacts with the patient, he or she can gradually return control to the patient by helping the individual understand the situation. If the patient feels that there is a degree of control over the environment and future, there is a greater willingness to channel energies toward participation in the surrounding world.

The health team realizes that a patient's behavioral response is directly related to intake and output of matter and energy. The nurse, as a vital member of the health team, acknowledges the patient's behavior and assesses its origin, realizing that behavioral responses can be manifestations of biological problems. By assessing behavioral responses of one patient, the nurse is in a position to anticipate and prevent similar responses in other patients.

Intake and Output of Matter and Energy

The intake system   The nurse, together with other members of the health team, assesses the variables or influencing factors, also called

[24]*Ibid.*, p. 94.

praxis, within the patient's environment that contribute to the patient's behavioral problems. The influencing systems as discussed earlier are economic, educational, health, and social. The cost of hospitalization is a top priority concern to most patients, and therefore should be a major concern for the health team. Critical care, highly sophisticated surgical procedures, and long term disability can create a tremendous economic overload for the patient and the patient's family. Since insurance may only pay for a portion of the hospitalization, a desire exists to leave the hospital as quickly as possible. Thus, the health team has the ultimate responsibility to expedite the discharge and minimize the expenses in a realistic way. Quality of care is most imperative for economic reasons. Quality signifies that the patient receive the exact tests necessary to diagnose particular biological problems. It does not imply extraneous tests which reflect defensive rather than quality medicine. Economic overload can make the patient angry if one realizes that a discharge is delayed due to a laboratory error or accidental deletion of a vital test. Needless to say errors can not always be prevented but organized and goal directed care can prevent accidental deletion of a particular diagnostic test, and excess emotional stress due to economic overload will be reduced.

A patient's knowledge of himself or herself and the current illness can influence emotional reactions to the hospitalization. If one believes that the professional team is not telling all the facts, he or she becomes angry or hostile, and this is a justifiable behavior. To avoid such a behavioral response, the health team can develop and utilize standardized teaching packets. Once the nurse assesses the patient's readiness to learn, the material can be explained to the patient. These packets can be taken home and continually referred to by the patient and his or her family. The patient should not be charged for the teaching material. Instead there should be payment to the patient for participation in the teaching program.

If the professional team considers health to be an influencing system, it should assess its significance to the patient. Illness, as a new experience, can be threatening. This is especially true if the patient has always been independent, aggressive, and active. To the patient, illness signifies a loss of mobility and forced dependence, both of which affect his image as a healthy individual in control of one's being and future. The health team helps such a patient incorporate a slightly different image into his or her being. Such an image need not be negative but rather realistic according to what changes are deemed necessary after a particular biological crisis. For the individual with repeated debilitating illness, realization of necessary changes in image are nothing new as he is forced to accept continual loss due to biological crisis. What becomes difficult is the threat of continued loss resulting in total disability or death. Regardless of the severity of illness, the health team assesses realistic changes in one's life style that may be necessary. Furthermore, the professional team realizes that the changes may only be temporary, and when realistic, fosters a positive adaptation towards the illness.

The last influencing system is a social one. It was mentioned earlier that the social system consists of the environment and supportive subsystems such as family, friends, and health team. The patient's immediate environment should be conducive to emotional stability. In other words, unnecessary and insignificant stimuli should be avoided. This is particularly true for critical care units, where the environment is noisy due to various supportive devices. It must also be remembered that the health team itself is a source of unnecessary stimuli. In some areas of the hospital, patients experience sleep deprivation, which can be responsible for behavioral responses such as depression, anger, hostility, and confusion. The health team therefore needs to assess a patient's environment and delete stimuli which could contribute to a negative behavioral response.

The patient's family may or may not be a supportive system. If the patient's behavior is that of depression, the family may become overly concerned. Family members draw energy from the patient by seeking explanations for depression or withdrawn behavior. In addition they dissipate their energies to the patient by becoming anxious. The energy received may not be constructive and only serves to make the patient more anxious. The nurse and health team in general should give the family feedback regarding the patient's behavior, explaining that this patient simply does not have the energy to become involved with them.

The health team can be a significant influencing system on the patient's environment and progress. The health team must realize that the hospitalized patient is in an unfamiliar environment, one that may limit activities in a manner which is neither understood nor accepted. The nurse and physician together must patiently explain and reexplain their purposes to their patient. According to Levine, the nurse-patient interaction depends on the perceptual systems of both persons. The nurse's presence within the patient's receptive environment immediately influences information input. By the same process, the nurse's perceptual system filters sensitivity to the patient's requirements.[25] By being aware of and sensitive to the patient's anxieties, the nurse is open to what may be going on inside. If the nurse is insensitive to the closed system of the patient's needs, he or she will be unable to channel the patient's energy output or behavior toward more positive goals. In general the closed health team or one which fails to listen to the patient allows achievement of a steady-state that will not necessarily be beneficial.

[25]*Ibid.*, pp. 97–98.

The living open system receives input from a variety of sources within its boundaries. The health team's goal is to keep the boundary open in a state of interaction. This is accomplished through open communication between the patient, family, and health team. Such communication prevents either living system from arriving at temporary closure. External threat can also lead to temporary closure as a protective defense, but the patient's boundaries remain open if there are non-threatening feelings about the environment and health team.

The output system   The health team first intervenes to anticipate and prevent negative behavioral response that depletes a patient's energy system. Second, if negative behavioral response should occur, the health team helps the patient and family cope with their behavior. Naturally the ideal situation is to anticipate those conditions in which an individual might experience negative behavioral responses such as depression, anger, hostility, and withdrawal. If the health team takes the influencing systems or variables into consideration and utilizes them in a positive manner, it is possible that negative behavior can be reduced. This implies that the team assesses its patient's educational needs and readiness for learning and provides meaningful teaching input that requires patient-family participation. It is also sensitive to the economic concerns of the patient and his or her family. If insurance forms or papers need a physician's signature, it should be obtained in an expeditious manner, thus facilitating the process of paper and/or claims. The patient's and family's attitude toward health and illness should be assessed to determine how they will relate to current illness. Individuals with previous experience know what is expected of them. However, the health team needs to assess the patient's expectations of them. Frequently patients hospitalized in different hospitals for the same problems compare the care received in each. If the care in the second institution is different, the patient feels he or she is not receiving quality care. Therefore a patient's previous experience and expectations of the health team need to be incorporated into a care plan. Finally, the social influencing system including environment and family support system can be evaluated for its influence on preventing negative behavioral response. A tense, anxious environment can only be communicated to and cause the patient to become tense. Likewise a patient's family, if overly anxious, contributes to a patient's anxiety. An anxious family needs the support of the health team, who must absorb the family's anxiety and help them to cope with the illness.

When negative behavioral responses do occur, the health team assesses the origin according to energy excess or deficit. Behavior resulting from energy excess is in response to anxieties and fears, and may be manifested as anger or hostility. The nurse is open to the anxieties, frustrations, and threats to existence experienced by the hospitalized patient. As previously discussed, the patient may be anxious about an aspect of care or the losses associated with illness, injury or surgical alteration. Excess energy is absorbed and constructively channeled by the nurse. The excess energy is channeled by encouraging the patient to physically or verbally participate in his or her own care. Physical activity gives the patient a feeling of progress and accomplishment and the patient senses personal fluidity rather than personal stasis.

Just as some patients and their families experience energy excess, others can experience energy deficit. The patient with a low energy level is directing energies internally. Behavior is manifested as depression and withdrawal, and what energy remains must be conserved. The health team, on the other hand, represents a high-energy system contributing some of its energy to the patient. The nurse in particular achieves this goal by temporarily assuming certain responsibilities and making certain decisions for the patient. Initially, the patient may not have enough energy to carry out activities of daily living, while the nurse as a high-energy system can perform those functions, thus conserving the patient's energy. In addition, the patient's family, physician, or friends serve as other high energy systems. The energy derived from such subsystems augments the patient's low energy system. The nurse receives feedback from physicians, social workers, pharmacists, dietitians, psychologists, and ministers to help formulate a plan of care.

Feedback

The health team has a responsibility to provide feedback regarding the patient's internal biological progress. In many instances the results of diagnostic studies and laboratory tests are neatly filed away in the patient's chart. Patients see their blood being taken away; however, no one bothers to tell them the significance or results of the test. Naturally the information provided from laboratory results must be assessed for its appropriateness to the individual patient's situation. As the patient is ready to accept information regarding serum enzymes, EKG, electrolyte panel, chest x-ray, and blood gases, he or she develops a sense of relatedness to the various treatment procedures and/or supportive devices within the environment. If the patient is kept informed regarding internal biological progress, there might not be the need for certain behavioral responses pertaining to educational deficit. Biological feedback helps the patient to see progress or to understand reasons for a temporary biological plateau.

Adaptation: Establishment of
Steady-State

Hopefully, the health team helps the patient achieve a positive balance by helping to evaluate the hospital experience and to formulate a realistic plan for the future. The individual looks forward to going home and adapting to necessary social role changes. The nurse, together with other members of the health team, plays a significant role in the patient's overall adaptation to the illness.

In summary, it is only through openness, the health team's warm and human expression or concern, that the patient may escape feelings of denial, depression, withdrawal, anger, or hostility. Because the team is open, it gets to know the child, adult, or aged individual for whom they care. In this respect the health team is able to anticipate and prevent negative behavioral output. Openness on the health team's part becomes the most significant factor in the emotional atmosphere of a strange hospital environment.

REFERENCES

Allport, Gordon, "The Open System in Personality Theory," *Modern Systems Research For the Behavioral Scientist*, (Chapter 42), Chicago: Aldine Publishing Company, 1968.

Ashby, Ross, "The Set Theory of Mechanism and Homeostasis," *General Systems*, 9: 83–97.

Buckley, Walter, *Modern Systems Research for the Behavioral Scientist*, Chicago: Aldine Publishing Company, 1968.

George, Frank, "Toward A General Theory of Behavior," *Methods*, 7: 24–44.

Grinker, Roy, "Open System Psychiatry," *American Journal of Psychoanalysis*, pp. 115–128.

———, *Toward A Unified Theory of Human Behavior*, New York: Basic Books, Inc., 1967.

Herbst, P. G., "Situation Dynamics and The Theory of Behavior Systems," *Behavior Science*, 2: 13–29.

Krech, David, "Dynamic Systems As Open Neurological Systems," *Psychological Review*, 57: 345–361.

Miller, James, "Toward A General Theory for the Behavioral Scientist," *American Psychologist*, 10: 513–531.

Nadel, S. F., "Social Control and Self-Regulation," *Social Forces*, 31: 265–273.

Powers, William, *Behavior: The Control of Perception*, Chicago: Aldine Publishing Company, 1973.

Skinner, B. F., *About Behaviorism*, New York: Alfred A. Knopf, 1974.

2
Anxiety

Everyone has experienced anxiety at some point in life. Anxiety is usually felt when confronting stress situations, whether new ones conjuring up fears of the unknown or familiar ones arousing feelings of avoidance. We live in a stress-oriented culture. According to Portnoy, "Anxiety producing factors in our culture grow progressively more numerous and intense, while anxiety relieving agencies have become sharply and increasingly less effective. Perhaps more fundamental are the increasing strains and pressures experienced by individuals living in a period characterized by great complexity, and instability, rapid change and the mingling of varied and differing cultures."[1]

Psychoanalysts believe that anxiety begins at birth and continues until death. An internal feeling, anxiety is sometimes difficult to identify and pinpoint. It is diffuse and may know no boundaries. Fischer points out that, "Anxiety is the intermittent, occasionally chronic sense of being a failure as a human being. Thus it is tied to the fact that one lives with other human beings in a culture that, among other things, presents criteria of humanness."[2] Sometimes anxiety may serve to protect us —warning us of a yet unexperienced situation. People refer to this as a feeling of "impending doom." On the other hand, there are times when a person feels anxious but is unable to identify the source of the anxiety. Moreover, he or she may be unable to function within this situation.

Anxiety can be caused by external environmental threats. Such is the case of a new situation over which the individual has no control of the outcome. Anxiety is really, "a multidimensional phenomenon, meaning that the total organism is involved in every aspect of it—the individual's perception of threat, his interpretation of it which involves his uniquely human capacity to symbolize and abstract, the role of the past in the

[1]Isadora Portnoy, "Anxiety States," *American Handbook of Psychiatry*, (Ed: Silavano Arieti), (New York: Basic Books, 1959), p. 307.

[2]William Fisher, *Theories of Anxiety*, (New York: Harper and Row, 1970), p. 34.

present as well as the capacity to evaluate future possibilities, conscious and unconscious decision concerning his way of coping with the threat, all within the context of interpersonal and cultural milieu."[3]

Patients experience anxiety upon arriving in a hospital setting. The child, adult, or aged individual's anxiety focuses on fear of the unknown environment and the threat to physical and/or emotional integrity. Once the threat to this physical or emotional integrity subsides, the individual becomes less anxious and more comfortable within familiar surroundings. In addition to familiarity within his surroundings, one also becomes more familiar with the staff providing the care. Regardless of developmental level, the nurse and the patient become involved with one another. The severity or duration of an illness may require that the patient be continuously exposed to health personnel. The goal is consistency of patient care and staff involvement. "Consistent patient assignments minimize the number of superficial relationships that patients must form and provide the reassurance fostered by seeing familiar faces. Not only does this facilitate orientation, but it also augments the development of effective therapeutic relationships."[4] Depending upon the patient's clinical problem, the nurse may spend his or her time in the here and now, implying a focusing of attention on recognition of complications associated with the patient's biological or emotional crisis. Furthermore, the nurse attempts to recognize and understand the patient's behavior and its psychological meaning as it affects coping with the illness.

Anxiety, whether conscious or unconscious, has the potential to become a problem for the child, adult, or aged patient. We will first discuss its definition and meaning. Since anxiety is such a broad concept, it will be broken down into three components identified by Bowlby, an these will be applied to patient's in various clinical settings.

ANXIETY: DEFINITION AND MEANING

It must be remembered that, "any attempt to define the nature and meaning of anxiety must begin with the statement that anxiety is a natural phenomenon which the individual experiences when values essential to his existence, his sense of being and his identity are threatened."[5] One cannot define Bowlby's components without first examining the general attributes of anxiety as a whole concept.

[3]Portnoy, *op. cit.*, p. 311.

[4]Kathleen Andreoli, *Comprehensive Cardiac Care*, (St. Louis: C. V. Mosby Company, 1971), p. 147.

[5]Portnoy, *op. cit.*, p. 307.

Anxiety

May has defined anxiety as, "apprehension cued off by a threat to some value which the individual holds essential to his existence as a personality."[6] Anxiety is a reaction to the threat of coping. As the individual learns to depend upon this, a threat to the individual's security produces anxiety. According to Peplau, such threats fall into two main categories: threats to biological integrity and threats to the self-system.[7] In the first instance, there are threats to the maintenance of homeostasis by temperature control and vasomotor stability, and through action to meet bodily needs. Threats to the self-system are threats to the maintenance of established views of self and to the values and patterns of behavior one uses to resist changes in self-view.

Threats to the patient's biological or emotional integrity occur the moment one experiences an illness or crisis. The threat and anxiety aroused continue until the patient learns that the biological or emotional system has reached stability. Even afterward, there are fleeting moments of anxiety. The patient who experiences a first myocardial infarction becomes anxious when thinking about the possibility of another insult to the heart. The child who is hospitalized for the first time experiences a special type of anxiety; separation anxiety. The surgical patient who is hospitalized for additional surgery becomes anxious when reflecting on the surgery, postoperative pain, and potential need for additional surgery. The adolescent or adult alcoholic patient hospitalized for bleeding esophageal varicosities realizes that without adequate rehabilitation he or she will return to the hospital in an even greater state of crisis and debilitation. The schizophrenic patient may live in a world of anxiety, since what is seen as normal anxiety by one individual is experienced as intense anxiety by the schizophrenic patient.

Threat to the individual's self-system occurs as the individual views relationships to past, present, and future changes. Such threats focus upon psychological integrity. Anxiety experienced by the patient when biological or self-system integrity is threatened can be perceived indirectly, by its effect. According to Freud, "Anxiety is in the first place something felt. We call it an affective state, although we are equally ignorant of what affect is. As a feeling it is of most obviously unpleasurable character, but this is not by any means a complete description of its quality; not every state of unpleasure may we call anxiety. There are other feelings of unpleasurable character (mental tension, sorrow, grief) and

---

[6]Rollo May, *The Meaning of Anxiety*, (New York: Ronald Press Company, 1950), p. 191.

[7]Hildegard Peplau, "A Working Definition of Anxiety," *Some Clinical Approaches to Psychiatric Nursing*, (New York: Macmillan, 1963), p. 324.

anxiety must have other characteristics beside this quality of unpleasure."[8]

We expect individuals who experience threats to their biological integrity and self-system to be anxious. This is normal anxiety: "It is man's nature to have anxiety in the face of certain kinds and degrees of threat. In brief, it is the ultimate expression of our being human. We experience normal anxiety in the face of death, old age and illness as we recognize our factual helplessness."[9] Because anxiety is multidimensional, it assumes many forms. Three of these forms or conditions have been identified by Bowlby as primary anxiety, fright, and expectant anxiety.[10] He identified them as components of separation anxiety; however, they have broader implications for patients in varying stages of development.

Primary Anxiety

Bowlby also refers to primary anxiety as separation anxiety. Therefore, for the purpose of this chapter, primary anxiety will primarily apply to the infant and/or child. Primary anxiety, "is thought of as an elemental experience and one which, if it reaches a certain degree of intensity, is linked directly with the onset of defense mechanisms."[11] In discussing primary anxiety, Bowlby refers to the instinctual system, composed of both behavior and the hypothetical internal structure that, when activated, causes the behavior. The behavioral response includes the motor behavioral pattern and its physiological and psychological concomitants. Whenever an instinctual system activates and is unable for any reason to reach termination, a form of anxiety results. Initially for the infant, anxiety is a primary response resulting from the separation of mother and infant.

Primary anxiety becomes a major nursing care problem when, due to illness, the child must be hospitalized thus separating him or her from the attachment figure. If this is the child's first experience with separation, anxiety may be built-in rather than learned. Thus, primary anxiety may be built-in or inherited. It can be detected on the basis of hospital interpersonal experiences, in which termination is a part of the eventual outcome. Anxiety is learnable, especially if the child experiences frequent separation. According to Martin, "Anxiety also possesses the property of

---

[8]Sigmund Freud, *The Problem of Anxiety*, (New York: Norton, 1963), p. 69.

[9]Portnoy, *op. cit.*, p. 310.

[10]John Bowlby, "Separation Anxiety," *The International Journal of Psychoanalysis*, March–June 1960, p. 92.

[11]*Ibid.*, p. 92.

being highly learnable: that is, the hypothetical response becomes readily conditioned to stimuli that do not innately elicit the response. This characteristic renders difficult if not impossible any attempt to define anxiety on the basis of stimuli that elicit it, since the stimuli that elicit it will vary widely from person to person."[12] The child becomes bound to the new attachment figure, the nurse. Without realizing it, the child may be bound to the nurse by a number of instinctual response systems, each of which is primary, and which together have high survival value.

Fright

Fright is the second condition of anxiety identified by Bowlby. It is an emotional experience shared by patients in all developmental stages. For the purpose of this chapter, it will be treated as a transitory condition between primary anxiety of the child and expectant anxiety of the adult or aged patient. Fright is the subjective experience accompanying at least two related instinctual response systems—those leading to escape behavior, and those leading to immobility or freezing. Like all instinctual response systems, those governing escape and freezing are built into the organism and perpetuated by heredity due to their survival value. Patients admitted into the hospital because of an emergency, surgical intervention, or diagnostic evaluation to rule out the possibility of cancer all experience fright. The patient enters a foreign world filled with strange pieces of equipment and strange noises. Instead of feeling secure in such a protective environment, the child or adult may be instinctively motivated to escape.

The individual may escape by withdrawing, but more often escapes by initiating his or her own termination on a verbal or nonverbal level. The patient may verbally express a readiness or desire to return to the haven of security, home. Patients may tell their nurse how well they feel, how much they feel they have improved, or how ready they are to leave the hospital. The patients may be seeking reassurance that they are in fact improving and will be leaving the hospital shortly. But whether realizing it or not, the patient is verbally initiating his or her own termination process.

The patient may be so frightened that one initiates termination on an action level. The adult patient may feel improvement to the point that there is no longer a need to remain in bed, to use an oxygen mask, to use intravenous therapy, or to use a cardioscope. Consequently, the patient removes the EKG leads or climbs out of bed. These clues are more obvious than verbal ones and can be handled directly.

[12]Barclay, Martin, "The Assessment of Anxiety By Physiological Behavioral Means," *Psychological Bulletin*, 58, May 1961, p. 235.

Expectant Anxiety

Bowlby also discusses expectant anxiety. As soon as the individual, whether infant or adult, has reached a stage of development in which some degree of foresight is possible, that individual is able to predict dangerous situations and can take measures to avoid them. Expectant anxiety applies primarily to the adult or aged individual who has current knowledge of previous experiences with illness and hospitalization. Therefore, that individual anticipates what might happen, experiencing expectant anxiety. For example, patients with recurring angina, pulmonary edema, respiratory distress, diabetic coma, glomerulonephritis, or emotional instability realize the implications of their illness or disease. They fear that they are likely to lose additional biological and/or emotional integrity. Expectations may vary with each subsequent hospitalization.

APPLICATION TO VARIOUS CLINICAL SETTINGS

Anxiety can be a positive and constructive force. It serves to motivate the individual toward improvement of adaptation or maturity. However, anxiety that has not been resolved becomes unconstructive and can have a damaging effect upon the individual. The individual's anxiety may cause a retreat to previous states of security. In this instance anxiety motivates one away from making decisions that would alleviate or resolve the anxiety state. Anxieties are numerous for the hospitalized child, adult, or aged patient. Significant anxieties for the child revolve around separation from attachment figures and fear of intrusive procedures. For the adult or aged individual, anxieties stem from the illness and its implication for the future. The anxieties experienced by all three age groups are normal. As we, "move from the old, the sheltered, the known, the tested and the certain into the new, the unknown, untested and uncertain; that is, whenever we stretch, expand and move forward we experience normal anxiety. In this view, normal anxiety is an inevitable accompaniment of healthy growth and change in the direction of greater freedom, autonomy and creativity as we move toward increasing fulfillment of our innate constructive potentialities."[13]

The patient moves away from a familiar home territory into an unknown and unfamiliar clinical setting and all too often, nurses place emphasis upon the illness itself without taking into consideration the meaning hospitalization has for the individual. Focus is on the shock of

[13]Portnoy, *op. cit.*, p. 310.

diagnosis, anxiety over illness and survival, total dependency, fear of equipment failure, and fear of rejection by significant others, while we place little, if any, attention upon successful emotional admission into the hospital environment. As a result, the patient experiences primary anxiety, fright, and expectant anxiety.

Primary Anxiety

The child is bound to the attachment figure, the mother, by a number of instinctual response systems. Initially the infant utilizes crying to bring about a close proximity between the infant and the mother. Later on in development, clinging and following activates closeness with the mother figure. If crying, clinging, or following does not lead to closeness, the infant will experience primary anxiety. Likewise when close proximity is maintained he or she experiences comfort. When infants or children become frightened they look toward the attachment figure for security. When she is unavailable or missing, they experience the dual anxiety of missing security and comfort.

The significant mother-child relationship which evolves during infancy becomes a basic factor in the child's overall attitude toward security and interpersonal relationships. The child whose anxieties have been promptly alleviated will have a positive adaptation to the surrounding world, while the child whose relationship with the attachment figure has been unsatisfying will have difficulty entering into trust relationships with others, thus hampering the ability to relate with others less significant than parents. The basic mother-child relationship can facilitate or alleviate feelings of primary anxiety. These early experiences have clinical implications for the hospitalized child. The hospital experience may be the infant's or child's first encounter with separation and may not be planned, as in emergency admissions due to sudden illness or injury.

Abrupt separation from attachment figures creates primary anxiety, as the sequence of events in a normal temporary separation process are blocked. The child and parents do not have an opportunity to discuss fears, anxieties, or expectations regarding hospitalization. The prepared child has an opportunity to clarify misconceptions thus casting aside any fantasies. Furthermore, the child knows his parents are aware of his or her insecurity and the child feels accepted by the parents. The child, who is hit by a car while playing might experience both guilt and rejection, fearing the accident might displease the attachment figures. This may be especially true if the parents warnings went unheard, leading to an accident. Not only does the child experience primary anxiety associated with the injury itself but also fear of rejection. To avoid feelings of rejection, both the nurse and the parents need to help the child adjust to the temporary separation, minimizing primary anxiety.

Younger children, particularly the two to three year olds, are most sensitive to primary or separation anxiety. Mother has been the most significant person in their small world and now she has left him or her with total strangers. Children at this age are vulnerable in that they want "Mommy" but cannot conceptualize or verbalize their need beyond the crying or demanding level. The nurse may assess certain bahaviors which are diagnosed as regression due to primary anxiety. Regressive behavior is exemplified by loss of bladder or bowel control, demanding bottle feeding, refusing to chew solid foods, and/or sucking the thumb. The nurse may assess the child to be restless, hyperactive, and unable to sleep because of nightmares or fear of the dark, when this regressive behavior is an attempt to bring the attachment figure to the bedside. These behaviors, including crying, have worked in the past and the child uses them again to see if they work in the present. The only difference is that the attachment figure is a stranger. As strangers, they have never been tested to see if their actions will alleviate anxieties. If the nurse understands the young patient's behavior, she or he will intervene to lessen primary anxiety resulting from separation. The nurse will become involved with the child and through this involvement become a substitute attachment figure. The child, who is able to move through a hospital environment, may demonstrate attachment to the nurse by following or clinging behavior. "These so-called 'attachment behavior(s)' serve to provide the child with an affectional tie to one person who will meet his physiological and psychosocial needs."[14] Affectional attachment of the child to the nurse is necessary for emotional adaptation to the hospital environment.

As the child continues to grow and develop, the frequency of regressive behavior diminishes. Of course there are clincial situations of severe biological crisis which may, once again, force the child into regressive behavior. Most children by age four to six or even older shift the focus of their anxieties. Within this latter age group, primary anxiety shifts from anxieties due to separation from attachment figure to anxieties over hospital routines, diagnostic studies, or intrusive procedures. Unlike the adult or aged patient, the child does not mask feelings regarding the various healing procedures that seem to encompass illness, disease, or injury. Children are very expressive in their dislike of certain members of the health team and certain procedures.

The health team needs to realize that some of its diagnostic or treatment procedures can be more frightening and painful to the child

[14]Elise Wear, "Separation Anxiety Reconsidered: Nursing Implications," *Maternal and Child Nursing Journal*, September 1974, p. 11.

than his or her physical illness or injury. In fact, the child may experience greater primary anxiety from a particular treatment than from temporarily refraining from riding a bike or skate board. Children are usually particularly anxious when dealing with hypodermic needles and injections. Kassowitz found that relative to the use of hypodermic needles children up to six months of age showed no evidence of apprehension; those from one to four showed the highest incidence of more-or-less violent fear and resentment; and after five there was a steady decline of frightening defense.[15]

It seems that many nursing interventions are naturally intrusive. According to Aasterud, "Nursing practice involves intrusive procedures which are capable of eliciting many primitive fantasies of mutilation and punishment, notably the use of gastric tubes, enemas, douches, catheterization and rectal temperature."[16] The child's only defense against intrusive procedures is through aggressive behavior such as crying, arm thrashing, hitting, kicking, and biting. Working against more powerful people, the child's behavior eventually proves ineffective. The health team needs to support its anxious patient through the frightening experience and the child needs to realize that these anxieties are normal. If parental assistance is possible, the mother or father may be the one to actually support the child during the intrusive procedure. Naturally the appropriateness of such an intervention must be assessed by the nurse.

There are times when a family member is in greater need of support than the child. The child attempts to control events in the environment through aggressive behavior, originating from primary anxiety. Control of biological integrity is not possible through aggressive behavior. Like the adult, the child relinquishes control over his or her body. Davis says, "The very nature of the illness requires that all, or nearly all, bodily functions and care be assigned to others. It requires little imagination to appreciate that when a patient is suddenly and completely divested of control of his body, he may experience this as a fundamental threat to his ego, even when he 'knows' that it is being done to help him."[17] The child may relinquish that which is not understood.

For the child, primary anxiety originates out of an apprehension to separation from significant attachment figures in the home environment. Later this fear is projected onto the substitute attachment figure, the nurse. Anxiety associated with attachment figures revolves around the child's fear of disapproval. The child may fantasize that illness or injury will bring disapproval from the parents, making him even more insecure.

[15]Karl Kassowitz, "Psychodynamic Reactions of Children to the Use of Hypodermic Needles," *AMA Journal of Diseases of Children,* 95, 1958, pp. 253–257.

[16]Margaret Aasterud, "Defenses Against Anxiety," *Nursing Forum,* Summer 1962, p. 44.

[17]Marcella Davis, "Socioemotional Component of Coronary Care," *American Journal of Nursing,* April 1972, p. 707.

Disapproval from attachment figures is threatening because the relationship with them is the most important of all relationships. Their positive attitude is important at this time, and can help to alleviate feelings of primary anxiety. Improper handling of these primary anxieties can eventually lead to a child's experiencing fright.

Fright

Fright is an emotion shared by patients in all developmental stages of life, varying with severity and duration of illness. Feelings of fright arise when the child or adult does not know what to expect in a given situation. Depending upon the patient's age or severity of illness, injury or disease process, the individual may not be able to physically escape the immediate environment. The child utilizes a unique escape behavior. "Escape responses share with crying, clinging and following the same terminating situation. The frightened baby, it might be said, is both 'pushed' toward his mother by his escape responses and 'pulled' toward her by his following responses."[18] The adult who is critically, chronically, or terminally ill may escape verbally by seeking information regarding a transfer and discharge. Emotionally there is escape through the utilization of various defense mechanisms such as denial, compensation, displacement, or rationalization.

Fright may be particularly alarming to the child and the schizophrenic patient since each is vulnerable to individual anxieties. For the schizophrenic patient, anxieties are diffuse and seem to know no boundaries, making the schizophrenic patient most susceptible to a fright response, escape behavior. Since physical escape is difficult for the schizophrenic patient, he or she escapes emotionally by turning within and becoming noncommunicative to surrounding others.

Beside escape response, the individual may react by demonstrating immobility or freezing behavior. Such may be the case with the schizophrenic patient who is so immobilized by fright that he or she becomes catatonic. Less obvious behaviors by adult or aged patients are the freezing responses of depressive and withdrawal behavior. The patient may be so frightened by the strange hospital environment and the illness, injury, or emotional crisis that there is an avoidance to any discussion. Instead the focus is on peripheral topics such as family, dog, toys, flowers, or the nurse. These topics arouse less anxiety within the individual and the patient may not recognize his or her own behavior. "The individual flees or remains immobile not because he has any clear awareness of danger but because his flight or 'freezing' responses have been activated."[19]

[18]Bowlby, *op. cit.*, p. 97.
[19]*Ibid.*

Patients use both obvious and subtle means to escape the fright of their immediate clinical situations. Take, for example, the patient who frequently uses the call light. It may appear, on the surface, that the patient has many needs. The nurse assesses the patient's surface behavior as inappropriate since the specific biological status does not necessitate frequent attention. As the nurse further assesses the meaning behind the patient's behavior, the diagnoses is fright due to anxiety response. The health team may feel that the patient's biological status has reached stability; however, the patient might not agree. It is possible that the patient correlates less attention by the nurse to avoidance rather than improvement. This elicits rejection and the individual expresses fright by increasing the frequency of using the call light. The staff needs to prepare all patients, regardless of age, for gradual improvement, alleviating anxiety in the form of fright behavior.

As the patient steadily improves, the staff can reduce treatments and remove pieces of equipment, serving to reassure the patient that he or she is getting well. If the termination process has taken place gradually, the patient may accept the improvement. This is usually the case with the respiratory patient who is gradually weaned off the volume respirator. Another patient may question having wires or tubes removed seconds before a transfer and may wonder why his or her need for the cardioscope and other devices is suddenly terminated. In all probability, this procedure could have occurred earlier.

The cardiac patient has a personal attachment to the cardioscope. "The monitoring device becomes a significant object to the acutely ill cardiac patient and he is very dependent on it for a sense of security. The exact purpose of the monitor should be clarified to the patient so that his fear of his heart not functioning without it will be dispelled."[20] The respiratory patient, if transferred with a tracheostomy tube, may become anxious about the frequency of being suctioned, feeling the need for the same amount of suctioning as was administered in intensive care. This patient has to be taught how to expectorate his or her own secretions, and should be told that there will be very little if any secretion. In other words, the patient, regardless of clinical problem, must be informed of individual progress and here is where the nurse plays a vital role in sharing information.

Expectant Anxiety

Expectant anxiety can apply to the child who experiences frequent hospitalization resulting in separation from significant others and intru-

[20]V. J. Shannon, "The Transfer Process: An Area of Concern for the CCU Nurse," *Heart and Lung,* May–June 1973, p. 366.

sive procedures. This child becomes conditioned and anticipates anxieties. Expectant anxiety has greater implications for the adult or aged patient. Therefore, the discussion of expectant anxiety will focus on the latter two developmental stages, the adult and the aged. Bowlby believes that, "As soon as the individual has reached a stage of development in which some degree of foresight is possible, he is able to predict situations as dangerous and to take measures to avoid them."[21] Expectant anxiety revolves around those clinical situations in which the individual feels he or she will be assailed by external stimuli. The external stimuli can be perceived as originating from either objects or people in the environment which remind the patient of the illness, injury, or disability. To the individual the external stimuli are disagreeable and activate instinctual response systems of escape or freezing. There are clinical situations in which the patient believes there will be a loss of control and a thrust into a world of insecurity. The critically ill, disabled, terminal, or emotionally disturbed individual represents such clinical examples.

For the adult patient, expectant anxiety revolves around two basic threats. These threats cause questioning of security within the boundary of the patient's own body and interpersonal relationships. The threats are of two categories: threats to the biological integrity and threats to the self-system. The first threat to biological integrity applies to the critically, chronically, and terminally ill patient. Illness forces the individual to realize a loss in degree of biological control. Such loss of control forced entrance into the unfamiliar territory known as a hospital where the patient must depend upon total strangers for care. In adapting to this new territory, the individual must learn the meaning of strange noises emanating from new neighbors as well as those coming from his or her own immediate environment. The patient must also adapt biologically to a higher level of wellness or to the physical level dictated by one's disability. The patient must adapt to the care assigned to others until gaining the ability to be less dependent. According to Shannon, "Adaptation to disease does not end when the acute phase of the illness is over, but rather this adaptation process is continuous and complicated. In the convalescent phase, the individual is mentally and physically more free to carry the burden of making a change by himself, but in the acute phase of his illness he must rely on the nurse to help him make the necessary adjustment."[22] Illness threatens the patient's sense of biological and psychological integrity. He or she must side track past expectations and formulate new and possibly more meaningful ones. The nurse must remember that this internal struggle may force the patient to consider oneself ill longer than is necessary.

[21]Bowlby, *op. cit.*, p. 98.
[22]Shannon, *op. cit.*, p. 364.

Adult patients, who frequently are readmitted into the hospital, experience expectant anxiety. Their past experiences lead them to anticipate present and future problems. Diagnostic studies and/or intrusive procedures are not new to them, nevertheless, this does not negate the anxieties they produce. Take for example the critically ill patient. Because of the severity and recurrency of his or her illness, the patient may find wires and tubes attached to every aspect of the body, some of which are intrusive. Likewise, a patient admitted for diagnostic procedures may also be subjected to procedures of an intrusive nature. Each individual experiences anxiety associated with threats to biological integrity. The critically ill patient realizes that the procedures or treatments are vital to survival or restoration. The supportive devices around the bed become support systems. The patient who submits to various diagnostic procedures is anxious over the outcome, fearing a stomach pain will be diagnosed as cancer. The patient may not verbalize these fears thinking that verbalization will make them true.

It was mentioned earlier that children do not mask their anxieties regarding intrusive or threatening procedures. The adult, however, does mask anxieties, fearing that behavioral response demonstrating the anxieties will bring staff disapproval. Adult anxieties may then manifest themselves on a physiological level. Therefore, the nurse must assess the anxieties' effect upon a patient's physiological systems. This is particularly significant to the patient whose biological integrity may already be severely compromised. The nurse may assess the following physiological responses to anxiety: increased heart rate, increased rate and depth of respiration, chest pain, frequent urination, diarrhea, anorexia, nausea, vomiting, excessive perspiration, increased blood pressure, or headache. Naturally there are other physiological responses; however, these seem to be the most significant to assess. The nurse must assess which intrusive or diagnostic procedures have the greatest threat. Aasterud believes that, "Certain nursing practices and procedures should be recognized as being threatening to the patient, either consciously as a source of pain and discomfort, or unconsciously reactivating childhood fears of mutilation, abandonment, deprivation and other parental punishments."[23]

It seems that adult surgical patients receive the brunt of various intrusive procedures. Their surgical sites or wounds are drained, probed, swabbed, taped, or cultured. Furthermore, at the peak of their pain experience they are instructed to turn, cough, and breathe deeply. Medication may only temporarily alleviate the pain. Besides, the patient's anxiety may surpass the effectiveness of medication. Therefore, with each request by the nurse to turn, cough and breathe deeply, the patient experiences expectant anxiety. Previous experience leads to expectations of

[23]Aasterud, *op. cit.*, p. 55.

future pain. This is particularly true for those patients who have suffered long periods of intermittent pain. Take for example the patient with peripheral vascular insufficiency who experiences intermittent claudication. The anticipation of the next episode of pain may be more devastating than the moments of pain itself. The patient's expectant anxiety is then due to anticipation of the pain experience.

The second threat causing expectant anxiety involves two components. The first component consists of threats to the self-system, while the second deals with threats to interpersonal relationships. These components have significance to all adult patients; however, they have even greater application to the patient in emotional crisis, who has difficulty with a faltering self-system and the ability to relate to others. An individual's self-system seems to represent the essence of being. Any threats to this basic system leads to anxiety within the individual. Sullivan says, "The self-system is an organization of views of the self and of patterns of behavior which operate to prevent and/or reduce anxiety."[24] It consists of the values, wishes, and images the individual internalizes. In other words, the individual has certain internal expectations and when these expectations are blocked he or she experiences anxiety. Repeated hospitalization due to illness or complications resulting from an illness threatens the individual's self-system. The threat is centered on a sense of a precarious future in which certain expectations must be altered. The alterations and an inability to foresee the unknown create anxiety. The individual hospitalized for biological problems probably has a basically strong self-system which will help in coping with the present and future, whereas the schizophrenic patient's self-system is weak.

The schizophrenic patient ". . . in a period of personality disturbance feels the threat of a neurotic trend which was his only method of coping with earlier basic anxiety, and hence the prospect is one of renewed helplessness and defenselessness."[25] The anxiety originates from a weakened self-system. Schizophrenia is a specific reaction to an extreme state of anxiety, which originates in childhood and is reactivated by psychological factors in adulthood. The nurse realizes that anxiety is a common denominator in all manifestations of emotional crisis but the anxious schizophrenic patient can be a particular nursing care problem. The already threatened self-system has no provisions for the confidence necessary to cope with current emotional crisis. Before the nurse can solidify the patient's weakened self-system, he or she must attempt to reduce the anxiety and teach alternative ways of coping with it. If not, the individual will continue a pattern of intense anxiety with each crisis,

[24]H. S. Sullivan, *Conceptions of Modern Psychiatry*, (New York: Norton, 1953), pp. 19–24; 46.

[25]May, *op. cit.*, p. 142.

anticipating an anxiety state whether or not one is warranted. The schizophrenic patient knows no other way to adapt to a potentially threatening situation because all situations are seen as threatening. Solidification of a weakened self-system can be a difficult task for the nurse because the schizophrenic patient may become threatened by his or her involvement.

The nurse who has not established a trust relationship with a schizophrenic patient will be ineffective in teaching alternative ways of coping with anxiety. Furthermore, the nurse realizes that, "the self is created by the ensemble of social relations that the child has with the significant adults in his life, by the reflected appraisals (verbal and nonverbal) of these significant adults. If these interpersonal relations are unhealthy and create an excessive amount of anxiety, the psychologic development is disturbed and the process of socialization is altered. This sequence of events may lead to schizophrenia."[26] The patient's failure to relate to people in a present environment is a result of past failures with significant others; the attachment figures. The nurse keeps in mind that a schizophrenic patient's most important anxiety initiating factors are those originating from interpersonal relationships. Besides teaching a patient acceptable ways of coping with anxiety, the nurse must also teach how to relate successfully with the new environment and the people therein. The nurse tries to help with the patient's integration into the ward environment. The schizophrenic patient may have difficulty integrating into the new hospital environment. How one succeeds in this protective environment may determine how he or she responds to the larger community. If there is no awareness of what to expect from the nurse and ward environment, one may fantasize on expectation of failure, resulting in anxiety." Anxieties are cued off when tension develops beyond the mean due to the organism's attempt to integrate in an environment for which it is not adequate and which is not adequate for it. Anxiety appears in the phase of disintegration of the natural cycle, disintegration-reintegrating as aspects of integrity."[27] The nurse's calm, accepting attitude can be the stabilizing force in a patient's emotionally unstable world.

The adult patient experiences expectant anxiety in two areas, illness and interpersonal relationships. The aged individual experiences expectant anxiety over an uncertain future. Kurzweil believes that, "This is the stage when the general basis of life is gradually shrinking, when physical vitality is reduced and the zest for life diminished. Few indeed are the individuals who can enjoy good health and preserve their vital physical and intellectual functions to a ripe old age."[28] Besides biological failings

[26]Roberta Cohen, "Anxiety As A Manifestation of Associated Drives and Events in a Female Schizophrenic Patient," *Journal of Psychiatric Nursing*, May–June 1973, p. 17.

[27]Portnoy, *op. cit.*, p. 309.

[28]Z. E. Kurzweil, *Anxiety and Education*, (New York: Thomas Yoseloff, 1968), p. 138.

and a sense of generalized weakness, the aged individual is also confronted with the anxieties of loneliness. He or she may be forced to depend upon others at a time when developmentally one should be independent and self-sufficient. However, illness or chronic disability has weakened the biological system. With each illness and subsequent biological loss, there is greater anxiety about the future. Support systems are limited and constricting. In addition, the aged patient experiences expectant anxiety regarding fears of not being wanted, of being useless, or of being a burden to his or her children. Many aged patients experience a feeling of helplessness, powerlessness, and overall emptiness. Those individuals who have sustained numerous insults to their biological integrity feel compelled to simply wait out the rest of their lives in what they perceive to be a limited future.

It is interesting to note that the aged patient has greater expectant anxiety regarding changes in life style or future than about death. According to Kurzweil, "acute fear of death is comparatively rare in elderly people, as recent researchers have tended to establish . . . the cares and worries of old people gradually undermine their will to live to the point when they regard death not with fear but as a welcome release. To most people, not life as such is of the highest value, but life permeated by a feeling of well-being and unimpaired functioning of body and mind."[29] The nurse intervenes to help an aged patient have a meaningful and worthwhile self-perception. If he or she feels life has meaning, there will be motivation to survive the current biological crisis. Of course the nurse must assess those areas in which she or he can realistically motivate the patient.

THE NURSE'S ROLE IN MINIMIZING ANXIETY

In order to minimize anxiety, the nurse in all clinical areas should begin work the moment a patient arrives in the hospital. We usually become so involved in the immediate admitting process that we sometimes fail to assess the patient's anxiety level. Such a reaction on the nurse's part is understandable. However, sometimes the nurse continues to perceive the patient on a biological level long after admission. Like the patient, the nurse fails to move beyond the threat to biological integrity. The nurse may see the patient as a biological entity, rather than as a human being with a biological problem. The nurse should begin to reduce the conditions that lead to primary anxiety, fright, and expectant anxiety.

[29]*Ibid.*, p. 139.

Primary Anxiety

Primary anxiety can be reduced if the nurse assumes that an infant or small child separated from attachment figures will experience anxiety. The nurse must also realize that separation at an early age can be a traumatic emotional experience, and must assess ways to alleviate the feelings of anxiety. Nursing care becomes of utmost significance. The nurse must skillfully intervene in three basic areas, providing for continuity of care, parental involvement, and play therapy which will allow the child to express feelings in a nonthreatening environment.

The child needs to have a continuing relationship with one person. Sometimes because of staffing problems or emergencies this is not always realistic. However, when possible the principle should be applied. As the same nurse becomes involved with a young patient, she or he becomes the substitute attachment figure. The child invests in the nurse the most precious possession, a sense of trust. Sudden unavailability will elicit the primary anxiety, rejection. This may have been the same regressive behavior assessed in early separation from mother. The nurse's goal is to provide individualized and personalized care. The nurse realizes that, "the traumatic effect of separation seems to be a function of multiple caretakers and the resultant lack of individualized care. The provision of a substitute mother can alleviate the child's anxieties."[30]

The second aspect of care revolves around parental involvement. Whenever realistic, the parents should be encouraged to remain as an influencing factor in their child's care. Of course the nurse must assess the parent's readiness for active involvement. As mentioned earlier, the parents may be in greater need of supportive care than the child. The nurse through discussions with the parents can assess each's relationship to the other. If the child's primary anxiety will be reduced by their involvement, the nurse establishes areas of care in which they can safely intervene. Research shows that involvement by the child's mother reduces primary anxiety and thus regressive behavior. Parents should be invited to share in the care of their child. The validity of such intervention has been documented by Claire Fagin.[31] Her investigation focused upon sixty hospitalized children, one and one-half through three years of age. Half of the children had their mothers with them during the hospitalization; the other half were hospitalized alone, although their mothers visited daily. Fagin found that, after discharge, the children whose mothers remained with them during hospitalization showed significant

[30]Wear, *op. cit.*, p. 14.

[31]Claire Fagin, *The Effects of Maternal Attendance During Hospitalization on the Past Hospital Behavior of Young Children: A Comprehensive Survey,* (Philadelphia: Davis, 1966).

changes, in a progressive direction, in appetite and manner of eating, emotional dependence, reaction to brief separation, and in the use of special toys. The children who were separated from their mothers during the hospitalization experience showed mild to severe regression in the same areas. Involvement by the attachment figure can have a beneficial effect upon reducing the child's primary anxieties of separation.

The last area in which the nurse intervenes is in play therapy. Through the media of play activity, the nurse can encourage young patients to share feelings regarding hospitalization, separation and illness, disfigurement, or injury. The nurse's attitude conveys understanding and acceptance. The child may not realize that his or her anxieties are normal and shared by other children of the same age or younger. Such reassurances by the nurse will help to lessen the child's anxiety. Furthermore, play therapy becomes a safe and nonthreatening area in which the child may express anxieties. For example, a child may be playing with a doll or stuffed animal and suddenly assume the parental role, scolding the doll or animal for becoming ill or injured. On the other hand, the child may talk as himself through the doll. Again the nurse may hear the child say, "I am sorry, Mommy. I didn't mean to get sick. I want to go home." The observant and sensitive nurse is able to gather insight into a young patient's feelings. Without realizing it, the child works through conflicts in the activity of play. The nurse helps the child by making a wide range of toys available. With older children, the nurse may use symbolic language as a means of facilitating external expression of internal anxieties. Symbolic language is possible through the media of painting and drawing. The nurse intervenes to reduce primary anxiety through continuity of nursing care, encouragment of parental involvement, and facilitation of play activities. In addition, the nurse demonstrates confidence and respect in the child's ability to cope with his or her own anxieties. Furthermore, the nurse's confidence in the child is demonstrated by encouraging endeavors with other people and his or her own care.

Fright

The nurse must assess those factors which are perceived as frightening to the child, adult, or aged patient. For these patients, fright originates from their immediate environment. The patient goes from a very protective yet independent home environment into one of unfamiliarity and dependency. The patient is placed in a strange room sometimes with a vast array of supportive devices attached to the body. Strangers move in and out of the environment. Each seems to have a purpose but their actions have no meaning to the patient. Instead of providing support they frighten and make the patient more anxious. The nurse intervenes to carefully explain events in the patient's immediate environment, explaining the purpose behind the various supportive devices and/or actions of the health team.

Depending upon the severity of the illness, injury or disease of the patient, he or she may require intense or close nursing surveillance. Initially this may be threatening because it reinforces anxieties that a severe biological crisis has occurred. Fright leads to two responses, escape and freezing. As discussed earlier, the child reacts with regressive behavior by crying or clinging to the nurse. The nurse should provide a structured time in which the child is held, talked with, or read a favorite story, all of which facilitate closeness and comfort rather than fear. Likewise, the adult patient may appreciate a nurse spending time quietly sitting at the bedside, holding a hand, or listening to fears and anxieties. As the patient's biological status reaches stability, the nurse may spend less time with the patient. Patients, regardless of the developmental stage, may have difficulty accepting reduced surveillance, mistaking it for avoidance behavior or rejection. Even though the nurse assesses biological improvement, the patient is unable to comprehend this and continues to see himself or herself as ill and in need of mechanical surveillance. The patient feels that the "life line" or "umbilical cord" is being abruptly severed. In order to avoid fright associated with reduced nursing and/or mechanical surveillance, a patient's nurse should gradually prepare the patient for their removal. The nurse attempts to make the patient's environment as conducive to anxiety reduction as possible.

Expectant Anxiety

The nurse must assess those factors which lead to expectant anxiety in the adult or aged patient. For the hospitalized patient, expectant anxiety revolves around two basic areas. The first involves threats to his biological system, and the second, threats to his self-system. Threats to the patient's biological system consist of two components, the illness and the various diagnostic or intrusive procedures.

Illness that has come to be a frequent event is frightening. Recurrent illness resulting in continual biological loss is possibly the most threatening. Take, for example, the emphysema patient whose pulmonary status is such that in time there will be total dependence upon a volume respirator. His or her future becomes frightening, knowing that eventually there will be dependence upon support systems—family and machines. The severely disabled arthritic patient may become dependent upon the family and, if alone, has no one. If not emotionally supported, the patient with terminal cancer can become frightened at the loss of the future. Each patient's fright can be dealt with if the nurse is able to assess its existence.

As discussed earlier, the nurse may only assess fright through the patient's behavioral response. The patient may utilize defense mechanisms as a means of coping. Depending upon the defense utilized, the nurse can only support the defense until the patient is able to progress to a new level of adaptation. The nurse helps adaptation by pointing out areas of improvement and strength. Granted the patient with terminal cancer may not improve, he nevertheless has strength that can be used at this time. For the patient who will reach some level of biological stability, the nurse helps that patient recognize improvement. However, those areas of improvement such as blood gases, enzyme levels, hemoglobin, hematocrit, EKG, liver profile, or electrolytes should be shared and explained to the patient. In this respect, the patient develops a sense of relatedness to his or her own improvement. Last, the nurse assesses the patient's readiness to learn about the illness and its future implications. In this respect, the illness becomes a less frightening experience.

The various intrusive procedures that seem to be a routine part of diagnosis and treatment are the second threat to the patient's biological system, causing expectant anxiety. Even though intrusive procedures are accepted by members of the health team as relatively normal or routine, they become threatening to the child, adult, or aged patient. It seems that the best time to explain an intrusive procedure, particularly with children, is at the time of institution. If the patient is told too far in advance, he or she may become more frightened than necessary. Furthermore, it is difficult to conceptualize what one has never seen or experienced. Therefore fantasies regarding the intrusive procedure makes the individual even more anxious. In addition, only the necessary details regarding the procedure are given. This becomes an influencing factor in enhancing or reducing anxiety. Too many details make the procedure seem more complicated and frightening than is realistic. Too few details make the adult patient feel that the staff is not being honest. The patient fantasizes the intrusive procedure will document what he or she fears to be the biological problem. It is a difficult task but the nurse must assess the patient's anxiety level in relationship to the procedure. This goal is accomplished by listening to the patient's questions. The questions usually revolve around duration of procedure, discomfort involved, and significance of results. Furthermore, the nurse assesses the patient's previous experience with the same or similar procedure. For example, it may be necessary to do a lumbar puncture on an arthritic patient. Due to the arthritic changes in the spinal cord, the procedure may seem to go on for a prolonged period of time. The arthritic changes make it difficult for easy insertion of the needle. Therefore, the doctor may make several attempts. As a result, the patient's anxiety level continues to rise. The nurse and physician who anticipate this problem can better support their patient throughout the procedure.

The second overall threat causing expectant anxiety is threat to the individual's self-system. Coupled with self-system is the individual's ability to relate with others in the environment. The nurse assesses and supports the patient's strengths. This enhances internal confidence enabling the patient to better cope with external crisis. "Striving to help the patient feel reassured, to increase his self esteem and to help him build confidence in himself so that he once again wants 'to be,' will enable both nurse and patient to take the first steps toward finding effective ways to cope with the stress that continues to bring about anxiety episodes."[32] This has specific significance for the schizophrenic patient. The nurse therapist assists in identifying more appropriate ways of coping with anxieties and threats to his or her existence. As the nurse helps the patient move through anxiety provoking situations, the patient learns about the evolving self-system. In this respect, the patient's freedom to move in the environment is increased. With supportive assistance, fears and anxieties in interpersonal relationships are also enhanced. How the nurse/therapist succeeds in alleviating the patient's interpersonal anxieties in a one-to-one relationship has implications for the patient's relationship with others. Therefore, the nurse intervenes in those areas in which the patient will achieve success. In time they move toward problem solving in larger areas of significance. As the schizophrenic patient learns to respond with courage, he or she endures the threats of individual anxieties. Success or failure with others in the hospital community equip the patient for similar experiences in the larger social community. The aged patient has expectant anxiety regarding a precarious future. The nurse helps this patient identify those areas in which the patient does have a future, including family, friends, and social activities. As with the schizophrenic patient, the nurse identifies strengths, namely the support-system family or friends.

Anxiety can be reduced. The reduction involves an organized plan to control primary anxiety, fright, and expectant anxiety. The nurse assesses the patient's anxiety level according to behavioral and physiological responses. The nursing interventions involve assessing the effect of separation from attachment figures for the child and the ability to find a substitute attachment figure. The nurse further assesses those events within the child, adult, or aged patient's environment which lead to fright. Lastly, expectant anxiety, as seen in the adult or aged patient, is assessed as a threat to biological and self-system. Each component of the general concept anxiety can be assessed shortly after the patient is admitted to a particular clinical setting. Once the presence or absence of anxiety is assessed, the nurse formulates a unique plan of care designed to alleviate the patient's anxieties. The nurse evaluates the effectiveness of

[32]Cohen, *op. cit.*, p. 20.

the intervention in an attempt to measure success. Proper assessment and organized care, including teaching, will enable the patient to move through a hospital stay with normal anxiety.

REFERENCES

Bateson, Jackson, *Toward A Theory of Schizophrenia*, Philadelphia: Saunders, 1964.

Baxter, James, "Anxiety and Avoidance Behavior in Schizophrenics in Response to Parental Figures," *Journal of Abnormal and Social Psychology*, 1962, pp. 432–437.

Beigler, Jerome, "Anxiety As An Aid in the Prognostication of Impending Death," *AMA Archives of Neurology and Psychiatry*, 77, February 1857, pp. 171-177.

Bowlby, John, *Attachment and Loss*, Vol. I, New York: Basic Books, 1969.

Branstetter, Ellamae, "The Young Child's Response to Hospitalization—Separation Anxiety or Lack of Mothering Care," *American Journal of Public Health*, LIX, 1969, pp. 92–98.

Burkhardt, Marti, "Response to Anxiety," *American Journal of Nursing*, October 1969, pp. 2153–2154.

Cassem, Ned. "What is Behind Our Masks?" *AORN Journal*, July 1974, pp. 79-92.

Cattell, R. B., and Scheier, I. N., "Theory and Research on Anxiety," *Anxiety and Behavior*, (Ed: Spielberger), New York: Academic Press, 1966.

Dye, Celeste, "Self-Concept, Anxiety, and Group Participation," *Nursing Research*, July-August 1974.

Eissler, K. R., "A Note on Trauma, Dream, Anxiety, and Schizophrenia," *Psychoanalytic Study of the Child*, XXI, 1966, pp. 17-50.

Johnson, Dorothy, "The Meaning of Maternal Deprivation and Separation Anxiety for Nursing Practice," *ANA Clinical Sessions*, 1962, pp. 22-33.

Levine, Gene, "Anxiety About Illness: Psychological and Social Bases," *Journal of Health and Human Behavior*, pp. 30-34.

Mechanic, David, "The Concept of Illness Behavior," *Journal of Chronic Disability*, 15, pp. 189-194.

Menzies, Isabel, "A Case Study in the Functioning of Social Systems As A Defense Against Anxiety," *Human Relations*, 13, 1960, pp. 95-121.

Powers, Maryann and Storlie, Frances, "The Apprehensive Patient," *American Journal of Nursing*, January 1967, pp. 58-63.

Prugh, Dane and Others, "A Study of the Emotional Reactions of Children and Families to Hospitalization and Illness," *American Journal of Orthopsychiatry*, XXIII, 1971.

Robertson, James, *Young Children in Hospitals*, New York: Basic Books, 1958.

Sarbin, Theodore, "Anxiety: Reification of a Metaphor," *Archives of General Psychiatry*, 10, June 1964.

Sarnoff, Irving, "Anxiety, Fear, and Social Affiliation," *Journal of Abnormal and Social Psychology*, 62, 1961.

Schulman, Sam, "Basic Functional Roles in Nursing: Mother Surrogate and Healer," *Parents, Physicians and Illness*, (Ed: Gartly Jaco), Illinois: Free Press, 1958.

Spitz, Rene, "Hospitalism," *The Psychoanalytic Study of the Child*, New York: International Universities Press, 1945.

Sutton, Helen, "Emotional Reactions to Medical Procedures and Illness in a Hospital Child Psychiatry Unit," *American Journal of Orthopsychiatry*, 28, 1958, pp. 180–187.

Yarrow, Leon, "Separation from Parents During Early Childhood," *Review of Child Development Research*, (Ed: Martin and Lois Hoffman), New York: Russel Sage Foundation, 1964.

3
Pain

Most people have had some experience with pain. Pain knows no age or cultural boundaries. Our modern culture seems to be preoccupied with pain and its elimination. If we watch the many television commercials, we are encouraged to fight the pain of headache, hemorrhoid, corns, warts, backache, joint stiffness, sore eyes, or indigestion with a variety of pills, ointments, eye drops, or liquids. Pain is expressed in various forms, several of which are not physically or bodily related. It surrounds us as the emotional and cultural entity of poverty, death, wars, starvation, disasters, suicides, violence, and illness. Pain then, is a multidimensional concept. According to Melzack, "Pain, we now believe, refers to a category of complex experiences, not to a specific sensation that varies only along a single intensity dimension. The word 'pain,' in this formulation, is a linguistic label that categorizes an endless variety of qualities. There are the pains of a scalded hand, a stomach ulcer, or sprained ankle; there are headaches and toothaches. Each is characterized by unique qualities."[1]

Pain has different implications and significance to each individual. For the most part, pain is a "perceptual experience whose quality and intensity are influenced by the unique past history of the individual, by the meaning he gives to the pain-producing situation and by his 'state of mind' at the moment. We believe that all these factors play a role in determining the actual pattern of nerve impulses that ascend from the body to the brain and travel within the brain itself. In this way pain becomes a function of the whole individual, including his present thoughts and fears as well as his hopes for the future."[2] As an experience, pain incorporates the total individual.

This first involves childhood encounters with pain and how parents handled the child's reaction. For example, a child may receive a scratch

[1]Ronald Melzack, *The Puzzle of Pain*, (New York: Basic Books, 1973), p. 41.
[2]*Ibid.*, p. 49.

while playing. To the child, the scratch is the most significant event of the moment. Mother or father cleans the small wound and covers it with a bandage. If the child's parent makes a tremendous fuss over the scratch, the child can become an adult with a low pain threshold. The individual's current pain experience includes not only childhood encounters but also adult experiences. The individual who has suffered severe trauma or chronic disability knows the all encompassing world of pain. Because of its many facets, vast amounts of research have been devoted to the relief of pain. Pain clinics exist which have been established for the sole purpose of directly treating the pain or helping the individual learn to cope with it.

For those individuals experiencing chronic long term pain, the pain itself becomes a way of existence. The outer world becomes monitored by internal pain experiences. LeShan believes that, "Pain permits personal existence to continue with little assistance from our usual orientations, defenses, safeguards and associations. It attenuates our relationships with the outer world at the same time that it weakens the inner structure. In painless consciousness, we are filled with images, associations, and thoughts. In the loud loneliness of pain, only our existence is real. We float alone in space, conscious only of the suffering."[3] The individual in pain, regardless of age, reaches out to those people in the external world who one feels can help him or her cope with the pain. There is hope in their ability to lessen fears and anxieties regarding pain. The health team realizes that fear and anxiety increase the individual's pain and that the mere anticipation of pain can magnify it.

Unfortunately, pain is primarily a patient experience rather than a dual experience shared by both the patient and members of the health team. The staff has a tendency to treat an individual's pain rather than assessing the various aspects of pain such as its duration, intensity, location, meaning, description, and/or previous experience. These are areas in which the health team must make pertinent assessments. Before applying its concept to various clinical settings, it would be beneficial to first define pain and then briefly examine theories related to pain.

DEFINITION AND THEORIES OF PAIN

Pain is a difficult concept to define because of its multidimensional aspects. It becomes whatever the individual says it is and what is experienced at the time. The diversity of pain experience makes it almost impossible to obtain a definition which members of the health team can

[3]Lawrence LeShan, "The World of the Patient in Severe Pain of Long Duration," *Journal of Chronic Disease*, 17, February 1964, p. 121.

apply. "Pain is not a single quality of experience that can be specified in terms of defined stimulus conditions. It may be agreed that pain, like vision and hearing, is a complex perceptual experience."[4] Pain has many causes all of which are equally important.

Pain represents a number of experiences each of which can be categorized and represented by unique events for each individual. In other words, what is perceived as pain by one individual is not perceived in the same manner by another. Pain, according to Melzack, can then be "defined in terms of a multidimensional space comprising several sensory and affective dimensions. The space comprises those subjective experiences which have both somatosensory and negative-affective components and that elicit behavior aimed at stopping the conditions that produce them."[5] Pain is not purely a stimulus response. Other factors must be taken into consideration. Physical pain involves a noxious stimulus of varying degree in intensity and duration. Psychological pain becomes more of a perceptual experience. Physical and psychological pain are closely interrelated. As has been discussed in various definitions pain involves both physical and psychological experiences of the individual. "It is a psychological experience of events occurring within the patient's body, always unpleasant and associated with the impression of damage to the tissues. This blend of physiological and psychological events has to pass through the patient's powers of expression and speech before being described and made comprehensible to a nurse or doctor."[6]

There are several different theories regarding the evolution of pain. Each attempts to explain pain in terms of its origin and the individual's physiological and/or psychological response. The theories are categorized as pattern theory, affect theory, specificity theory, and gate-control theory. Of the four theories, specificity and gate-control seem to be the most significant. Before discussing these latter theories, a brief definition of pattern and affect theory will be given.

Melzack believes that "Goldscheider's pattern, or summation, theory proposes that the particular patterns of nerve impulses that evoke pain are produced by the summation of the skin sensory input at the dorsal horn cells. According to this concept, pain results when the total output of the cells exceeds a critical level as a result of either excessive stimulation of receptors that are normally fired by nonnoxious thermal or tactile stimuli, or pathological conditions that enhance the summation of impulses produced by normally nonnoxious stimuli."[7] Affect theory

[4]Melzack, *op. cit.*, pp. 45–46.

[5]Melzack, *loc. cit.* p. 46.

[6]Kenneth Leele, "Pain: How It Varies From Person to Person," *Nursing Times*, July 20, 1972, p. 890.

[7]Melzack, *op. cit.*, p. 140.

implies that pain has more than only a sensory quality. Instead it also has a negative affective quality. This quality drives an individual into activity. An individual is compelled to do something about a negative situation and will take the most effective course of action to stop the event. Therefore, the behavior is in the realm of motivation. Affect theory then, has to do with emotion and behavior.

The more traditional theory of pain is known as specificity theory. "Specificity theory proposes that a specific pain system carries messages from pain receptors in the skin to a pain center in the brain."[8] This theory then indicates that there are special nerve fibers that respond to different stimuli. These stimuli can be pain, temperature changes, touch, or even position changes. Each stimulus is transmitted through different nerve fibers. Take for example an individual who, while running, steps on a nail. The pain in the foot tells him or her immediately that a problem exists. In this respect, the pain has a specific origin, the foot. The stimulus from the nail travels up nerve fibers in the foot, leg, back and finally into the head where an alarm system is triggered. The individual feels pain and responds by ceasing further running. The overall result is that the person feels pain and responds to it.

The last theory is possibly the most recent and popular of all theories. In addition, it has the greatest significance to members of the health team. The gate-control theory was proposed by Melzack and Wall. The most significant difference between gate-control and specificity theory," . . . is that pain impulses transmitted from nerve receptors through the spinal cord to the brain can be modulated or altered in the spinal cord, brain stem, and cerebral cortex. The potential blocking ability of certain cells along the transmission route can result in little or no pain perception regardless of the intensity of the noxious stimulus. The gate control theory also helps explain the influence of psychological factors on the pain experience, including perception and interpretation."[9] Melzack and Wall have defined a functional unit of densely packed cells called *substantia gelatenosa*. It extends the length of the spinal cord and becomes the site of a transmission blocking action which closes the gate to entering impulses. These impulses then are not conveyed to the transmission cells. When the gate opens, sensory input is allowed to reach the transmission cells in the dorsal horn of the spinal cord. According to Segele, "The gate-control theory supports the hypothesis that pain is a complex perceptual experience in which sensory input is altered by a distinctive but interacting neural system before that input evokes pain perception and response."[10]

[8]*Ibid.*, p. 126.

[9]Dorothy Siegele, "The Gate Control Theory," *American Journal of Nursing*, March 1974, p. 499.

[10]*Ibid.*, p. 501.

To the individual a pain producing situation has only self-meaning. The current situation may be related to a history of pain and the present state of psychological being. All these variables influence not only reaction to pain but also the perception of the experience. Pain as applied to various clinical situations can be divided into two overall categories. The first is the physiological component of pain which includes physiological manifestations and variables. Second, there exists a psychological component of pain which takes into account psychological manifestations or behavioral responses and variables.

APPLICATION TO CLINICAL SETTING

The child, adult, or aged patient may or may not be experiencing pain upon entering the hospital. Due to the nature and severity of the illness, pain may become the presenting complaint. Other patients who originally enter the hospital free of pain may at some point in time develop it. For some patients pain becomes a temporary way of life, an example being the burn, arthritic, or terminally ill patient to whom pain becomes a primary concern. In these instances it becomes the concern of the health team. In most clinical settings the relief of pain is not always the primary concern of the nurse. The staff in critical care or emergency room may be more interested in diagnosis and emergency care than the patient's pain. Furthermore, the individual's pain may be a result of the health teams actions. Unfortunately, pain becomes a by-product of various diagnostic studies, intrusive treatments, or surgical procedures. The accompanying pain is not intentional, it is simply a by-product.

Pain as it applies to the child, adult or aged patient will be discussed according to two categories or components, physiological and psychological. Each component will be further categorized into manifestations or behavioral responses and influencing factors.

Physiological Component

Melzack[11] believes that two terms are significant in the attempt to understand the physiology of pain. These terms are specificity and specialization. Specificity implies that a receptor, fiber, or other component of a sensory system subserves only a single specific modality (or quality) of experience. Specialization, on the other hand, implies that the components of a sensory system are highly specialized so that particular types and ranges of physical energy evoke characteristic patterns of neural signals, and that these patterns can be modulated by other sensory

[11]Melzack, *op. cit.*, p. 74.

inputs or by cognitive processes to produce more than one quality of experience or none at all. The entire brain is considered to be the pain center. It seems that the thalamus, hypothalamus, brainstem reticular formation, limbic system, parietal cortex, and frontal cortex are all involved in pain perception. A stimulus produces neural signals that travel through an active nervous system. In the adult, the neurological system is a combination of past experiences, culture, anticipation, and anxiety. These brain processes play a vital role in the selection, abstraction, and synthesis of data from the overall sensory input.

Pain viewed as overwhelming, demands the individual's immediate attention because it disrupts ongoing behavior and thought. Pain serves as a motivating force which drives the person into activity aimed at stopping it. In this respect, pain becomes more than a sensory response and acquires motivational-affective properties. Physiologically there are central cells which monitor the input of stimulus for long periods of time. Intense stimuli can prolong neural activity which persists long after stimulation ceases. This process plays an important role in the pain process. Physiological or bodily pain is a signal to the individual of physical harm. It tells the individual that a breach in the protective barrier has taken place. Pain serves a purpose as a protective mechanism. The individual experiences pain whenever any tissue is being damaged and causes the person, by reflex, to remove himself or herself from the pain stimuli.

Guyton[12] gives the example of sitting for a long time on the ischia which can cause tissue destruction because of lack of blood flow to the skin where the skin is compressed by the body's weight. When the skin becomes painful as a result of the ischemia, the person shifts the weight unconsciously. This has implications for the nurse working with the immobilized child, adult, or aged patient. The infant or small child is unable to verbalize the need to be moved thus relieving ischemia associated with a pressure point. Instead the nurse observes the small patient crying or thrashing his or her arms and legs. The adult, due to paralysis, severe injury, or supportive devices, may be immobilized and unable to change position. Likewise the aged CVA or comatose patient is unable to independently change position. Each patient, particularly the paralyzed or comatose, depends upon the nurse to provide a protective environment in which the protective barrier, the skin, is maintained by turning. The individual who has lost the sense of pain due to a spinal cord injury becomes a unique problem for nurses. The inability to feel ischemia pain and respond by moving leads to ulceration at the area of pressure.

Guyton has classified pain according to three different types: pricking, burning, and aching. A description of each is important for the nurse who attempts to assess the type of pain a patient is experiencing. A

[12]Arthur Guyton, *Textbook of Medical Physiology*, (Saunders, 1971), p. 577.

pricking pain is felt when a needle is stuck into the skin or when the skin is cut. It is also felt when a widespread area of the skin is strongly irritated. Burning pain is the type of pain felt when the skin is burned and can be the most severe in terms of suffering. Aching pain is not usually felt in the surface of the body. Instead it is a deep pain with varying degrees of intensity.

Physiologically, pain can originate from a noxious stimulus within the patient's body. Tissue damage can cause pain. Guyton[13] has divided the origin of tissue damage resulting in pain into two further categories. First, he feels that bradykinin and histamine function to stimulate pain endings thus contributing to pain experience. The exact mechanism is not known; however, it is believed that bradykinin may be the principle substance that stimulates pain endings. Cell damage releases proteolytic enzymes that almost immediately split bradykinin and other similar substances from the globulins in the interstitial fluid. In addition, damaged cells also release histamine in lesser amounts. Like bradykinin, it can also elicit a pain response.

The second origin of physiological pain involves tissue ischemia and muscle spasm. When blood flow to the tissue ceases, the tissue itself becomes painful. The greater the rate of metabolism of the tissue involved (such as the arm), the more rapidly will pain appear. The cause of pain in ischemia is not completely understood. It is believed that pain might be due to accumulation of lactic acid in the tissues. Lactic acid forms as a consequence of the anaerobic metabolism (metabolism without oxygen) that occurs during ischemia. Muscle spasm is also a cause of pain. The contracting muscle compresses intramuscular blood vessels and either reduces or cuts off blood flow. Next, muscle contraction increases the rate of metabolism of the muscle. Consequently, muscle spasm causes a degree of muscle ischemia which results in ischemic pain.

There are many stimuli to an individual's body which pose threats to its tissue integrity. These stimuli are called noxious stimuli. They can originate externally or internally to the body. External stimuli may take the form of a blow from a blunt object, cut, or prick. Internal noxious stimuli arise from within the body itself. It may result from tissue ischemia by a myocardial infarction; inflammation from abscess in a finger or deep within the pleural or visceral cavity; or, from muscle spasms such as cramp or renal colic. Of significance to the nurse working with hospitalized patients is visceral pain from various organs. The viscera have sensory receptors for no other modalities of sensation besides pain. The specific areas of significance to nurses are cardiac, esophageal, gastric, biliary, pancreatic, renal, and uterine pain. The patient in describing and locating a pain may think the pain is epigastric; however, it is really

---

[13]*Ibid.*, p. 579.

cardiac in origin. An understanding of the various visceral pains helps the nurse to more accurately locate the pain.

Physiological manifestations   Physiological manifestation of pain involves assessment of visceral pain and the overall signs and symptoms of pain. As mentioned earlier visceral pain is the most difficult pain to assess. Physiological manifestation of pain in terms of signs and symptoms takes into account intensity, duration, and meaning of the pain experience.

For the patient entering coronary care, cardiac pain originates from ischemia secondary to coronary ischemia. In assessing the pain's location, the nurse observes its origin in the base of the neck, over the shoulders, over the pectoral muscles, and down the arms. Furthermore, the nurse observes that the patient's pain is more frequently noted on the left side than the right. This occurs because the left side of the heart is more frequently involved in coronary disease. Guyton points out that, "when coronary ischemia is extremely severe, such as immediately after a coronary thrombosis, intense cardiac pain sometimes occurs directly underneath the sternum simultaneously with pain referred to other areas . . . skeletal nerve endings passing from the heart through the pericardial reflection around the great vessels conduct this direct pain."[14] In addition, the nurse may assess other pain symptoms associated with coronary thrombosis. The cardiac patient complains of tightness in the chest. The exact mechanism behind the manifestation is unknown. However, it is believed that a reflex spasm of blood vessels, bronchioles or muscles in the chest contribute to the pain. This may explain such related symptoms of the cardiac patient as shortness of breath and diaphoresis.

Esophageal and gastric pain can be easily confused with cardiac pain. Esophageal pain is usually referred to the pharynx, lower neck, arms, or to midline chest regions beginning at the upper portion of the sternum and ending at the lower level of the heart. The nurse must realize that irritation of the gastric end of the esophagus may cause pain directly over the heart. The patient may believe this pain is cardiac in origin while in reality, the pain is caused by spasm of the cardia. The cardia is the area where the esophagus empties into the stomach. Gastric pain, on the other hand, originates in the fundus of the stomach and is caused by gastritis. The patient complains of pain in the anterior surface of the chest or upper abdomen from below the heart to the xyphoid process. Patients describe the pain as a burning sensation. The health team who suspects peptic ulcer will assess the patient's pain to be located on either side of the pylorus in the stomach or in the duodenum. As with gastric pain, the

[14]*Ibid.*, p. 585.

patient complains of intense burning. The significant difference between gastric and ulcer pain lies in accurate assessment of the pain's location.

Biliary and gallbladder pain may be confused with peptic ulcer pain. Pain from the bile duct and the gallbladder is localized in the midepigastrium. This is almost coincident with pain caused by a peptic ulcer. Furthermore, the pain is described as burning although cramps due to spasm often occur. Biliary disease also refers pain to a small area at the top of the right scapula. Such pain is transmitted through sympathetic afferent fibers that enter the ninth thoracic segment of the spinal cord. Due to its proximity with the biliary and gallbladder, pancreatic pain must also be considered here. Acute or chronic pancreatitis causes pain in areas both anterior and posterior to the pancreas. The pain may be due to lesions in which pancreatic enzymes eat away the pancreas and surrounding structures. The nurse should recognize that the pancreas is located beneath the parietal peritoneum and that it receives many sensory fibers from the posterior abdominal wall. Such pain is localized behind the pancreas in the back and is described by the patient as a burning sensation. A skilled nurse is able to assist the patient in accurately locating a pain and assessing its significance.

The last two visceral pains of clinical significance to the nurse consist of renal and uterine pain. Renal pain is better localized than those pains already discussed. Guyton points out that the kidney, kidney pelvis, and ureters are all retroperitoneal structures and receive most of their pain fibers directly from the skeletal nerves. The patient usually experiences pain directly behind the ailing structure. Occasionally pain is referred via visceral afferent to the anterior abdominal wall below the umbilicus. Pain from the patient's bladder is localized directly over the bladder. Such localization helps the nurse in assessing bladder pain due to distention or cramp. Uterine pain may be more complex. Both parietal and visceral afferent pain may be transmitted from the uterus. Dysmenorrhea is associated with low abdominal cramping pains. Depending upon the patient's particular physiological problem, the pain may be described as cramping, aching, or burning.

The nurse needs to know physiological origin and thereby manifestations of pain to assess its location and true meaning. Therefore, pain in the tip of the scapula can either signify scapular or biliary pain. Lack of knowledge regarding the physiological component of pain may cause the nurse to overlook the possibility of biliary pain. The same knowledge is required of other organs which manifest problems in terms of visceral pain. The nurse who does not have knowledge of the various visceral pains is unable to accurately assess the significance of a patient's pain. Furthermore, the nurse must be able to assess signs and symptoms of pain.

The nurse must be able to recognize the presence of pain in a child, adult, or aged patient. Therefore, the nurse assesses various physiological parameters. The nature of physiological responses seems to be dependent upon two factors; the duration of pain experience and degree of anxiety occurring with it. The nurse may observe the following signs and symptoms: increased pulse, increased respiratory rate, increased blood pressure, pallor, dilated pupils, diaphoresis, nausea, vomiting, diarrhea, and muscle aches. These physiological manifestations are the result of increased sympathoadrenal activity. Each sign or symptom has clinical significance. For example, the patient in hypertensive crisis should not experience pain for a prolonged period since it could increase an already elevated blood pressure. Likewise, the patient in coronary care with supraventricular tachycardia does not need to have the pulse rate increased further. The list of examples could continue.

Physiological parameters may be the only means of assessing physiological pain in the patient who is unable to verbalize pain because of limited cognitive ability, comatose state, or speech impairment. The patient, regardless of age, may adapt to physiological pain. Adaptation takes place when the stimulus for activation is repeated frequently or over a long period of time. The adaptive responses are compensatory, resulting from prolonged sympathetic responses. It is interesting to note that adaptation is the result of a decrease in sympathetic response. It can be assessed by only a slight increase in the pulse rate and blood pressure.

Variables   Besides knowledge of physiological origins of pain and an ability to assess physiological parameters for manifestations of pain, the nurse must also recognize factors or variables which influence a patient's pain response or experience. McCaffery[15] has identified physiological and physical factors influencing the individual pain experience. These include the following variables or influencing factors: the neurophysiological processes underlying the sensation of pain; duration and intensity of pain; alterations in the level of consciousness; cutaneous versus visceral sites of pain; environmental conditions; sensory restriction; and physical strain and fatigue. Neurophysiological processes underlying pain and visceral sites of pain have already been discussed.

The duration and intensity of pain work together and have a direct effect upon the patient. Intense pain can lead to activation of the sympathetic nervous system. If the pain continues, adaptation followed by stress reactions can occur. Furthermore, pain of long duration can establish pain memories in the nervous system which contribute to the persistence of pain after the noxious stimuli are removed. The adult or aged

---

[15]Margo McCaffery, *Nursing Management of the Patient With Pain*, (Philadelphia: Lippincott, 1972), p. 15.

patient may view encounter with pain of any intensity as an isolated event. After the painful experience of diagnostic test or intrusive procedure is completed, the pain receives little attention. Instead the individual transfers the focus of attention toward something else. The child, on the other hand, may not shift his or her attention. For example, the child who receives repeated venapunctures or other intrusive procedures will anticipate pain. In other words, for these children each painful encounter will assume a cumulative significance. The patient in chronic pain represents the other end of the duration continuum. Chronic pain is not localized to one area of the body. Arthritic pain, for example, consumes the entire body. The individual focuses his attention on the pain, to the exclusion of everything else. The pain becomes all consuming to the point of physical and emotional exhaustion. Consequently, the patient's body movements and verbal communications decrease in intensity and frequency. He begins to ask why the pain occurred to him and what its effect upon his future will be.

The patient's level of consciousness can influence reactions to pain. Level of consciousness can be altered to the point whereby the patient is insensitive to pain. Factors contributing to reduced sensitivity are head injury, infections of the central nervous system such as meningitis or encephalitis, sedation, narcotics, and conditions that reduce oxygenation of the brain. The patient who is unconscous obviously will not respond to painful stimuli. Response to pain may be a significant diagnostic test for the neurological patient. The nurse may assess a patient's decreasing level of consciousness by a growing inability to respond to pain. Patients unable to verbalize pain may be analogous to those who overreact to pain.

The patient's immediate environment can be an influencing factor. The nurse should be aware of temperature changes in the patient's hospital environment. The adult or aged patient with musculoskeletal problems, such as arthritis, experience pain in a cold environment. The cold leads to muscle tension followed by pain. Similarly, patients with arteriosclerosis or peripheral vascular insufficiency may not tolerate a cool environment. In addition, the nurse may need to place a small heater by the patient's bed or place additional blankets on the bed. Lights may be a painful environmental stumulus to the patient with glaucoma or cataracts. Therefore, the nurse needs to darken the patient's environment by dimming the lights and closing the blinds. Excessive noise might be a source of pain for those individuals accustomed to silence.

Sensory restriction refers to the child, adult, or aged individual's environment in which the stimulus is not adequate to maintain an optimal level of cortical arousal. The stimuli may be of insufficient amount, pattern, or variation, causing the hospitalized patient to experience sensory deprivation and perceptual monotony. To counteract a situation of sensory restriction, the centrally regulated threshold for sensation is lowered. Thus, the amount of sensory input required to achieve optimal cortical arousal is reduced. As a result, the individual may be more sensitive to pain and other stimuli than usual. Nurses frequently see sensory deprivation in adult patients with bilateral eye patches or children with full body casts. Perceptual deprivation is a common problem in critical care units in which the patient's environment is filled with various machines and supportive devices each making its own unique hum, buzz, or beep. The monotonous environment is one without variation. This may be a nursing care problem for patients on bedrest, in full body casts, with burns over their face, hands, and chest, or in complete isolation, involving all the senses.

Lastly, prolonged fatigue and sleep deprivation are variables which alter the patient's response or sensitivity to pain. Hospitalized patients confronted with sleep deprivation are usually those in critical care units. Here the environment is noisy and patients are frequently awakened for various treatments or procedures. Fatigue has a tendency to slow down transmission of nerve impulses. The individual's reaction time is reduced and there is difficulty maintaining a normal train of thought. The fatigued patient has little energy remaining to cope with pain. Normal coping mechanisms of distraction or varying the stimuli are diminished.

In terms of physiological pain, the nurse should have knowledge of the pain's physiological origin, purpose, and type; assess physiological manifestations of pain; and finally, assess those variables or influencing factors which apply or contribute to the physiological component of pain.

Psychological Component

The psychological component of pain involves two types of perceptions. The first is perception of past experiences such as early encounters with pain and the role significant others played in its alleviation. The second is perception of pain as a threat to the individual's physical or emotional integrity. In other words, the latter threat involves loss in varying degrees. Each individual varies in the perception of pain. It is thought that the variation in perception is due to a difference in pain threshold. "That is, people are assumed to be physiologically different from one another so that one person may have a low threshold (and feel pain after slight injury), while another has a higher threshold (and feels pain only after intense injury). There is now evidence that all people, regardless of cultural background, have a uniform sensation threshold —that is, the lowest stimulus value at which sensation is first reported."[16] Even though each individual has a low stimulus threshold at which he or she experiences pain, the perception of pain is nevertheless influenced by other factors.

[16]Melzack, *op. cit.*, p. 24.

A patient's current perception of pain takes into account early childhood experiences which are greatly influenced by his or her parents' perceptions and attitudes toward pain. Parents may make an unrealistic fuss over a simple cut or bruise, or, on the other hand, may demonstrate little sympathy toward a more serious injury. The child who receives an overwhelming amount of attention may, as an adult, develop a low stimulus threshold to pain. Likewise, the child whose injuries are minimized may develop a higher stimulus threshold. Therefore, childhood experiences with pain shape adulthood attitudes regarding it.

The child's experiences include the attitudes and beliefs of significant others who either enhance or alleviate the pain. Consequently, parental influence, cultural background, and the individual's attitude contribute to a concept of pain and influence reactions to it. According to Mastrovito, "If parents give little heed and few rewards to the hurt child, one might expect the emerging adult to bear in relative silence and with a certain degree of stoicism. On the other hand, some children who receive a great deal of attention, reassurance, and care when hurt but little when comfortable may subsequently use pain as a way of dealing with life stresses or to gain support and affection from others."[17] The hospitalized child may try to use pain to gain sympathy from both parents and substitute parents. The health team and small patient may enter into a web of emotional events. The staff, at times, must implement treatments that inevitably cause pain. Knowing pain will be a factor during a procedure (such as venapuncture, lumbar puncture, or injection), the staff members may experience their own discomfort. They realize that the child is dependent upon them for restorative treatment and overall protection. Nevertheless, the child still blames the nurse for pain associated with intrusive procedures. The child screams, kicks, and cries only to have the substitute parent, the nurse, become angry. The nurse's behavioral response of anger is due to a negative perception of the pain situation. The nurse perceives failure in the intervention. Therefore, the internal anger is projected onto the child. Understanding this behavior will help the nurse to assist a young patient's coping with a painful situation.

The second perception of pain involves a perceived threat. The threat may be a diffuse or specific feeling. The individual experiencing mental or nonbodily pain is aware of an uncomfortable feeling which he is unable to localize to any one part of his body. Mental pain causes the individual to realize that his psychological protective barrier has been broken. In this respect, the individual feels a loss or injury to his emotional wholeness. Psychological pain that is diffuse involves emotions

[17]Rene Mastrovito, "Psychogenic Pain," *American Journal of Nursing,* March 1974, p. 514.

such as grief, mourning, fear, anxiety, guilt, or painful ideas. These emotions are not confined to any one part of the body or particular experience. Consequently, this type of pain knows no boundary. The nurse can help a patient localize diffuse emotions by helping to identify those events that occurred prior to the anxiety or guilt state. In this respect, the nurse focuses the patient's emotions. Once he or she knows what contributed to the psychological pain, the patient can anticipate and cope with it.

Perception of specific threats involves loss of all or part of a function. The myocardial infarction patient perceives the threat of pain involving loss of myocardial function and potential loss of life. The fear of pain focuses specifically upon the heart whose function has been temporarily or permanently altered. Likewise, the renal patient perceives a threat of loss to involve loss of independence and financial security. This is especially true if he or she must be totally dependent upon hemodialysis. The patient may suffer the pain of role changes which threaten the sense of personal integrity and self esteem. The patient, for his or her own reasons, may deny the existence of-pain. Another patient may complain of severe pain yet refuse therapy designed to alleviate the pain. The latter individual may feel the threat of pain due to curative procedures or treatments to be greater than the illness or injury itself.

A stimulus may be painful in one situation and not in another. The more anxious the patient, the less the ability to cope with pain or the threat of pain. In other words, the patient's stimulus threshold to pain is reduced. Given another time, the same individual may not react to the same painful stimuli. Therefore, the nurse must be sensitive to those environmental factors which serve to lessen the patient's pain threshold. The patient's anxiety and fear regarding an illness and placement within a strange highly technical environment are examples of stimuli which reduce the patient's threshold. Anxiety and fear become psychological variables which contribute to a high degree of variation between stimuli and its perception.

Another example of pain threat involves the losses experienced by the cancer patient. Cancer patients vary in their description of pain. Some describe their pain as mild, aching, or dull. According to Hillebroe, "It is difficult to appreciate what pain of this nature does to a person when it persists continuously for months or even a few years. However, we can observe how such pain wears out the emotional and physical reserves of a person, robbing him of any rest for life. At progressive stages, the malignancy invades pain-sensitive nerves of the bodily tissues, intensifying suffering."[18] The cancer patient's perception of loss is greater than most

[18]Herman Hilleboe, "Care of the Advanced Cancer Patient," *Patient Care,* February 1972, p. 19.

patients. It must be remembered that this loss encompasses life itself, since the threat to existence is death. Aged cancer patients may not concern themselves with the threat of death as they are sometimes more concerned with the threat to their psychological integrity in terms of independence and social autonomy. As physical illness progresses, they relinquish valued mobility, autonomy, and independence. The same applies to other aged patients not confronted with cancer but with physical illness associated with declining years.

The psychological component of pain consists of past experiences and threats, diffuse or specific, to the individual. The adult and aged patient's pain experience is a result of childhood encounters with pain. The adult and aged patients are more cognizant of threats involving pain than are children. Each individual regardless of age is capable of manifesting pain on either a nonverbal or verbal comminication level.

Psychological manifestations Psychological manifestations of pain involve affect changes such as excitement, irritability, withdrawal, hostility, depression, rigidity, unusual posture, knees drawn up to abdomen, rubbing, or restlessness. These behavioral responses can be categorized according to nonverbal or verbal manifestations of pain.

Nonverbal response to pain is manifested as vocalization, facial expression, and body movements. The nonverbal clues are particularly significant for the small child who is unable, due to limited cognitive and communicational skills, to verbalize pain. Likewise, the aged patient may have similar problems of expression. Aphasia may limit the ability to accurately communicate pain. With other patients, a nonverbal response helps the nurse assess the validity of a patient's verbal denial of pain. Verbally the patient denies pain, while nonverbally giving clues indicating pain. Assessing nonverbal manifestations of pain can be a difficult task for the nurse especially if she or he relies only on the patient's verbal denial or admission of pain.

Vocalization becomes a nonverbal manifestation of pain. Vocalization consists of emitted sounds other than language and cannot be comprehended as verbal symbols. Vocal behaviors can be used by the verbalizing patient to indicate the presence, severity, duration or meaning of pain. The child vocalizes pain by whining, crying, screaming, or whimpering. The nurse may unintentionally think the small child is only seeking attention. Therefore, the nurse may not assess that these vocalizations are pain related. An assessment should include the length of time the child cries; the frequency or number of times the child cries in a given period of time; and the type of cry. A vocalization that begins as a whine and progresses into a definite cry may indicate pain. The nurse will then need to assess physicological parameters in an attempt to validate a problem.

An adult or aged patient vocalizes pain through screaming, groaning, grunting, or gasping. The adult patient who experiences a myocardial infarction or pulmonary embolism may vocalize pain before verbalizing its occurrence, location, duration, and intensity. These patients may make a sudden sharp gasp or groan. Other nonverbal responses follow shortly thereafter. The patient who experiences a painful intrusive procedure usually vocalizes a small scream or grunting noise. This vocalization occurs at the onset of the procedure (such as venipuncture or intravenous therapy) and then diminishes after the initial prick of skin.

Like vocalization, facial expressions become significant nonverbal clues that the patient is in pain. Patients vary in their facial expressions. For example, a patient may have a very sober expression with opened eyes and no facial grimaces. Other facial expressions consist of clenched teeth, tightly shut lips and eyes, wrinkled forehead or biting of the lower lip. Needless to say, the nurse may see many other facial contortions. If facial expressions are assessed as indicating pain, the nurse must validate whether or not the patient is really experiencing pain. Next, the nurse assesses those factors which contribute to the pain experience, thus alleviating them. One patient may wrinkle the forehead in anticipation of a painful experience while others use facial expressions throughout the entire pain experience.

There are patients who use neither vocalizations or facial expressions to communicate their pain. Instead they communicate their pain with body movements. We have all witnessed the self-imposed immobility of postoperative surgical patients. They immobilize the part of their body altered through surgery. For example, the patient who experiences abdominal aneurysm resection may be observed holding the abdomen while gently trying to change position. Another individual with the same type of surgery may resist any type of movement in anticipation of pain. The patient with an injured arm or leg may request that the nurse immobilize that part of the body until he or she turns. The above patients immobilize primarily the surgical site or injured part. On the other hand, the patient who has sustained trauma or injuries may immobilize the entire body. Regardless of the reason, each individual is in essence splinting as a means of protection against the threat of pain. Small children are not unlike adults in their attempt to sustain one position in order to lessen pain. After a massive trauma, young children have a tendency to immobilize the entire body. When a portion of an extremity is injured, the child usually fails to move the entire extremity.

Besides immobility, the nurse may assess other body movements indicating pain. A patient in pain can be observed to have inappropriate or inaccurate body movements. The patient seems to thrash around the bed in a restless manner or frequently moves the legs or arms around in bed while tossing and turning. The patient is attempting to find relief from pain. It may take an observant nurse to assess what the patient's behavior signifies. Rather than scolding the patient for tearing apart the bed, pulling the tubes and wires, or sitting on the edge of the bed without assistance, the nurse verbally identifies this as nonverbal behavior. In this respect the pain can be verbalized according to its location, duration and intensity. Psychologically the patient feels relief in knowing that the health team is aware of the pain he or she attempted to endure alone.

Other body movements consist of rubbing the affected body part. The nurse frequently sees an arthritic patient rubbing the tender joint prior to ambulation or while quietly sitting in the room. The patient with peripheral vascular insufficiency may also rub the legs in an attempt to facilitate circulation and soothe pain. Even the cardiac patient may be observed rubbing the chest during or in anticipation of angina. Children often rub an injured body part due to a bump or bruise. Psychologically a rubbing body movement seems to soothe the affected site and possibly close the gate to pain.

The second major category of psychological manifestation consists of the patient's verbal response to pain. Verbalization involves certain cognitive abilities such as how the patient thinks and the manner in which thoughts are organized. The individual possesses the ability to communicate through language.

The small child is unable to depend upon verbal input from members of the health team. Instead he or she seems to observe the pain response of other children in the environment and uses this as a guide to his or her own pain. Furthermore, the child observes the origin of pain such as procedures or treatments involving needles. If confronted with the same or similar piece of equipment, the child anticipates pain and verbalizes anxieties accordingly. The nurse assessing pain in the child must keep in mind that a young child of less than two years is unable to express his thoughts and feelings verbally. The four- or five-year-old child's language ability and large vocabulary can mislead those who provide care. At this age, the child is able to organize sentences and communicate in such a way that the adult may think he or she understands the child's message. The adult or aged patients may have similar problems. Their cognitive ability may be altered by drugs, brain damage, verbal ischemia, or hypoxia. Therefore, the nurse must take into consideration a patient's physical problem and cognitive reliability when assessing pain.

Assessment of pain through verbalization involves both the nurse and patient. The nurse observes existence of pain, tolerance to pain, and factors affecting the pain. The patient, on the other hand, verbalizes location, quality, duration, intensity, rhythmicity, and meaning of the pain. The patient with reliable cognitive abilities locates a pain according to the body part involved and depth of involvement. Duration involves the length of time spent in pain. One patient may experience pain of long duration and low intensity. Another patient experiences the same pain; however, his or her reduced tolerance makes the experience seem to be of greater intensity.

A last component of the patient's verbalization of pain involves rhythmicity or patterning of pain. The four components (location, duration, intensity, and rhythmicity) are significant to the obstetrical patient. The latter two verbalizations help the nurse time a patient's contractions. The meaning of pain varies with each patient and becomes a variable. Adults or aged patients have a well-defined sense of body image. Children, on the other hand, do not have a complete concept of their body image. A child may tell the nurse that an arm hurts when the pain is located in a sprained finger. Those patients unable to verbalize the duration of their pain can be encouraged to identify factors contributing to pain. In other words, the events prior to the pain experience.

Variables   McCaffery[19] believes that the factors influencing a patient's psychological response to pain include the degree of powerlessness experienced by the patient; the presence and attitudes of other people; the amount of information given the patient; the degree of threat the pain imposes on the life situation; personal and past experiences with pain; cognitive level; and the extent to which the patient has used pain for secondary gains. The last three variables are most important. Each adult or aged patient is a product of past experiences, including those of childhood. Individuals unable to cope with emotional pain on a verbal basis may internalize conflicts thus causing physical pain associated with gastritis, ulcerative colitis, or peptic ulcer. The nurse, through discussion with the patient, and the patient's family or parents, assesses the significance of past pain experience as a variable in the patient's current pain experience. If he or she has been previously hospitalized, the nurse must assess whether or not it was a traumatic experience associated with intrusive procedures, complications, or threat of death.

The child, adult, or aged patient's cognitive ability has already been discussed under psychological manifestations. It is significant to mention that associated with cognitive ability is the patient's understanding of the pain experience or events circumventing it. Of course, understanding is dependent upon knowledge input. The patient with indigestion who simultaneously experiences chest pain may think he or she is having a coronary, not realizing that the pain is not cardiac in origin but referred from the epigastric region. Furthermore, knowledge input gives the

[19]Margo McCaffery, "Patients in Pain," *Nursing, 73,* pp. 42–50.

patient a sense of power. The patient understands what is happening internally to the biological systems and relates it to the various diagnostic procedures or supportive devices surrounding the bed. The child may require a simple explanation of events whereas the adult might require more lengthy explanations. These factors are assessed by the nurse.

The last variable to be discussed briefly involves the extent to which pain provides secondary gains. Pain may become a way of gaining attention and/or recognition. The individual confronted with feelings of loneliness may temporarily have them alleviated during a pain experience. People in the immediate environment respond to the pain state and their response lessens the loneliness. Other individuals feel they can control people through their expression of pain. Whatever their reason, pain becomes a defense mechanism. As with all defense mechanisms, the nurse must assess its significance to the patient. Also, the nurse must assess the degree to which the patient depends upon pain for attention, when seeming to experience pain, and what effectively alleviates the pain. It is possible that structure and visits from family members or staff members may reduce a patient's complaint of pain. If attention and freedom from loneliness is what the patient really deserves then the presence of significant others may alleviate the need to gain attention through pain.

NURSING INTERVENTIONS

The health team's goal is relief of pain. Total relief may not be possible for all patients. Nevertheless the nurse attempts to lessen the patient's pain as much as possible. This goal is accomplished by dividing interventions into three categories, referred to by McCaffery as anticipation, presence, and aftermath of pain. For the purposes of discussion, I choose to define the categories as follows: pre-pain experience, actual pain experience, and post-pain experience.

Pre-Pain Experience

If the nurse has knowledge that a particular diagnostic study, surgical procedure or other intrusive treatment will cause pain, she or he must prepare the patient for the pain experience. Part of preparation consists of assessing the absence or presence of anxiety. Patients vary in their manifestation of anxiety, therefore, behaviors directly related to anxiety may be difficult to assess. The nurse can assume that the child, adult, or aged patient who faces diagnostic studies which might reveal a terminal illness, intrusive treatments involving needles, or a surgical procedure will experience a degree of anxiety. Studies by Janis indicate that a degree of anxiety is necessary to get the patient through a traumatic experience. McCaffery relates this principle directly to pain. "During the anticipation of pain, pain relief is enhanced if the patient experiences a moderate amount of anxiety and this anxiety is channeled into methods of coping with pain. When a pain sensation is felt, the reduction of anxiety associated with pain tends to decrease the perceived intensity of the sensation and/or increase the tolerance for pain."[20] The nurse must assess whether or not the patient's anxiety state is related to pre-pain or post-pain experience. The patient may be anxious regarding the outcome of the pain experience. The outcome may validate fears and fantasies. Therefore, the nurse intervenes by identifying the focus of the anxiety.

Another aspect of preparation in pre-pain experience includes providing the patient with information about what to expect. If pain is a part of an experience, the patient must be told. The patient needs to know the intensity and duration of pain. In this respect, the patient knows what to expect and can even assist during the experience. It also gives the patient an opportunity to share, with the nurse, previous pain experience involving the same procedure. For example, a patient during a previous admission had a lumbar puncture. Due to arthritic changes in the spinal cord, multiple needle insertions were necessary before the procedure was successfully completed. For the patient, the experience was traumatic in that he or she sustained intense pain of long duration. The trauma was not anticipated by the health team or patient. With the current lumbar puncture, pain and difficulty are again anticipated. The patient may react with greater anxiety because of the previous experience. However, the health team's awareness of arthritic changes can lead to more precise insertion of the needle.

The child may be unable to articulate past experiences with pain. The nurse can use play therapy as a means of encouraging the child to express feelings. For example, a doll might become a substitute for this or another patient. If the child has witnessed a painful situation, the doll can be used to describe the events.

The nurse also plays a significant role in setting the stage for pain reduction. Prior to the pain experience, the nurse might decide to restrain the patient with hand restraints, posey belt, or another nurse. Such intervention only reinforces the fact that the experience will be painful and the child or adult patient interprets the procedure as punishment. If possible, restraining, as an alternative intervention, should be of low priority, reserved for the patient with an altered cognitive ability who must be restrained for his or her own protection. For children, crying

[20]*Ibid.*, p. 82.

during a painful experience is normal behavior and it should not elicit scolding. Instead, the child should be supported.

Actual Pain Experience

During the actual pain experience, the nurse intervenes to facilitate meaningful sensory stimulation and reduce noxious stimulation. Meaningful sensory stimulation involves distractions. Distraction through a number of ways decreases intensity of pain and hopefully increases the patient's tolerance to it. Distracting can be accomplished through any of the following: counting, word games, physical activity, and autostimulation such as singing and visualization.

Counting and word games may be helpful in distracting children. These distractive activities are initiated during a pleasant experience. For example, the nurse and child may play word games during a bath. The nurse can think of a word and allow the child to choose a word which is similar. The nurse could choose the word red to see what the child's response will be. The child may respond with another color like yellow, a fruit associated with the color, like an apple, or something associated with blood or pain. The nurse may then progress from safe words to words involving hospitalization. The nurse can learn about a young patient according to word association. Once a pain experience begins, the child and nurse begin their word game and continue, if possible, throughout the procedure.

When possible, physical activity can be a distraction technique. Pain has a tendency to immobilize the patient, regardless of age. The arthritic patient fears pain associated with initiating physical activity. However, once ambulation begins, the intensity of the pain seems to be reduced. Likewise, a patient with epigastric pain seems to find relief when ambulating. Patients on complete bed rest can still utilize physical activity as a means of distraction. For example, a patient with peripheral vascular insufficiency finds relief when exercising the legs in bed.

Another form of physical activity applies the principle involved in gate control theory. The patient and/or nurse uses touch. Touch involves stroking, rubbing, or massaging. The nurse, while sitting at the patient's bedside can soothe an affected arm or leg by gently stroking it. Of course the nurse has assessed the origin of the patient's pain in order to further assess the appropriateness of the intervention. Rubbing an extremity with a thrombophlebitis would not be appropriate. Frequently stroking the forehead of an anxious patient in pain seems to lessen the pain by increasing the patient's tolerance. A backrub also has a soothing effect upon the patient and can be a meaningful form of sensory input. It also gives the patient and nurse an opportunity to get to know one another.

Furthermore, the patient can be taught to rub the affected body part at the onset of pain. This becomes a type of autostimulation.

Autostimulation involves many things, including singing or visualization. The patient may feel embarrassed by singing alone, therefore, the nurse can sing along. Children may actually enjoy singing their favorite songs or reciting favorite nursery rhymes. The adolescent's nonhospital world consists largely of autostimulation through verbal communication and music. We are all familiar with the loud rock music enjoyed by many adolescents. Realizing this the nurse can see that a tape recorder, radio, or record player are available for this patient's use, perhaps obtaining one through the parents.

Verbalization, as a form of autostimulation, is possible through a variety of ways, such as reading stories, telling stories, or watching television or movies. A small child is delighted when someone reads to him or her. Most children love stories, especially those with large colorful pictures. It gives the nurse an opportunity to hold the child, if possible, and together look at colorful pictures while a story is read. The nurse can also utilize the time to assess a patient's duration for distraction and developmental appropriateness. For a short period of time the child is distracted from any pain. Adults may also enjoy having their nurse read to them. Again it provides a close interactional time in which the patient has the nurse's undivided attention. Such an intervention may be most beneficial to the patient with cataracts, facial burns, or multiple fractures which necessitate total immobilization.

Television becomes a means of escape for all patients regardless of their age. Children and adults have favorite programs they enjoy watching. Television also becomes a companion to those who otherwise have limited autostimulation abilities. For example, the tracheostomy patient is unable to hum, sing, or talk. If hospitalized in respiratory care, the nurse may be unable to spend time reading to this patient. Therefore distraction becomes possible through television. Naturally, the appropriateness of its use must be assessed for each individual patient. Movies are often shown in chronic care facilities where patients are hospitalized for a long time. However, it is possible to show movies on a ward for short-term patients who need temporary distraction from pain.

The nurse helps to reduce pain by decreasing the amount of meaningless input. Meaningless sensory input can unintentionally occur from members of the health team. Therefore, the nurse intervenes to control and/or eliminate unnecessary noise in the patient's environment. The nurse must carry out certain procedures which are necessary but painful. The nurse contributes to the patient's already existing painful state. The nurse should attempt to intervene in the least offensive manner possible.

The nurse, while intervening in the patient's actual pain experience, attempts to distract through another dimension. This dimension involves the use of waking-imagined analgesia as a type of distraction. According to Siegele, "The person is taught to influence pain perception by imagining a pleasant situation involving the painful part and trying to recapture and relive the pleasurable sensation whenever he has pain."[21] Unlike distraction, in which, the patient uses objects or events in the immediate environment to lessen pain, WIA involves a pleasant experience. The patient is requested to recall the memory of a previous pleasant event like sailing into a beautiful sunset or a scenic vacation. If unable to recall a pleasant event, the patient can create one by using the imagination. Psychologically, the patient separates himself or herself from the mind and body, utilizing all senses to recreate all the original sensations associated with the event while simultaneously experiencing a painful situation. WIA involves a degree of concentration and imagination. For the adult or aged patient who has never used WIA, the nurse must intervene to stimulate the memory of previous pleasant sensations. The nurse helps the patient recall meaningful events in a general fashion. Depending upon the intensity and duration of the pain, the nurse helps the patient expand the memory from general to more specific. In other words if the actual pain experience will be prolonged, the patient should have sufficient pleasant details to mentally sustain him or her throughout the pain state. WIA is difficult for children, therefore the other types of distraction, which have already been discussed, must be utilized.

The second major way in which the nurse intervenes during actual pain experience is to decrease noxious stimulation. Noxious stimulation is a result of internal physiological changes and external environmental conditions. Naturally, it is impossible to alleviate all pain resulting from both internal and external noxious stimulation. The nurse intervenes to make the child, adult, or aged patient as comfortable as possible. Those noxious stimuli resulting from internal physiological changes may be difficult to alter or reduce.

The patient experiencing pain due to a muscle spasm finds temporary relief in medication, traction, or hot-wet packs. The nurse assesses which intervention is the best for the patient, basing the decision upon evaulation of the reduction in pain and/or increase tolerance to pain. Such a patient experiences pain associated with movement. Pain of movement may surround the severely disabled arthritic patient, the burned patient, or the postoperative patient with abdominal or chest surgery. The pain of each must be accurately assessed before movement begins. In other words, the arthritic patient's pain is joint related, needing, therefore, careful range of motion to maintain what limited joint mobility remains.

[21]Siegele, *op. cit.*, p. 502.

The burn patient's pain is related to exposed or sensitive nerve endings. The nurse therefore changes the dressings as quickly as possible in an attempt to reduce pain associated with exposure to air. For patients with abdomen or chest injury, the nurse teaches them the less painful ways of turning. In addition, the nurse might teach them how to utilize accessory muscles for the purpose of coughing and deep breathing. Pain associated with internal physiological disease, injury, or illness is difficult to alleviate. The nurse's most effective intervention may be to help the patient cope with this pain.

Noxious stimulation can originate in the patient's immediate environment. For example noise may originate from equipment, other patients, or the health team itself. Equipment or supportive devices, especially in critical care units, are sometimes distracting and noisy. The machines hum, beep, and buzz at varying levels of intensity making sleep impossible for some patients. Sleep deprivation leads to reduction in the individual's tolerance to pain. The nurse needs to remove unnecessary supportive devices as soon as possible. Likewise the nurse may need to separate the noisy patient from other patients. In addition the health team members must be sensitive to the noxious stimulation created by their voices. Some clinical areas are noisy simply because of the staff. Nurses must be aware of the various noxious stimuli originating from the environment.

Post-Pain Experience

This is the period of time immediately after the pain experience. Normally once the pain experience or situation has been completed (that is, procedure or treatment) the nurse leaves the patient alone completing other responsibilities. The child, adult, or aged patient remains with the fears and anxieties regarding the experience. The patient may think that the health team will return to complete the painful procedure, not understanding that the experience has been terminated. Consequently, the nurse must inform the patient when the situation is over. The nurse remains to alleviate the post-pain fears and if necessary discuss the actual pain state. In this respect, the patient learns from the experience and the next time he or she will be able to cope more effectively.

In summary, pain affects all patients in varying degree. A major variable is the patient's tolerance to pain based upon previous experience. The nurse assesses characteristics of pain such as intensity, location, duration, and type. From the assessment and observations of the patient's nonverbal and verbal behavioral responses, the nurse is able to formulate a plan of care designed to relieve pain. The nurse realizes that total relief is, in many instances, impossible. Therefore, the goal is to help the patient find relief. The effectiveness of the intervention is then based upon the attainment of relief. Nurses can and do creatively intervene to help the child, adult, or aged patient cope with pain.

REFERENCES

Alexanger, L., "Differential Diagnosis Between Psychogenic and Physical Pain," *Journal of the American Medical Association,* 181, 1962.

Armstrong, D., "Pain-producing Substance in Human Inflammatory Exudate and Plasma," *Journal Physiology,* 135, 1957.

Beecher, H. K., "Relationship of Significance of Wound to Pain Experienced," *Journal of the American Medical Association,* 161, 1956.

———, "Generalization from Pain of Various Types and Diverse Organs," *Science,* 130, 1959.

Blaylock, J., "The Psychological and Cultural Influences on the Reaction to Pain: A Review of the Literature," *Nursing Forum,* 7, 1968.

Bronzo, A., "Relationship of Anxiety with Pain Threshold," *Journal Psychology,* 66, 1967.

Bruegel, M. A., "Relationship of Preoperative Anxiety to Perception of Postoperative Pain," *Nursing Research,* 20, 1971.

Collins, L. G., "Pain Sensitivity and Ratings of Childhood Experience," *Perception Motor Skills,* 21, 1965.

Copp, Laurel Archer, "The Spectrum of Suffering," *American Journal of Nursing,* March 1974, pp. 491–495.

Dodson, H. C., "Relief of Postoperative Pain," *Am. Surg.,* 20, 1954.

Drakontides, Anna, "Drugs to Treat Pain," *American Journal of Nursing,* March 1974, pp. 508–513.

Gaumer, William, "Electrical Stimulation in Chronic Pain," *American Journal of Nursing,* March 1974, pp. 504–505.

Goloskov, Joan, "Use of the Dorsal Column Stimulator," *American Journal of Nursing,* March 1974, pp. 506–507.

Hackett, Thomas, "Pain and Prejudice: Why do we Doubt that the Patient is in Pain?" *Resident and Staff Physician,* May 1972, pp. 101–109.

Hardy, J. D., "The Nature of Pain," *J. Chronic Dis.,* 4, 1956.

Hodges, W. F., "Effects of Ego Threat and Threat of Pain on State Anxiety," *J. Personality Soc. Psychol.,* 8, 1968.

Janis, I. L., *Psychological Stress*, New York, Wiley and Sons, 1958.

Johnson, Jean, "Sensory and Distress Components of Pain," *Nursing Research*, May-June 1974, pp. 203–209.

Jones, A., "The Reduction of Uncertainty Concerning Future Pain," *J. Abnorm. Psychol.*, 71, 1966.

Loewenstein, W. R., "On the Specificity of a Sensory Receptor," *J. Neurophysiol.*, 24, 1961.

McCabe, G. S., "Cultural Influences on Patient Behavior," *American Journal of Nursing*, 60, 1960.

McLachlan, Eileen, "Recognizing Pain," *American Journal of Nursing*, March 1974, pp. 496–497.

Moss, F. T., "The Effects of Nursing Interaction Upon Pain Relief in Patients," *Nursing Research*, 15, 1966.

Ramzy, Ishak, "Pain, Fear, and Anxiety," *Psychoanalytic Study of the Child*, 13, 1958, pp. 147–189.

Sternbach, R. A., *Pain: A Psychophysiological Analysis*, New York, Academic Press, 1968.

Way, E. L., *New Concepts in Pain and Its Clinical Management*, Philadelphia, F. A. Davis, 1967.

4
Sensory Deprivation

We have a tendency to take our relationship with the immediate sensory environment for granted. It is assumed, until a crisis occurs, that the interaction will remain a constant. Rarely do we differentiate among the vast multitude of sensory stimuli confronting us. Even more so, we do not question the effects of such sensory stimuli on our cognitive abilities or behavior. Throughout the past fifteen years there has been a growing interest and rapidly expanding literature on the subject of sensory deprivation. Researchers began to gather more knowledge about new techniques, reviewers noted its similarities to other areas of scientific knowledge, and theorists started to integrate the findings into a systematic explanation. According to Suedfield," ties appeared between more established lines of investigation and new approaches. With continual research and thinking, it has become obvious that these ties are vitally meaningful and that a greater integration of related approaches in many areas is necessary for the adequate understanding of any one approach."[1]

It has long been a fact that restricting the sensory environment may have profound effects on behavior. This was demonstrated through experiences of polar explorers, shipwrecked sailors, and prisoners of war. These individuals were noted to have changes in mood, perception, and thinking. Data is still being collected as to changes, if any, that occur in space flight. Historically, research in sensory deprivation consisted of the effects of long term sensory and/or social deprivation during development, and reports of relatively brief deprivation of organisms. The first of these dealt mostly with experimental treatments of infrahuman species, while the latter typically involved human beings who were isolated in natural situations. Advances were applied to work on boredom and vigilance, and the increasingly popular theories of activation and arousal.[2]

[1]John Zubeck, ed., *Sensory Deprivation: Fifteen Years of Research,* (New York: Appleton-Century Crofts, 1969), p. 3.

[2]*Ibid.,* p. 4.

Zubek has pointed out that, "During the last decade considerable attention has been paid to the experimental study of the effects upon human behavior of a reduction in the level and variability of stimulation from the visual, auditory and tactile-kinesthetic sense modalities. The attempts to achieve such a reduction in environmental stimulation are usually referred to by such terms as sensory isolation, sensory deprivation and perceptual deprivation."[3] Suedfield believes that "one way to identify the conceptual ancestors and relatives of experimental sensory deprivation is to analyze its significant features, each of which turns out to be the main focus of other lines of investigation. These main characteristics include the reduction of stimulus input levels, the reduction of stimulus variability, social isolation and confinement."[4]

Traditionally, sensory deprivation has been studied in relatively healthy individuals. The effects of altered sensory input, using volunteers, has been a successful means for obtaining research data. These individuals were placed in environments where they could be isolated from sensory input or patterned visual or auditory responses. Today, interest needs to be generated toward the relationship between hospitalization and sensory deprivation. Studies have examined these relationships on a specific basis, such as studies of patients with eye surgery, neurological disorders, casts, tractions, or those confined to a tank respirator. We need to broaden these studies to better understand the relationship between the patient and the sensory environment. Studies need to concern themselves with whether or not a certain kind of environment can cause deprivation. A significant way of studying the sensory status of the patient is to formulate an assessment hierarchy and identify those variables or factors that influence whether or not a patient experiences sensory-perceptual deprivation. These are the major areas in which the nurse can intervene.

The nurse needs to be aware of contributing factors that could lead to sensory deprivation. Once an awareness exists, the nurse can look to the patient's environment and discover creative ways of avoiding or alleviating the potential problem. First, it would be helpful to define the concept deprivation and some of its related terms.

DEFINITIONS

The broad term sensory deprivation is known by a variety of names including technological deprivation, perceptual deprivation, isolation,

---

[3]John Zubek, "Effects of Prolonged Sensory and Perceptual Deprivation," *British Medical Bulletin*, 20, 1969, p. 38.

[4]Zubek, *op. cit.*, p. 4.

sensory restriction, and confinement. It deals with the phenomena which result from reduction in the absolute level and/or degree of structure in sensory input.

Sensoristasis

According to Schultz, "Sensoristasis can be defined as a drive state of cortical arousal which impels the organism (in a waking state) to strive to maintain an optimal level of sensory variation. There is, in other words, a drive to maintain a constant range of varied sensory input in order to maintain cortical arousal at an optimal level. Conceptually, this sensory variation-based formulation is akin to homeostasis in that the organism strives to maintain an internal balance, but it is a balance in stimulus variation to the cortex as mediated by the RAS (Reticular Activating System)."[5] Some activities require a greater degree of cortical arousal than others. For example, driving a car requires more cortical arousal than riding a bus. While driving a car, the individual can vary sensory input by changing lanes, turning on the air conditioner, singing, honking the horn, or listening to the radio. If sensory stimulation falls below an optimal level, the individual seeks alternative stimuli or alternative ways of varying the stimuli. In this respect the individual restores sensory equilibrium.

There are times when patients are unable to seek alternative stimuli. Their illness or limitations may limit contact on an action level with the environment. On the other hand, there are times when the patient's sensory environment contains excess stimuli. In this instance the patient seeks to reduce additional cortical arousal or input. Mitchell points out that, "A decrease in optimal sensory level appears to affect the development or normal perception and response in the growing organism. For example, children reared in extremely restricted environments demonstrate abnormal social and perceptual behavior when placed in a 'normal' situation."[6]

Perceptual Deprivation

In recent years, two labels, sensory deprivation and perceptual deprivation, have been used systematically or interchangeably in some laboratory investigations. Absence or reduction of stimulus variability is referred to as "perceptual deviation" or "perceptual isolation." It is the

---

[5]Duane Schultz, *Sensory Restriction: Effects on Behavior*, (New York: Academic Press, 1965), p. 30.

[6]Pamela Holsclaw Mitchell, *Concepts Basic to Nursing*, (New York: McGraw Hill, 1973), p. 198.

result of environment stimulus remaining constant. In addition there is reduced patterning present with imposed structuring and homogenous stimulation. Perceptual deprivation occurs in an environment where sound is muffled, light is diffused, and bodily sensations are nondistinct.[7]

The hospital environment with its unique noises, equipment, procedures, rules, and regulations, has little or no meaning. Depending on the patient's illness or injury, the environment may also be monotonous. For example, the patient immobilized due to multiple fractures or neurological disease can suffer perceptual deprivation. Besides the monotony resulting from immobilization, the patient's immediate environment, with its dull colors and unchanging pictures, can further contribute to feelings of monotony.

It must be remembered that as we move through our daily encounters, we are aware of bodily sensations. Our bodily sensations help us to perceive our environment; whether it is raining, hot, cold, damp, or potentially dangerous. The patient who is immobilized due to illness or injury is unable to spatially perceive the environment. At one time he or she was able to physically move through space and perceive the surrounding world. Now, there is dependence on other sensory modalities, ears, eyes, mouth, or nose, reducing sensory input. Perceptual deprivation also refers to the reduction in stimulation from some previous conditions.

Sensory Deprivation

Sensory deprivation is defined as "an absolute reduction in variety and intensity of sensory input, with or without a change in pattern. An environment of silence and darkness, for example, would be considered an instance of sensory deprivation."[8] To deprive is to divest, to take away. The sensory process is not completely taken away and the individual is not divested of the sensory experience. The experience of sensory deprivation can be described as a situation in which reception or perception of stimuli is blocked or altered. It also implies that the environmental stimuli themselves are blocked or altered. According to Chodil, "All cases of sensory deprivation will exhibit an alteration of sensory input in the form of sensory underload. Stimuli in the environment may be below normal level for attention purposes. Therefore, the stimuli do not find the body receptors 'at tension' or ready to respond. Repetition, lack of change, or cues of inadequate intensity exist. Poorly

[7]Judith Worrell, "Nursing Implications in the Care of the Patient Experiencing Sensory Deprivation," *Advanced Concepts in Clinical Nursing,* (Philadelphia: Lippincott, 1971), p. 133.

[8]Worrell, *loc. cit.*

functioning receptors will block adequate stimuli and result in sensory underload. Perception altered by an anxiety state will allow the body to attend to a normal stimulus received by a healthy receptor."[9]

Sensory deprivation is not a unitary condition; singly or together, immobilization, confinement, and interpersonal isolation are implicit in the deprivation; and each is stressful. Sensory isolation and sensory deprivation refer to reduction in the quality, with or without a change in pattern. The deprivation may be of single modality. For example, one sensory channel is blocked due to the aging process or injury. An individual may, due to cataracts or trauma to the eyes, lose his or her sight. Furthermore, deprivation can exist as multimodality. The three major senses become involved . . . sight, hearing, or touch. Again, the cause can be similar to those of singular modality.

Isolation represents a degree of sensory deprivation or stimulus property. Isolation takes place when the individual is separated from his normal environment causing a feeling of distance from others. This has been referred to as aloneness. When the individual experiences perceptual isolation and deprivation, the patterning of stimuli is reduced. For example, decreased auditory stimulation causes perceptual deprivation in individuals who are socially isolated, that is, removed from people. On the other hand, confinement reduces the freedom of movement that the individual normally enjoys. Confinement implies motor restriction and is frequently termed "immobility." Confinement has a tendency to reduce both the quality and quantity of sensory information available to the organism. The ability of the organism to react and interact with the environment is reduced.[10] There are degrees and combinations of isolation and confinement to which the individual can be subjected and a variety of ways in which these can be achieved.

In order to assess a given deprivation situation, one might look for certain significant characteristics of the setting and of the person involved. Jackson believes important characteristics of the setting include: "reduction in the amount of intensity of stimulation in each sensory modality (vision, hearing, touch, internal body sensation, taste and smell); reduction in the patterning of meaningfulness of stimulation in each sensory modality; changes in stimulation other than decreases, such as the many new stimulations associated with hospitalization; restrictions imposed upon movements and body positions; degree of social isolation; duration of deprivation; and the realistic dangers, if any, which are present in the deprivation situation."[11] Jackson's description of the set-

[9]Judith Chodil, "The Concept of Sensory Deprivation," *Nursing Clinics of North America*, 5, September 1970, p. 456.

[10]Worrell, *loc. cit.*

[11]Wesley Jackson, "Sensory Deprivation As A Field of Study," *Nursing Research*, 20, January-February 1971, p. 46.

ting leads to the formulation of an assessment hierarchy. The assessment hierarchy involves assessing each sensory modality for intensity of input, patterning of input, and variation in input. The sensory modalities are visual, auditory, olfactory, tactile, visceral, and kinesthetic. With sensory deprivation, the patient experiences a reduction in intensity of input, patterning of input, and variation of input. Therefore, the nurse, using the three criteria, assesses the amount and type of sensory input received by each sensory modality. Illness or injury can alter any one of the sensory modes.

DEPRIVATION AND THE PATIENT

A depriving environment provides insufficient stimuli to maintain optimal cortical arousal. In examining deprivation each sensory modality must be individually assessed. According to Carter, "All sensory modalities have collateral connections with the reticular activity system. When stimulated, this system leads to arousal and facilitation of perceiving, attention focusing, learning, and motor activity. An unchanging stimulus pattern and a reduced quantity of sensory input may minimize the functioning of this system and impair learning."[12] There are both external and internal sensory modalities. External modalities are visual, auditory, olfactory, and tactile. Internal modalities are visceral and kinesthetic. Sensation can be stimulated both internally and externally. This idea is important," . . . because stimuli from both sources contribute to the sensory information which is ultimately interpreted by the brain. An increase or decrease in stimuli from either the internal or external environment, therefore, only partially changes the total sensory input to the brain."[13]

Information about the sensory environment is a significant aspect of the assessment process. Because the assessment hierarchy focuses specifically on deprivation, the concept will be examined according to reduction of stimulation, meaningfulness, and patterning in sensory modalities.

Reduction of Stimulation in Sensory
Modes

Brawley believes that, "There is early evidence that a variety of pathogenetic processes (metabolic, toxic, degenerative, genetic, life-

---

[12]C. H. Carter, *Medical Aspect of Mental Retardation*, (Illinois: Charles Thomas, 1965).
[13]Mitchell, *op. cit.*, p. 197.

experimental, et cetera) may influence the sensory input regulating system in such a way that a state of internal sensory deprivation, an informational underload, ensues even in the presence of average external stimulus intensity."[14] In a normal environment, the individual experiences stimulus density and stimulus variability. The patterning of environmental stimuli is of great importance to adaptive behavior. Patients, regardless of their age or clinical setting, may be reacting to reduced intensity of some stimuli, to reduced patterning of stimuli, to increased intensity of other stimuli, to the addition of new stimuli, and to change in the meaning of stimulus. Mitchell points out that, "Sensory status is the person's situations in respect to all sensory modalities (specific sensory entities). It includes the functioning of the various sense organs and receptors, the normality or abnormality of perception of sensory stimuli, and the quality of the sensory-perceptual environment."[15] The patient's current sensory environment is assessed according to kind, quality, and quantity of stimuli. It is compared to the patient's usual environment. Depending upon the individual's usual sensory environment, hospitalization could represent deprivation or overload.

Children, adults, and the aged are all capable of experiencing a reduction in the amount or intensity of stimulation. Young children require an emotional climate that will facilitate a feeling of trust in oneself and others. A child needs and thrives on rich sensory and cultural experiences. The child's immediate environment should allow opportunities for exploration through the various sensory modalities. In exploring the sensory environment, the child gains valuable feedback which becomes helpful in developing and/or refining movements. Through touch, sight, and smell the child learns about the world. Sackett believes that, "there is growing evidence that the environment during infancy of animals and human beings affects their subsequent perceptual, motor and social abilities. The nervous system of human beings and of many animals is not completely developed at birth. Therefore, many investigators postulate that early sensory and perceptual experiences influence the anatomic development of the neural networks by which general arousal of the brain is translated into specific perception."[16]

Infants and young children, due to illness or injury, might necessitate frequent periods of hospitalization. Consequently, some of their sensory modes can suffer from rich sensory stimulation. Other children may experience temporary reduction in stimulation of some senses; for example, the child in a full body cast or halo traction. Because the child is unable to explore the environment, he or she may be deprived of visual

[14]Peter Brawley, "The Informational Underload Model in Contemporary Psychiatry," *Canadian Psychiatric Care,* 12, April 1967, p. 105.

[15]Mitchell, *op. cit.,* p. 195.

[16]*Ibid.,* p. 204.

and kinesthetic stimulation. Fleming[17] points out that sensory losses in children may be either congenital or acquired. They may result from psychological, biophysical, or sociocultural factors. Most is known perhaps about the biophysical causes, where specific changes are evident; less is known about the psychological causes, and least is known about the sociocultural causes. Biophysical causes of sensory losses include infection, injury, tumors, and hereditary factors. Social isolation can produce intellectual retardation due to reduction in learning experiences. Deprivation of sensations affects personality development and intellectual development.

There are times when a child must be isolated from other children to prevent transmission of pathogens or for protection from threatening pathogens. A child with leukemia is an example of the latter. His or her vulnerability is the result of sensory-perceptual and social restrictions leading to deprivation. Isolation also leads to social deprivation in the adult patient. When the child or adult is placed in a room alone, people who enter the room wear masks and bland-looking gowns. The only physical activity afforded them from the patient's view in bed is a pair of eyes. Depending upon other problems besides the immediate reason for being in isolation, the child or adult may or may not be left alone. He or she hears voices and foot steps quickly passing the room; however, due to their physical separateness they do not represent meaningful stimuli. The nurse may enter the environment only to perform necessary procedures. Once completed, she or he leaves the perceptual field, again, leaving the patient alone. Senses may be intact and capable of stimulation but the immediate sensory environment is void of such stimulation. Because of reduction in amount and intensity of stimulation, the patient withdraws into sleep. The nurse may discover that the patient is bored and deprived, and this is why there is a retreat into sleep.

The adult, especially, might have episodes of hallucinations, depending upon the degree of deprivation. Lilly suggests that isolation demonstrates how the brain stores energy that cannot be discharged through normal somatic channels. Under these conditions, the mind projects its contents outward in the form of delusions and hallucinations.[18] For the adult patient, illness itself creates reduced sensory input. This is especially true when one of the special senses has been affected by illness, but reduced sensory input also occurs in toxic and metabolic diseases that affect the central nervous system. Very often treatment procedures themselves result in a change or reduction in con-

[17]Juanita W. Fleming, "Sensory Losses in Children," *Current Concepts in Clinical Nursing*, (Ed: Betty Bergerson, et al.) (St. Louis, C. V. Mosby Company, 1967), p. 342.

[18]G. Ruff, "Isolation and Sensory Deprivation," *American Handbook of Psychiatry*, January-February 1971, p. 49.

tact with the environment and consequent functional changes in behavior.[19]

A patient may be immobilized by a particular illness or injury; immobility becomes a treatment procedure. Immobilization implies confinement, which produces stresses of its own. There are patients who are immobilized due to therapeutic approach to an illness or because they have lost mobility from injury or illness. For example, children and adults fracture various parts of their body in accidents or falls. As a result, they sometimes require drastic and prolonged immobilization. Treatments in body casts, tractions, or tongs are stressful mainly because they cause kinesthetic deprivation. In addition, the orthopedic patient is subjected to monotony. The traction limits the patient to one position—on the back. Due to the type of fracture and traction, visual awareness may be limited, seeing only the traction. The patient is confined to a territory of three feet. This becomes the only environmental frame of reference. He or she can look through the side rails and partially see other beds, patients, and staff.

As mentioned previously, the greatest constant visual stimulant is the ceiling. The same or similar problem confronts small children with tractions. The ceiling never changes and always remains in sight. If the patient's curtains are pulled, visual input is even further reduced. The primary reduction in stimulation that leads to deprivation is immobility. The patient is unable to gather sensory stimulation through ambulating around the bed. In addition, there is limited ability to physically extend one in social contact with other patients and staff. To a certain extent the patient is isolated. Patients, ". . . can be isolated without marked curtailment of sensation from their physical environment but the stimuli are those of inanimate or at least impersonal nature, with the whole range of sensory stimuli related to social interchange excluded."[20]

The deprivation due to prolonged immobilization sometimes leads to transient psychotic states. Both therapeutic and necessary immobility may cause a psychological reaction stemming from what the individual perceives to be changes in body image. Such changes result from sensory deprivation coupled with a modification in body image which may be secondary to the illness, injury, or disease. Immobility, because it reduces stimulation of senses, leads to a feeling of deprivation. Furthermore, "Perceptual deprivation and immobility (kinesthetic deprivation) produce greater cognitive deficits than sensory deprivation alone."[21] Accord-

[19]Patrick Linton, "Sensory Deprivation In Hospitalized Patients," *Alabama Journal Medical Science*, 2, 1965, p. 257.

[20]Eugene Ziskind, "A Second Look at Sensory Deprivation," *Journal of Nervous Mental Diseases*, 138, March 1964, p. 226.

[21]Mitchell, *op. cit.*, p. 200.

ing to Luckman, "Studies in sensory deprivation have established that when people are deprived of sensory stimulation they may develop confusion, inaccurate perception, faulty reasoning, impaired memory and even hallucinations."[22] Frequently, the confused patient is either whisked away to a private room at the end of the hall, curtains pulled around the bed, medicated, or restrained. Such treatments further decrease the patient's perceptual fields. The nurse, thinking she or he is protecting the patient from physical injury, may actually contribute to feelings of confusion. Other disorders or illnesses, such as complete or partial blindness from cataracts and/or deafness, also cause deprivation due to reduction in stimuli through visual and auditory modes. Confusion sometimes becomes the behavioral response of such patients. In addition to the above examples, the therapy of cardiac patients often produces prolonged immobilization. The regimen of prolonged immobilization from bedrest, in conjunction with possible cerebral hypoxia and fear of potential death, might precipitate behavioral changes.

The aged patient may experience deprivation in its multimodality form. Such patients have reduced visual, auditory, and taste sensations. To compensate for their reduction, the patient wears glasses and hearing aids. Taste might be reduced not only from the normal aging process but also through use of dentures. Tactile or kinesthetic sensory input can also be reduced if the aged patient is immobilized in casts or tractions. Fracturing a hip is a major problem facing the aged population. As with children and particularly adults, prolonged immobilization can lead to boredom, hallucinations, and disorientation in the aged.

It is not uncommon to find the aged patient's prosthetic devices such as glasses, hearing aids, or dentures in a drawer out of the patient's reach. Possibly the patient was confused and they were removed in anticipation of potential damage. The nurse fails to realize that the patient already experiences reduced intensity of sensory input due to the aging process. Further reduction by removal of prosthetic devices may actually contribute to the patient's confusion, hallucinations, and disorientation. The patient depends on these devices in order to communicate with the sensory environment. Without their use there is a further thrust into a world of aloneness with reduced intensity of sensory input.

Patients with partial or complete loss to any one of the sensory modes is capable of experiencing reduced intensity of sensory input through that mode. When stimulation is reduced through two modes, the patient has greater potential for sensory deprivation and subsequent behavioral changes. The degree of deprivation is dependent upon the length of time the mode is deprived and the sensory mode involved.

[22]Joan Luckman and Karen Sorensen, *Medical-Surgical Nursing: A Psycho-physiologic Approach*, (Philadelphia: Saunders, 1974), p. 78.

Reduced sensory input through visual and auditory modes might be more traumatic to a patient than visual and kinesthetic loss. Each mode must be assessed according to the meaning it has for the individual patient. The patient experiencing reduced sensory input from the environment might be unable to identify its meaning and significance. Because of perceptual deprivation the patient may become inattentive to the environment. In turn, decreased ability to sustain attention can cause an inability to accurately perceive this environment.

Reduction of Meaningfulness in Sensory Modes

It is important to note that in situations of sensory restriction there also exists a condition of reduced meaningfulness. Regardless of the patient's age or clinical setting, there are needs to make his or her world meaningful. There seems to be a need in all patients to order stimuli in the environment into a meaningful pattern. The experience of deprivation or restriction may not allow the patient to derive this meaning. When the deprivation barrier cannot be overcome, the unfulfilled need for sensory input leads to behavior characterized by regression, disorganization of sensory coordination, and cognitive difficulty. According to Flynn, "Emphasis has also been placed on the importance of meaningful contact with the environment in minimizing sensory deprivation. Some investigators believe that it is the restriction of meaning that is mainly responsible for the effects of sensory deprivation, rather than the quantitative physical limitation of stimuli per se."[23] The sensory environment must have meaning and the patient must see his or her place in that environment. Otherwise, the patient experiences perceptual deprivation.

Sensation and perception are closely interrelated. Even very minor alteration in sensations and perceptions can constitute significant changes in the patient's life. Furthermore, the changes could interfere with the ability to function. Mitchell points out that, "To be meaningful, sensations must be interpreted as well as perceived. The interpretation of sensations is the basis for response to the environment. Early response is primarily reflex. For example, the infant responds to hunger by moving his mouth toward any object which touches it (rooting)."[24]

A major concern of one's hospital environment is familiarity. Hospitalization to many patients, regardless of their age, is a new experience. The patient is removed from familiar settings—the home and the familiar

[23]W. R. Flynn, "Visual Hallucination in Sensory Deprivation," *Psychiatric Quarterly,* 36, 1962, p. 55.

[24]Mitchell, *op. cit.,* p. 195.

contents therein. The patient is taken away from a comfortable bed and pajamas; a favorite overstuffed arm chair; one's own private bathroom; favorite toys; the dog, fish, or cat; the dining room table on which many stimulating meals have been placed; a yard and garden where time is spent quietly meditating; and, above all the family, including wife, mother, husband, father, or brother and sister. At home the patient was master of an immediate but small domain. He or she had independence and personal freedom of choice and decided the hour to don pajamas and retire to bed (exception being with children); how long to sit in a favorite chair and watch television; the amount and type of food eaten at the dining table; the distance chosen to walk the dog; the time spent riding a bike; and how hard to work in the garden. There was a variety of stimuli around at all times. The patient could increase or decrease the stimulus as he or she wished.

Familiar sights, sounds, and smells are left behind, and no longer is there close tactile contact with the family. The exception might be with small children whose families are encouraged to remain nearby. Once in the hospital, someone else assumes the decision-making responsibility. The familiar is exchanged for the unfamiliar. Personal possessions such as money, jewelry, papers, and clothes are either locked up, sent home, or neatly placed in a closet elsewhere. Familiar, comfortable, and colorful pajamas are replaced by a loose white gown and tight or loose fitting pants. A comfortable king size bed is replaced by a narrow bed with bars called side rails. The private bathroom is replaced by a urinal, catheter, external condom catheter, bedpan, or commode, none of which insure privacy. Activity is limited to the bed or bedside commode. Of course, this depends on the patient's physiological problems.

The patient is not free to walk or run around the immediate environment as he or she would normally do with a dog or playmates. Therefore, freedom to ambulate and obtain meaningful environmental sensory stimulation is reduced. The familiar overstuffed chair or bean bag chair is replaced by a hard straight chair. The familiar dining room table and chair are replaced by a bed and overside table. Meals are no longer shared with family members. Familiar tasty food is replaced by bland institutional food, reducing oral stimulation. Again, depending upon the problem, the patient may not be allowed food. Depending upon the age of the patient, the familiar family members may be replaced by rules and regulations of visiting hours. This alone creates both sensory and perceptual deprivation.

In addition, meaning must also be derived from words and actions. The messages received from staff regarding the patient's illness, progress, and future must be on a comprehensive level. Members of the health team who talk to and/or over the patient in a technical level will only force withdrawal. The incoming verbal stimuli have no meaning as the technical language is foreign. Instead of listening to the nurse's and doctor's discussion, he or she assumes they are talking in symbolic language to each other. Therefore, attempts are made not to eavesdrop on their conversation even though the patient is involved. Again, absence of meaningful stimulation produces the effects of sensory deprivation.

Each patient will attempt to organize meaning in the environment and the messages received from it. Ludwig believes that, "It seems reasonable to assume that men possess different perceptual styles which not only permit them to organize and interpret their sensory input in characteristic ways, but which also induce them to choose a sensory environment most conducive to their optimal functioning or feeling of well-being."[25] Out of fear the patient may wrongfully misinterpret or perceive what he or she is told about his or her illness and progress. The patient attaches his or her own meaning to the technical language. What results is a self-perception of greater or lesser illness.

Certain patients, because of their placement in a special setting such as critical care, are more vulnerable to reduction of meaningfulness through the sensory modes. The critically ill patient, due to the nature and severity of illness, is anxious. The anxiety reduces or distorts self-perception. Perception can be reduced by means other than anxiety or fear. Various drugs can affect the patient's ability to perceive meaning in the environment. The nurse must take this into account while assessing a patient for perceptual deprivation. According to Mitchell, "If sensory-perceptual restriction or overload is added to this state, it is reasonable to predict that he may exhibit many of the perceptual distortions, problem-solving difficulties, anxieties, or even hallucinating behavior reported in experimental sensory and perceptual restrictions. If this is the case, raising or lowering the level of sensory stimulation or providing meaningful pattern to the sensory input should decrease these symptoms in time."[26]

Successful adjustment of the critical care patient during illness requires maintenance of integrated, coordinated functioning with the ability to interpret the environment correctly. If one only sees the familiar being replaced by unfamiliar, there will be difficulty adjusting. Linten believes that the older patient seems to be especially vulnerable to changes in the environment. The removal of the older individual from familiar surroundings to the hospital results in abnormal behavior that is not directly related to the illness. He further suggests that adequate social and sensory contacts are especially important in the care of the physically

[25]Arnold Ludwig, "Self-Regulation of the Sensory Enviornment," *Archives General Psychiatry*, 25, November 1971, p. 413.

[26]Mitchell, *op. cit.*, p. 203.

ill patient. Because of this one should not restrict visitors, maintain a dark room, or forbid the use of telephone or radio, unless these sensory stimuli are specifically contraindicated.[27]

The patient may be inclined to focus upon the negative aspects of the hospital environment. With each subsequent loss of familiar stimulation, the nurse needs to offer meaningful explanation in its place. Such interpretation or explanation is dependent upon input from the real environment. Providing appropriate and meaningful input is the role of the nurse in working with patients experiencing reduced meaningfulness of sensory input.

Reduction of Patterning in Sensory Modes

Repetition and lack of variation of meaningfully patterned sensory stimuli leads to perceptual monotony. The stimulus input may be normal for cortical arousal; however, it lacks variety. Staying in a windowless room creates feelings of perceptual monotony. In addition, social isolation produces perceptual monotony. According to Schultz, ". . . the optimal level of sensory variation of an individual is influenced by early postnatal levels of stimulation and the resulting level of cortical arousal as mediated by the reticular activating system. In other words, the level of stimulus variations to which the neonate is exposed functions to influence the optimal range of cortical arousal appropriate for adaptive behavior of the adult organism."[28]

Infants need variations in their sensory environment. Without adequate stimulation, meaning, and variety the infant might fail to thrive. Mitchell states that, "Variety of sensory-perceptual environment is essential for infants and children of all ages. The attention span increases as a child grows, but all children become bored rather quickly with an unchanging environment, that is, they experience perceptual monotony. During nap time, a monotonous, relatively nonstimulating environment may help a child get to sleep, but continuation of the same environment all day leads to apathy and fussiness."[29] The child needs rich sensory environment. Such an environment would facilitate the development of differentiation in each sensory mode. Likewise, an impoverished sensory environment prevents such differentiation within the modes.

Patients in critical care are particularly vulnerable to reduced variation of some sensory stimuli. The variety in environmental stimulus is diminished in some critical care units. "Here familiar visual cues such as

[27]Linton, *op. cit.,* p. 256.
[28]Schultz, *op. cit.,* pp. 25–26.
[29]Mitchell, *op. cit.,* p. 207.

windows and clocks are replaced by unfamiliar repetitious machinery, noise, and "routine" procedures such as having a light directed into the eye or a blood pressure cuff inflated. In an environment like the intensive care unit the patient experiences both stimulus deprivation and, at times, overload."[30] The sensory environment may contain enough stimulation for cortical arousal. However, the sometimes repetitious clicking IVAC machine, hissing oxygen unit, clicking intermittent suction, or the rhythmic noise produced by a volume respirator do not provide variety. As a result the patient experiences perceptual monotony.

DEPRIVATION AND THE NURSE'S ROLE

The primary therapy of sensory-perceptual deprivation is prevention. The nurse, regardless of the patient's age, facilitates deprivation avoidance by being aware of the patient's physical environment. The nurse identifies things within the environment that contribute to sensory or perceptual deprivation. The nurse systematically assesses the intensity of input, meaning and pattern, or variations. In assessing the various sensory modes, the nurse begins with the same mode each time. Furthermore, the nurse accomplishes the goal of avoiding deprivation through management of the patient's sensory environment and maintaining significant stimulation. Each major goal contains variables or influencing factors that can be manipulated by the nurse. The variables are of two types, internal and external to the patient.

Management of Environment

To successfully manage something, the individual must be aware of the variables or influencing factors involved in the management process. The nurse who manages a patient's internal and external environment must empathize psychological, situational, and interpersonal variables. It's as if the nurse enters a patient's physical-emotional being and sees the world through his or her eyes. There are aspects of the patient's total sensory environment that the nurse learns to turn off. The patient, if overloaded or underloaded, does not have this ability to differentiate. Instead, the patient may tune out many sensory stimuli and be left void or deprived.

Internal environmental variables   Variables internal to the patient are primarily psychological. Psychological sensory restriction alters the

[30]Chodil, *op. cit.,* p. 459.

patient's cognitive efficiency, emotional state, and attitude toward changes of conformity. Many times patients experiencing periods of sensory deprivation have difficulty concentrating, focusing attention, organizing thoughts, and solving problems. These behaviors apply specifically to immobilized patients and those in isolation. It is possible that a patient spends several hours of the day alone. The nurse may have difficulty reaching such patients because their ability to concentrate or organize thoughts is reduced. Cognitive efficiency may be reduced to the point that there is difficulty identifying stimulation or extracting meaning from the external environment. In addition, the nurse must assess whether a state of deprivation or fear of illness is causing the patient's behavior. Once assessed, the nurse intervenes on the patient's present cognitive level. In time the nurse provides appropriate stimulation to raise cognitive abilities.

Patients deprived of sensory stimulation can become confused or disoriented. Furthermore, their temporarily unstable emotional state might lead to anger, hostility, lowered self-esteem, or even paranoia. The nurse realizes that patients who become disoriented and confused or who experience fantasies, illusions, or hallucinations must be quickly reoriented. If not, the patient becomes agitated or panicked. A simple explanation may alleviate the problem and reassure the patient. Temporary confusion is frightening to the patient because of fears of loss of control over events affecting the patient. The nurse intervenes to gradually raise the level of less threatening stimuli. The nurse does this by replacing threatening stimuli with familiar ones. A family member may sit with the confused patient and attempt to aid orientation. If the patient's emotional instability continues, there may be need for psychiatric consultation.

External environmental variables   External variables in the patient's environment are situational variables, interpersonal variables, and a number of sensory restrictions. Situational variables are those barriers in the patient's immediate sensory environment that contribute to reduction in sensory stimulation. Depending upon the patient's age or clinical setting, the room or bed may be void of stimulation for normal cortical arousal. Whenever possible, the patient's physical environment should contain elements of his or her personality. The patient needs personal belongings such as a clock, glasses, toys, toilet articles, books, cards, and picture in close proximity. It is normal for the child or adult patient to miss a dog, parents, children, brothers, sisters, or grandchildren. If the patient or the family have pictures, the nurse can tape them to the adult patient's traction or to the child's crib. This keeps the patient in visual touch with the familiar.

Infants and small children seem to respond to colorful visual objects in their environment. The objects, if within reach, seem to foster visual and tactile stimulation. White discovered that, "A group of infants exposed to increased handling and to objects hanging overhead spent more time looking at objects and were able to purposefully grasp objects sooner than a group who spent their time in cribs with nothing to look at but their hands."[31] To provide visual stimulation, the nurse can hang colorful mobiles over the infant's crib. For the premature infant or infant in an isolette, the nurse can tape a colorful object to the isolation side. The nurse can then position the infant to see the object. In addition, the nurse can alter the number of bright objects the infant sees and feels. Mitchell believes that, "If the infant has begun to reach for things, hanging toys provide reinforcement for reaching and grasping—they move, make noise, or bounce. Reaching leads to normal eye-hand coordination."[32]

Another situational variable involves keeping the patient oriented to time. In order to accomplish this goal, the nurse must keep a clock or watch within visual or tactile reach of the patient. In conversations with the patient, the nurse can refer to the time. The nurse must consider the patient's ability to orient himself to time. An assessment must be made of the patient's ability to estimate the time lapse between events, to relate past events to present or future ones and to grasp the sequence of events. Within each area, the patient may become disoriented regarding reality. To the patient who is unable to estimate time intervals, two hours becomes five minutes or five minutes becomes two hours, not understanding why time seems to race by or stand still.

If the patient wears glasses or a hearing aid, these personal belongings should be worn by the patient. The hearing aid will reduce sensory overload for other patients. In other words, the nurse no longer needs to yell in the patient's deaf ear. If, however, the patient does not have a hearing aid, the nurse will need to raise the level of auditory stimulation. Likewise, the patient who has reduced visual ability and no glasses will need the nurse to compensate by describing the immediate environment or placing objects within easy reach. For patients with reduced visual acuity, the nurse must place the patient's call light within reach. If necessary, it can be pinned to the patient's pillow or gown.

During the day, the patient's room should have adequate light. If the room has windows, all shades or curtains should be pulled back during the day. Whenever possible, the child or adult patient should be encouraged to sit in a chair near the window. At night, all lights should be

---

[31]Burton, White, "An Experimental Approach to the Effects of Experience in Early Human Behavior," *Minnesota Symposia on Child Psychology*, 1, 1967, pp. 201–26.

[32]Mitchell, *op. cit.*, p. 207.

turned off with the exception of a small night light. The latter might be a familiar light to children.

Additional aids to orientation and stimulation are radios and/or televisions. Radios to be most effective should be clearly tuned into programs that are of interest to the patient. The sound should be at an auditory level that will provide sensory stimulation. It must not, however, overstimulate a roommate who might have a lower auditory threshold. Children seem to enjoy listening to loud music for long periods of time. Whenever possible, pediatric units might own several portable record players or tape recorders. In this respect, familiar music can be brought into the hospital. Patients also enjoy watching television. For the patient who spends several waking hours watching favorite programs, the television becomes an important form of sensory stimulation. Children enjoy cartoons; adolescents like movies; and, some adults and aged patients involve themselves in daily soap operas.

Both the television and radio can be used to orient the confused adult or aged patient. If the television set has its own private sound control, it can be placed near the patient's ear. The older patient, even though confused, may need both the glasses and a hearing aid applied while listening to the television. In this respect, both sensory modalities, visual and auditory, will be stimulated, whereas the radio offers stimulation of only one sensory modality. Regardless of the problem, the nurse must assess the appropriateness of their use. For example, stimulation through television or radio alone may not be sufficient. The patient also needs the human-to-human contact obtained through the nurse.

Children and adults enjoy playing games. The child who is isolated or immobolized due to multiple fractures is unable to go to the dayroom and participate in play activities. Therefore, the nurse enters into play activities with the patient. For the child with multiple fractures, other children can be encouraged to include the patient in their games. Adult patients who enjoy bridge might play together in the dayroom. Games for all ages will foster sensory stimulation through socialization. Besides games and toys, children enjoy playing with modeling clay. Clay provides visual and tactile stimulation. In addition, it can become a vehicle of channeling excess energy—beat the clay.

People themselves become variables in the patient's environment. The patient, regardless of age, needs to see all aspects of the environment. In this respect one can see the more viable and mobile aspects of the environment; people. The patient needs to feel the closeness of others. The sensorially deprived patient has a great need for security and protection against harmful stimuli. The nurse meets these needs by fostering a sense of closeness. Closeness involves touching the patient when it seems appropriate, as young and old patients respond to touching. The nurse's human touch helps to orient the frightened or confused patient to reality. The nurse also fosters closeness between the patient and his or her family. The nurse intervenes to teach and support family members in maintaining an adequately stimulating environment. For example, the family might read stories, verses, or articles to the patient.

The nurse can encourage forms of autostimulation such as singing, muscle exercises, or movement out of the room. Children and adults enjoy singing, especially if other people participate. All patients should maintain as much physical movement as physiologically possible. It has been discovered that patients become confused if they remain immobilized. Therefore, patients who are immobilized due to their illness should be encouraged to touch themselves, do isometric exercises, and permit others to touch them. Unfortunately, the confused patient is restrained, thus further reducing the ability to touch.

Maintaining movement is a significant nursing intervention. According to Sorensen, "Movement is helpful in maintaining orientation to body image; therefore, passive exercises, encouraging the patient to move, turning and positioning the patient, rolling the bed up or down for various periods, and getting the patient out of bed and out of his room as much as possible are essential nursing actions."[33] The small child who is unable to leave the crib can be moved into the hallway, dayroom, or nurse's station. As mentioned before, exercises will foster awareness of body parts and therefore, a sense of relatedness to those parts covered by casts or dressings.

Maintain Meaningful Stimulation

The nurse attempts to make the patient's environment meaningful by utilizing any measure available that will increase sensory input and make the pattern meaningful for the patient. The nurse realizes that sensory stimulation cannot be passive since passive input can become monotonous. Nurses facilitate this meaningful environment through identification and limitation of meaningless stimulation.

Internal meaningfulness The variable that fosters or facilitates internal meaningfulness for the individual is knowledge. Knowledge is provided when the nurse explains unfamiliar facets within the patient's sensory environment. The patient may have normal cognitive abilities and a healthy emotional state but be unable to derive meaning from the surrounding world. Immediately after the patient is hospitalized, he or she is subjected to diagnostic tests, treatments, and other intrusive pro-

[33]Luckmann, *op. cit.,* p. 79.

cedures. Each procedure or treatment must be explained to the child or adult patient. The nurse assesses the amount of knowledge input to be given. Too much information creates sensory overload and the patient psychologically closes the mind. Too little information oversimplifies a potentially dangerous situation and gives the patient a false sense of security. If possible, information given should be repeated by the patient in order to ascertain the level of comprehension. The fact that the patient is immobilized from bedrest, tractions, casts, or pieces of supportive devices needs to be explained. Critically ill patients who are surrounded by a variety of supportive devices need some brief explanation. Mitchell points out that, "Structure and pattern can be introduced into the world of the acutely ill, less aware persons by careful brief explanation of everything which the nurse is doing, by describing the surroundings, and by interpreting the various sounds and activities "[34]

The nurse can develop creative teaching strategies incorporating various visual aids such as diagrams or colorful charts. These will then raise the knowledge level of the patient. The various strategies can be reapplied to other patients with similar educational needs. This then becomes an exciting way in which the nurse enters imaginatively into the patient's internal world.

External meaningfulness   As the patient's biological status improves, the nurse can involve him or her in self-care. Participation occurs on both a verbal and physical level. The nurse encourages the child or adult to verbalize feelings. Studies show that people who are encouraged to verbalize their thoughts and feelings during prolonged immobilization or isolation have fewer manifestations of anxieties. Verbalization seems to lessen the trauma and increase the tolerance of confinement. The nurse encourages the patient to talk. For the tracheostomy patient, the voice becomes a form of sensory stimulation. When the blind patient talks, the nurse must remember to verbally respond so the patient knows she or he is listening. The patient is unable to see the nurse's nonverbal response, relying on the auditory mode for feedback.

Verbalization helps the patient cope with illness. If coping is not accomplished, aberrant behavior or depression results. The nurse helps the patient to cope through awareness of feelings, needs, and fears. The nurse who is aware of the inherent dangers from the physical and social environment mobilizes resources toward making the sensory input meaningful to the patient. Reassurance is also a vital necessity in avoiding deprivation. Reassuring the patient helps him to cope with illness, disease, or injury. Reassurance is based on mutual trust, understanding, respect given by the nurse, and the establishing of appropriate limits for

[34]Mitchell, *op. cit.*, p. 214.

the patient. The patient develops internal resources which foster confidence and self-esteem.

The nurse encourages the patient's participation on a physical level. Bathing oneself creates tactile stimulation and movement. Furthermore, the patient becomes encouraged that the biological status is stabilizing. Ambulating in the room facilitates a new sensory awareness of the immediate environment. The awareness extends to the hallway, dayroom, and nurse's station.

In conclusion, the nurse attempts to create an optimal physical environment for the patient. The environment created is one in which there exists enough sensory stimulation, meaning, and variation for cortical arousal. The nurse assesses each sensory mode for the intensity of input. The nurse then assesses the patient's internal and external environment and determines the number of sensory restrictions involved. Further, the nurse assesses the variables and intervenes accordingly to successfully alter the environment in an attempt to avoid deprivation. The nurse's overall task is a difficult one. However, it is possible to create a sensory environment that resembles the familiar and restores the meaningful stimulation to the patient. This is possible only when we as nurses, "stop considering the person only as his body and begin to understand the body as a person. We then open biological function and action to the personal, social and physical world around. What goes on between persons affects what goes on inside them."[35]

REFERENCES

Adams, Henry, "Sensory Deprivation and Personality Change," *The Journal of Nervous and Mental Disease*, 143, pp. 256–65.

Arieti, Silvano, "Isolation and Sensory Deprivation," *American Handbook of Psychiatry*, vol. 3, Chapter 24, 1966.

Biase, Vincent, "Anticipated Responses to Short-Term Sensory Deprivation," *Psychological Reports*, 1969, pp. 351–54.

Black, Sister Kathleen, "Social Isolation and the Nursing Process," *Nursing Clincs of North America*, 8, December 1973.

Burnside, Irene, "Sensory Stimulation An Adjunct to Group Work with the Disabled Aged," *Mental Hygiene*, 58, July 1969.

Burt, Margaret, "Perceptual Deficit in Hemiplegia," *American Journal of Nursing*, May 1970.

[35]Edward Stanbrook, "Architects Not Only Design Hospitals: They Also Design Patient Behavior," *Modern Hospital*, 105, December 1965, p. 100.

Charlton, M. H., "Visual Hallucinations," *Psychiatric Quarterly*, 37, 1963, pp. 489–97.

Conover, Mary, "Understanding and Caring for the Hearing-Impaired," *NCNA*, 5, pp. 497–506.

Davis, John, "Sensory Deprivation: The Role of Social Isolation," *Archives of General Psychiatry*, 5, July 1961, pp. 84–90.

Dayton, Gleen, "Overt Behavior Manifested in Bilaterally Patched Patients," *American Journal of Opthalmology*, 59, May 1955, pp. 864–70.

Dominian, J., "The Psychological Significance of Touch," *Nursing Times*, July 22, 1971, pp. 896–98.

Elmer, Elizabeth, "Failure to Thrive Role of the Mother," *Pediatrics*, 25, April 1960, pp. 717–20.

Filante, W., "Sensory Deprivation on an Eye Service—Its Significance and Management," *California Medicine*, December 1960, pp. 355–56.

Frank, L. K., "Tactile Communication," *Psychological Monographs*, 56, 1957, pp. 209–55.

Freedman, David, "The Influence of Congenital and Perinatal Sensory Deprivation on Later Development," *Psychosomatics*, 9, September–October 1968.

Katz, Violet, "Auditory Stimulation and Developmental Behavior of the Premature Infant," *Nursing Research*, 20, May–June 1971.

Kubie, Lawrence, "Theoretical Aspects of Sensory Deprivation," *Sensory Deprivation*, ed. Philip Solom. Cambridge: Harvard University Press, 1961.

Leiderman, Herbert, "Sensory Deprivation," *American Medical Association Archives of Internal Medicine*, 101, February 1958.

Lewis, Michael, "Cardiac Responsivity to Tactile Stimulation in Waking and Sleeping Infants," *Conceptual and Motor Skills*, 29, 1969.

Linnell, Craig, "The Hearing-Impaired Infant," *NCNA*, 5, September 1970, pp. 507–15.

Ludwig, Arnold, "Psychedelic Effects Produced by Sensory Overload," *American Journal Psychiatry*, 128, April 1972.

Mendelson, J., "Catechol Amine Excretion and Behavior During Sensory Deprivation," *American Medical Association Archives of General Psychiatry*, 2, February 1960, pp. 147–55.

Ohno, Mary, "The Eye Patched Patient," *American Journal of Nursing*, February 1971, pp. 271–74.

Parker, Donald, "Delirium in a Coronary Care Unit," *Journal of the American Medical Association,* August 28, 1967, pp. 132–33.

Payne, Peter, "Behavior Manifestations of Children with Hearing Loss," *American Journal of Nursing,* 70, August 1970, pp. 1718–19.

Segall, Mary, "Cardiac Responsibility to Auditory Stimulation in Premature Infants," *Nursing Research,* 21, January-February 1972, pp. 15-19.

Woods, Nancy Fugate, "Noise Stimuli in the Acute Care Area," *Nursing Research,* March-April 1974, pp. 144–49.

5
Stress

Stress is not unique to any one age, economic, or cultural group. There are individuals who experience daily stress because of their occupation, geographic location, or health status. Stress may or may not be specific. According to Selye, "Stress is therefore not the specific result of any one among our actions; nor is it a typical response to any one thing acting upon us from without; it is a common feature of all biological activities."[1] In many instances, stress involves a number of factors which can operate simultaneously or separately. Stress can be an influence whether it originates from the individual's internal or external environment. Whatever the influencing factor, it tends to alter the individual's stable equilibrium.

Furthermore, what constitutes stress is not perceived in a universal manner. Two individuals confronted with the same task or situation may react with varying degrees of stress. What is perceived to be stressful for one individual is not by another. The individual's perception of stress is most significant. "Because of man's nature, stress does not necessarily or always have an objective basis in reality. It may be provoked by threats and symbols of danger and deprivation as well as by actual danger or deprivation. Stress of this type is frequently insidious and as damaging as that from more concrete sources."[2] Nevertheless for the individual experiencing stress, it is real, and causes one to respond behaviorally. One's response may be viewed as inappropriate by those not directly involved in the stress situation. However, to the involved individual, the response is appropriate.

It is interesting to note that throughout one's life, an individual learns various ways of coping or adapting to a stressful state. Exposure to actual stress or what is perceived as actual stress for long periods of time, can endanger or even shorten an individual's life. Selye believes that,

[1]Hans Selye, *The Stress of Life,* (New York: McGraw-Hill, 1956), p. 255.

[2]Harry Martin, "Human Adaptation: A Conceptual Approach to Understanding Patients," *The Canadian Nurse,* 58, March 1962, p. 237.

"Anything that causes stress endangers life, unless it is met by adequate adaptive responses; conversely, anything that endangers life causes stress and adaptive responses. Adaptability and resistance to stress are fundamental prerequisites for life, and every vital organ and function participates in them."[3]

Each individual perceives and adapts to stress in a unique way. This means that everyone has the potential or ability to realize their limits within a stressful situation or to destroy themselves through failure to recognize these limits. It should be pointed out that like anxiety, some stress is necessary to mobilize the individual into action; however, beyond this point, stress becomes a concern for all members of the health team.

The health team is becoming more cognizant of the interrelationship between stress and disease. There is interest in understanding the mechanisms which maintain health and those which cause disease. Obviously there is a delicate balance between health and disease. "Health, in a positive sense, consists in the capacity of the organism to maintain a balance in which it may be reasonably free of undue pain, discomfort, disability or limitation of action, including social capacity. Disease corresponds to failure or disturbances in the growth, development, function, and adjustment of the organism as a whole or of any of its systems."[4] The balance between health and disease can be disrupted by stress.

Stress is a growing concern for nurses providing care in a variety of clinical situations. Stress will be defined before discussing how the concept applies to various developmental or age groups.

DEFINITION OF STRESS

Stress seems to represent a variety of responses manifested as anxiety, emotional tension or frustration, anger, inability to adjust to a situation, or difficulty with judgment and decision-making processes. Stress, as an experience can be temporary, recurrent, or continual. Recurrent or continual stress can cause physiological and psychological exhaustion. Each individual, at some point, is confronted with stressors. Stressors are defined . . . "as agents or factors that challenge the adaptive capacities of an individual, thereby placing a strain upon that person which may result in stress and disease."[5]

[3]Hans Selye, "Stress and the General Adaptation Syndrome," *British Medical Journal*, June 17, 1950, p. 4667.

[4]Selye, *The Stress of Life*, p. 459.

[5]Joan Luckmann and Karen Sorensen, "Stress and Disease: Major Causative Factors," *Medical-Surgical Nursing: A Psychophysiologic Approach*, (Philadelphia: Saunders, 1974), p. 41.

It is difficult to assess how much stress any one individual can endure. Measurement of stress tolerance has been accomplished inside a well defined and structured experimental setting. The amount of stress tolerance has not, on the other hand, been measured in a nonexperimental setting. Therefore, when an individual is confronted with a stressful situation no one, including the individual, knows how one will respond. One can frequently hear a spectator of someone else's stress say, "I wouldn't react that way if I were he." Unless the spectator has experienced the same stressful situation or crisis, this statement is unjustified. There are times when members of the health team make the same or similar judgments. Regardless of whether the stress is real to the spectator, it is real to the individual involved.

There are many definitions of stress as it relates to events within the individual's internal and external environment. "The definition of an event as a 'stress' can, in general, be made only after we know that it has had some disturbing effect on the person exposed to it. What we are really saying is that some events produce significant disturbances in the organism, and these may be so marked that they are a disease."[6] Many individuals define a stressful event as a threatening encounter, one that causes the individual to become insecure with himself or herself and the immediate environment. Each individual needs to feel secure with oneself, if not with the environment. If a stressful event causes the individual to react in ways unlike normal behavior, he or she becomes self-threatened. After a crisis has occurred in which an individual responds in a totally unique way, he or she may be heard to say "I even scared myself," or "I didn't know I was capable of acting that way." Psychologists define stress as, "a state where the well-being (or integrity) of an individual is endangered and he must devote all his energies to its protection."[7]

Selye, who has done vast research in the area of stress, provides one of its most practical definitions. "We can look upon stress as the rate of wear and tear in the body. When so defined, the close relationship between aging and stress becomes particularly evident. Stress is the sum of all the wear and tear caused by any kind of vital reaction throughout the body at any one time. That is why it can act as a common denomination of all the biological changes which go on in the body; it is a kind of 'speedometer of life.' "[8]

In some regions of the world, people live beyond the age of one

[6]David Graham, "Disease As Response to Life Stress," *Psychological Bases of Medical Practice*, 1963, p. 115.

[7]C. N. Cofer and M. H. Appley, *Motivation: Theory and Research*, (New York: Wiley, 1964), p. 463.

[8]Selye, *The Stress of Life*, p. 274.

hundred. In examining their culture, one notes a marked reduction in stressful situations; life seems to be tranquil and slow paced. In Western civilization, man is continually exposed to numerous daily stresses, including the growing stress of illness and disease. Stress, then, is the overall wear and tear on an individual's physiological and psychological being. Adaptive processes allow the individual to cope with stress. However, with prolonged stress even the adaptive process can become depleted and eventually fail. Nurses working with patients in various clinical settings should assess potential stressful situations and the patient's stress response. Stress will be discussed as it applies to the child, adult, and aged patient.

APPLICATION TO CLINICAL SETTINGS

Stress affects all hospitalized patients regardless of age or clinical setting. The idea of being hospitalized, separated from the familiar and secure, is stressful. When one is hospitalized, one relinquishes one's being to the control of others who manipulate the body in ways that are perceived to be intrusive. Of course loss of control depends upon the severity of the illness, injury, or disease process, and the causes and effects of psychological stress can vary with age. According to Luckmann, "The active tumultuous life of the adolescent makes him particularly vulnerable to infection and to accidents. The competitive, exhausting existence of the middle class adult makes him susceptible to such problems as stress ulcers, hypertension, heart disease, and alcoholism. The elderly person, his life lonely and his hopes diminished, often lapses into an inactive existence accompanied by various degenerative disorders."[9] In order for the health team to assist its patient cope with stress, regardless of age or clinical problem, a systematic means of assessment is necessary. For the purposes of stress assessment, the tool will be referred to as a stress framework.

Stress Framework

The stress framework, consisting of three components, is a way of assessing the severity of a patient's stress experience. The three components which will be applied to the child, adult, and aged patient are: (1) degree and/or duration; (2) the individual's previous experience; and (3) available resources.

[9]Luckmann, *op. cit.*, p. 44.

Degree-Duration of Stress

The degree and duration of stress can be further divided into two categories; psychological and biological. Depending upon the severity of the illness, injury, or disease, there are definite psychological implications. The resulting stress can cause the individual to behave in predictable ways. Likewise, biological implications imply how the individual's body must adapt to the acute or chronic biological changes. With acute biological changes, the individual experiences short term stress of tremendous magnitude. Because the stress is hopefully short term, adaptive responses will only be temporarily weakened and not depleted. However, chronic biological changes of a long nature can cause the individual's adaptive processes to become depleted. Such an individual may be unable to cope with even the simplest additional stress.

Child   Psychologically, stress causes each individual to react in a way that is unique to the individual and his or her stage in the developmental cycle. Children need more than an environment which is stimulating and which provides mobility through imaginative and creative play. In addition, "they also need a continuous relationship with a mothering person who can respond to them according to their individual needs and who can act as a source of continuity of experience which is the basis for those permanent inner images of outer people and things which the child builds up in the course of his first two years of life."[10]

Between the age of six months and three years, the child depends upon a familiar person for future emotional and cognitive development, including needs for affection and stimulation. The familiar person who knows the small child's needs is usually the mother. The mother knows a child as an individual with unique personality, cry, smile, or laugh. Hospitalization for the small child brings about a loss of mother. The familiar mother who knows the child is replaced by strangers in an impersonal setting. Such a change is likely to have a long term effect upon the child. According to Coleman, "Most, but not all, children show an initial response of acute distress and crying (the period of protest), followed by a phase of misery and apathy (the phase of despair), and finally a stage when the child loses interest in his parents (detachment) and appears relatively contented."[11]

A lack of awareness of such phases may cause the nurse to misassess and misdiagnose that a young patient is experiencing stress. The nurse

[10]Sula Wolff, *Children Under Stress*, (Maryland: Penguin Press, 1969), p. 18.

[11]James Coleman, "Life Stress and Maladaptive Behavior," *The American Journal of Occupational Therapy*, May-June 1973, p. 172.

must constantly keep in mind that each child reacts to stress in a unique manner. The nurse may assess that a toilet-trained young patient wets the bed at night. This behavior is assessed as regressive in nature. Labeling the behavior is not sufficient help for the young patient who already feels guilty for being ill and now for the accident. Such behavioral responses may be manifested even before the stress situation is apparent to the health team. A child may have overheard a nurse or doctor tell the mother that in two days he or she will undergo a special diagnostic procedure. The procedure constitutes stress and the child reacts to the anticipation of stress just as intensely as to the stress itself.

In other instances the environment itself becomes the source of stress. A small child may be frightened by the unusual and strange noise of the hospital environment. Such an environment is familiar to the staff but unfamiliar to the small child. Furthermore, the child at home has his or her own room and privacy. In the hospital the child may have to share a room with several other small patients. The new roommates physical problems and various supportive devices may further compound the young patient's feeling of stress. For example, a small child with a nasal gastric tube, Foley catheter, dressings, casts, and IV may initially be a curiosity to the observing young patient. However, if the observing young patient should need an IV, there may be fear that, in time, the other supportive devices will be applied. Even though the patient will not need other supportive devices, the small child is unable to verbalize these fears because the grossly appearing nasal gastric tube or casts are not a part of the vocabulary. We can only stabilize, with a label, those things for which we have a word in our vocabulary. To stabilize means to label something or place it in a category so it can be dealt with. The small child has a limited vocabulary and therefore is unable to conceptualize the object verbally. Instead, the observant nurse sees the crying child pointing to his or her own nose and then to the roommate. These nonverbal gestures indicate fears that the strange tube will be attached to his or her nose. Here the nurse attempts to assess the young patient's behavioral response, attach it to a situational stress, and, if possible, alleviate the child's psychological stress.

The small child experiences psychological stress due to separation from a familiar mother and sudden placement in a strange environment. The variable or influencing factor is the degree or duration of the separation and length of hospitalization. Additional psychological stress for children evokes from the degree and duration of dependency and physical restrictions imposed by their illness, injury, or disease. Some small children resent giving up their sense of independence. According to Wolff, "Some children, for whom the mastery of independent eating, washing and toileting was accomplished in the face of great longings for dependency and passivity, do not give up these achievements easily: they become difficult and intractable patients."[12]

The nurse should remember that small children take great pleasure in the accomplishment of such tasks as eating and toileting. These may seem like small accomplishments to the adult who has mastered skills of greater complexity, but to the child who is growing in autonomy, their loss is more significant. To suddenly have these areas of independence taken away causes the child to experience stress. The young child, in all probability, does not understand why he or she has to be separated from the mother or why he or she is suddenly deprived of the tasks they were actively encouraged to learn. The child is placed in a dilemma, of which there was no choice. Depending upon the actual biological problem and its emotional effects on the small child, the nurse may need to assume responsibility for these tasks. For example, for the child with renal problems, it is imperative that the health team be aware of hourly urinary output. To accomplish this goal, a Foley catheter may be necessary. Not only is the procedure intrusive, it also serves to limit the child's mobility. However, once the nurse assesses that the young patient's biological dysfunction has stabilized or the ability to appropriately handle certain tasks is regained, the nurse should encourage independence. The degree and duration of forced dependency play a significant role in the child's ability to reestablish independence. In other words, if the child is placed in a dependency situation for a prolonged period, there may be a refusal to regain autonomy.

Forced dependency involves not only temporary loss of certain tasks, but also loss of mobility. Physical immobility can cause the small child further stress. To a young child, movement through the environment is a form of motor and cognitive stimulation. The child learns about himself or herself while exploring the unknown. Hospitalization greatly reduces the child's mobility. Illness, disease, or injury of an acute or chronic nature further limits mobility. This is especially true with children who have an orthopedic problem and require prolonged immobilization in a cast. Again the duration of immobilization can cause psychological stress. The stress related to physical restraint can lead to behavioral responses of an aggressive nature. According to Wolff, "In general motor restraint increases expression of aggressive feelings both in toddlers and older children. There is more verbal aggression but also more restlessness and irritability."[13]

Biological implications, the second category, can also be related to the degree and duration of stress. Illness, injury, or disease have different implications to the small child. Many of the illnesses associated with

[12]Wolff, *op. cit.*, p. 53.
[13]*Ibid.*, p. 53.

childhood are mild. The child experiences temporary but limited inactivity. The child also receives intense concern from the mother. From this mild illness experience, the child learns illness behavior, including the sick role. Furthermore, the child is reassured that needs will be meant and the illness will disappear. Illness, injury, or disease of a more serious nature involves hospitalization.

A serious illness not only exposes the child to hospitalization in an unfamiliar setting, but also to intrusive diagnostic and treatment procedure. The child's previous experience with intrusive diagnostic and treatment procedures may be quite limited. Furthermore, the child has limited cognitive abilities. Both these circumstances cause stress. Any threat to the small child's body integrity can imply a threat to life. For example, an injection has unique connotations for the child. According to Erickson, "Puncturing the skin with a needle breaks the wholeness of the skin surface, and to a young child this makes a hole through which his blood may leak out. If blood is withdrawn he fears that all his blood has been removed. He is so primed for danger that when told his blood pressure is to be taken, he hears only the words 'blood' and 'take,' and responds with anxiety."[14]

The nurse should keep in mind that what seems to be a routine part of hospital life is not routine to the child. A child with major burns may react violently when confronted with treatments in the Hubbard tank. The health team may assess the behavior to be associated with the child's anticipation of pain. However, a closer assessment may reveal that the child associates the Hubbard tank with drowning, actually being afraid of the water. The tank, in relationship to his or her small body, seems overwhelming. Thus, besides the biological problem of infection and skin grafting, the child has the additional stress; fear of drowning. Another child may be limited or completely restricted from oral intake of food and fluids. Again, the procedure seems routine to the nurse; however, the child associates it with rejection or punishment.

Even other children on the pediatric ward can be a source of stress for the child. The child may be in close proximity to another child who is seriously ill and whose moaning, crying, or screaming can cause stress. Furthermore, if the roommate should suddenly die, the child becomes afraid that his or her own illness or disease may lead to the same result, again experiencing stress.

Chronic illness or disease constitutes stress of a different nature. It usually implies frequent hospitalization. Take, for example, those children with congenital or acquired cardiac, gastrointestinal, pulmonary, or renal problems. They may have multiple scars to show for their biological

[14]Florence Erickson, "Stress in the Pediatric Ward," *Maternal Child Nursing Journal*, Summer 1972, p. 113.

problems. According to Wolff, "All these children have been exposed to prolonged hospitalization and often to major surgery usually very early in their lives; their parents have at one time faced the possibility that their child may die, and many such children carry with them into later life some outward signs of their illness."[15] Chronic illness, such as diabetes, may also cause unique stresses for the child. This, of course, depends upon the age of onset. Older children, particularly adolescents, may have the greatest difficulty adapting to the illness. For the child, diabetes becomes a lifelong problem including dietary restrictions of certain foods frequently associated with youth such as candy, Cokes, and ice cream. The child or adolescent must assume the responsibility for restraining from eating such foods. In addition, "Diabetic children are generally subjected to a routine of daily injection of insulin, many must in addition keep to a diet and limit their intake especially of sweets, the foods which symbolize comfort and having a treat."[16]

Adult and aged   As with the child, the adult and aged patient can experience stress on either a psychological or physiological level. Janis,[17] in his research, has identified three phases of psychological stress. These are the threat phase, the danger impact phase, and the post impact victimization phase. During the threat phase, the patient anticipates an oncoming danger. Of significance is the degree of danger anticipated. This is also referred to as the severity of stress. Coleman points out that, "Severity of stress refers to the degree of disruption in the system that will occur if the individual fails to cope with the adjustive demands. The severity of stress is, in turn, determined primarily by three factors: the characteristics of the adjustive demand, the characteristics of the individual, and the external resources and supports available to him."[18]

The adult or aged patient may be confronted with both external and internal stresses, both implying a psychological traumatization for the individual. This is particularly significant if something of value is lost. External stresses are those associated with losses such as an important job, social role, forced retirement, values, or a loved one. Internal stresses are usually related to biological alteration in integrity. Biological alteration can also have a psychological effect upon the individual's self-concept and body image. Even though both types of stress imply a tremendous demand and can simultaneously affect the same individual, the nurse's intervention focuses more closely on the patient's internal stresses.

It is hard for the nurse to assess what factors determine how a

[15]Wolff, *op. cit.*, p. 65.

[16]*Ibid.*, p. 65–6.

[17]Irving Janis, *Psychological Stress*, (New York: Academic Press, 1974, pp. 7–8.

[18]Coleman, *op. cit.*, p. 170.

patient will psychologically cope with illness, injury, or disease. The factors may be highly individualized for the particular adult or aged patient, usually focusing on the significance, duration, and variation of the adjustive demands during the threat phase. "The importance, duration, and multiplicity of demands are some of the key characteristics of the stress situation that determine its severity. The longer the stress operates the more severe it is likely to become. Similarly a number of stresses operating at the same time or in a sequence that keeps the individual off balance are more stressful than if these events occurred separately."[19] Therefore, if the patient anticipates a continued exposure to a threat over a prolonged period of time, that patient will undoubtedly experience psychological stress.

The danger impact phase is the time during which the adult or aged patient realizes that the illness or disease is at hand. The patient is environmentally surrounded by evidence of an altered biological being. Such evidence takes the form of supportive devices which are attached to the body. It is at this time that the patient further realizes that success depends greatly upon the protective actions of his or her own biological adaptive system and the support of the health team in the immediate environment. The degree of stress, associated with the danger impact phase, may depend upon the specific biological system involved. To many adult or aged patients, their health represents life and the essence of their biological being. Therefore, any threat to this system is a threat to life itself. Likewise many patients fear renal problems or complication which might lead to dependency on a hemodialysis machine. A simple urinary tract infection may become a source of monumental stress for such a patient.

Patients may also experience stress if they are frequently hospitalized for the same biological problem. The aged patient, with chronic obstructive pulmonary disease, feels threatened with each recurrent respiratory infection. Each breath is exhausting and brings the patient closer to the things causing fears; dependency upon a ventilator and others to assume continued breathing. Both threats of potential dependency cause psychological stress.

Within the danger impact phase, the adult or aged patient behaviorally reacts in a unique way, directly associated with the degree and duration of stress. As stress increases, the patient experiences changes in cognitive functioning, including a reduction in objective thinking and adaptive efficiency. While experiencing stress, the individual also experiences a degree of emotional arousal. However, as the stress situation remains intense, the individual's emotional response may be inappropriate. These variables influence adjustment to stress and contribute to

[19]*Loc. cit.*

behavioral response. They include fear of loss to body integrity through damage and externalized anger. The adult or aged patient manifests fear of altered body image through apprehension, nervousness, and attempts to protect the weakening biological being. The patient attempts the latter by refusing intrusive diagnostic procedures or treatments.

Second, externalized anger is directly expressed toward members of the health team. The anger may be behaviorally manifested through resentment. As the illness, injury, or disease process becomes more of a reality during the danger impact phase, the patient resents forced dependency, as it becomes dependency without dignity. Throughout adult life the individual has moved independently making decisions, formulating alternative plans, and in general, recognizing himself as a controlling force over internal and external elements in life surroundings. Suddenly the patient is confronted with the reality of illness or injury only to realize that there is a loss of control of the being. The patient fears that total control may never be completely restored. Therefore, the expressed resentment or anger at others is really misplaced.

In reality the patient is angry at his or her own body or the situation which led to hospitalization. It is far easier and safer to express anger toward strangers than oneself or family. Thus, externalized anger as behaviorally manifested through resentment is to be expected during the danger impact phase. The difficulty lies in assessing the behavioral response, as it may be latent or disguised as sarcasm, negativism, or inappropriate humor.

The postimpact victimization phase is the time when the adult or aged patient perceives losses. The battle has ended and the casualties need to be assessed. In assessing the sustained losses, the adult or aged patient may experience deprivation. Depending upon the illness, injury, or disease, the loss can involve only a temporary loss of function or a permanent loss of part or whole.

Take, for example, the cardiac patient whose loss may be minor since only a small loss of myocardial function results from a myocardial infarction. Such a patient is free of complications and with proper supportive care can return to a somewhat curtailed life style. For the cardiac patient whose loss is major, complications such as congestive heart failure or cardiogenic shock may severely limit the patient's future. Each complication may signify a poor prognosis because a loss of a part exists. Therefore, the biological and psychological losses are great.

Patients can also experience loss of the whole. For the female patient who discovers a lump in her breast, the loss becomes a whole—surgical removal of her breast. Furthermore, she lives with the stressful fear that her body is in a time capsule in which cancer may manifest itself elsewhere. Another example of loss in whole is the diabetic patient who enters the hospital with a thrombophlebitis. The thrombophlebitis has severely diminished peripheral perfusion thus causing the loss of the leg. Each individual experiences a loss of varying magnitude. The loss, especially that consisting of part or whole, leads to deprivation. The cardiac patient may be deprived of an active life. For patients with an amputated body part, the deprivation focuses on altered body image and fear of future loss.

Realization of loss, together with various biological and/or psychological deprivation, causes the adult or aged patient to experience frustration. Frustration arising from altered or unfulfilled goals leads to psychological stress. The individual's frustration can compound an existing clinical problem, thus increasing stress related or induced illness. As psychological stress increases, biological process can break down. This can lead to biological and psychological disease.

Physiological stress is the second component to be assessed within the degree-duration of the stress framework. Ironically, physiological illness or disease can be the result of psychological stress. According to Kral, "It seems possible that under the impact of multiple severe stresses acting over a considerable length of time not only one, but all parts of the stress resistance mechanisms might suffer long lasting and even irreparable damage, although perhaps to a different degree."[20]

Illness and disease cause adult or aged patients ot feel as though they have an unknown thing inside their body. It becomes an entity with an existance of its own. Depending upon the severity of the illness, injury, or disease, the "thing" may render the patient a helpless victim. The nurse must keep in mind that stress affects people in different ways. "A very stressful situation that is short lived is often better tolerated by an individual than a less stressful situation that tends to be chronic. This is because chronic stress demands continuous adaptive efforts. Eventually, because of constant wear and tear of a chronic nature, the individual actually changes physically and psychologically, becoming more vulnerable to other stressors."[21]

Such is the case with patients who have chronic pain. A few examples are the arthritic, osteocarcinoma, or patient with peripheral neuropathy. The pain focuses the patient's attention to the affected body part. Likewise, after the patient has experienced an illness, there is a reduction in the adaptive capacity of the involved organ or system, although the same individual may be healthy in all other areas. An exception occurs when the individual strains the already altered organ

---

[20]V. A. Kral, "Long Term Effects of a Prolonged Stress Experience," *Canadian Psychiat. Assoc. Journal,* 12, 1967, p. 180.

[21]Luckmann, *op. cit.,* p. 41.

beyond its capacity. When this occurs other systems seem to become involved. The cardiac patient who sustains repeated myocardial infarction leading to a marked reduction in myocardial reserve and adaptable capacity further experiences other biological changes. The patient experiences pulmonary edema and possible hepatocongestion and acute tubular necrosis due to perfusion deficit.

Another example is the patient with mitral insufficiency due to rheumatic heart disease or papillary muscle dysfunction from myocardial infarction. If the patient's mitral insufficiency is due to rheumatic heart disease, the limitations are gradual and may not manifest themselves for years. Such individuals carry the potential threat with them for years and learn to adapt to its existence. Papillary muscle dysfunction may occur suddenly thus minimizing the individual's ability to adequately adapt. The former is an example of long term duration with less stressful significance. The latter, however, represents intense stress with short term duration. Engel summarizes the concept of physiological and psychological stress: "A person may satisfy all the criteria of health at any point in time simply because the adaptive capacity of a defective system—be it biochemical, physiological, or psychological—has not been exceeded . . . it may be a matter of time; eventually the system will breakdown under the impact of accumulated and repeated small stress."[22]

Previous Experience

The child, adult or aged patient's previous experience with hospitalization focuses upon two characteristics. These are stress tolerance and perception of stressful events.

Child   A child's previous hospital experiences may be numerous or nonexistent. The influence that hospitalization has upon the child, in terms of stress tolerance and perception, is dependent upon age and what happens while hospitalized. It has been observed that infants less than seven months of age are not affected by hospitalization. While they are generally quiet, they do seem to cry more than when at home. Nevertheless, they respond to unfamiliar nurses just as they would their own mothering figure. Furthermore, the infants do not seem bothered when their mother leaves. At this time hospitalization is more stressful to the mother who feels as if she is abandoning her own child when the child needs her the most. It is the mother who experiences separation anxiety

---

[22]George Engel, "A Unified Concept of Health and Disease," *Perspectives in Biology and Medicine*, 3, Spring 1960, p. 469. Published by The University of Chicago Press.

and fear of failure when she, once again, assumes total responsibility for her child. If hospitalization at this age has been prolonged, the nurse will need to reacquaint the small infant with the mother. In other words, the mother may have difficulty identifying with her own infant when well. Therefore, she needs to be included, as much as is realistic, in the care of her own infant. In this respect, she becomes reacquainted with the infant's likes and dislikes while simultaneously renewing her own confidence as a mothering figure.

After seven months of age, infants react to their new environment, including the strange nurses. They seem to have less stress tolerance than previously demonstrated. They manifest their stress intolerance through such behavioral responses as crying, overdependence, and clinging. As each strange health-related individual makes contact with the small child, stress level increases while tolerance for what they do to the child diminishes. When the child's mother arrives for visiting hours, the child clings to her and demonstrates frustration quite loudly when she must leave.

As the child gets older, there is a greater cognizance of the surroundings. Some children accumulate experiential knowledge regarding hospitalization and its frightening diagnostic procedures. Furthermore, their behavioral responses become more indicative of the tremendous stress they experience. Hospitalization leads to the most disturbed behavior in children between the ages of two and four. According to Wolff, "In this age group screaming and panic attacks are common, outbursts of anger occur whenever parents leave and some children become depressed, withdrawn and develop eating and sleeping disturbances."[23] It is possible that the child of two or four dictates what is seen and experienced within the immediate environment. Objects take on a strange form completely out of proportion to reality. A small 5 cc syringe may be perceived as a 50 cc syringe. It is no wonder that the child becomes anxious when the nurse approaches with an injection or a laboratory technician desires a blood specimen. The same imperception may occur with other diagnostic or treatment procedures as the child perceives health care people hurting rather than helping.

Illness, injury, or disease may immobilize a child forcing that child to lie on the back. It is from this position that the environment is viewed, invoking feelings of vulnerability. In addition, siderails, traction, wires, tubes, or casts contribute to feelings of vulnerability and dependence upon a strange environment. Like intrusive diagnostic procedures, surgery is also perceived to be stressful and potentially painful for the child who fails to see how the procedure can be helpful. "Between age 3-6 children are preoccupied with their bodily intactness and castration anx-

---

[23]Wolff, *op. cit.*, p. 58.

ieties are readily stimulated. . . . Illnesses are explained in moralistic terms; painful procedures are viewed as punishment and arouse more guilt and anxiety than at any later stages of life."[24]

Studies have also revealed that children who have had a traumatic experience prior to hospitalization reacted with greater stress than those who came from a secure home environment. According to Wolff, "The insecurity of a rejected child, for example, impairs his chances of an independent adjustment away from home. He does not carry with him the firm inner image of a loving mother which can reassure him while he is parted from her."[25]

Adult and aged   As with the child, previous experience for the adult and aged patient focuses on stress tolerance and perception. Stress tolerance refers to the degree of stress the individual can tolerate before becoming disorganized or decompensated. Each patient has a unique level of stress tolerance. Patients who have experienced continued biological crisis over a prolonged period of time seem to have a higher level of stress tolerance than others. Such is the case with chronic illness. The patient has had to learn to adapt to the continued stress. The observer, nurse or doctor, may not see the stresses in the patient's life or environment that contribute to the illness, injury, or disease process. The observer assesses the situation to be tolerable; however, the patient's assessment is different. For example, the schizophrenic patient may itemize events leading to a breakdown. To the health team, the events are tolerable but to the schizophrenic patient, the events are intolerable.

Stress tolerance also refers to the limitations and potentialities of the adult or aged patient for dealing with stress. These factors are dependent upon peer adaptation to stressful situations. For either patient, illness may be a new experience. Consequently, the individual has little previous experience with adapting to biological crisis. Stress tolerance is also influenced by the type of crisis involved. In other words, certain stresses have more significance and meaning to some individuals than others. The loss of a job may be less stressful to one individual than another. The fear of cancer may be more stressful to the individual who has a strong family history of cancer. Another individual may fear cardiac, pulmonary, or renal disease more than cancer itself. No one can predetermine what illness, injury or disease will have the greatest degree of stress for a particular individual or that person's ability to tolerate the stress. The adult or aged patient strives to maintain a balance or to reestablish a balance. According to Martin, "Meeting his needs and adapting to the stress which confronts him in life, the individual, including his body,

[24]*Ibid.*, p. 61.
[25]*Ibid.*, p. 59.

resorts to various measures—physiological, psychological, social—which tend to maintain a relatively stable balance between and among the various systemic parts."[26]

The second factor of previous experience deals with the adult or aged patient's perception of the clinical problem. For such patients the severity of the perceived stress is dependent upon interpretation of the clinical problem. For example, a patient may enter the hospital complaining of abdominal pain, distention, and constipation and in that patient's mind a tentative diagnosis is formulated. Diagnostic studies and X rays confirm what the patient fears; an abdominal tumor. The patient's doctor, in explaining the diagnosis, treatment, and prognosis may outline the possibilities of the tumor being benign or malignant. In all probability the adult or aged patient's attention focuses on the term malignant. For that patient, life has ceased with the diagnosis. Possibly this patient has known someone with a similar clinical problem who, in fact, did have a malignant tumor. Thus, the severity of perceived stress is tremendous. Unless the patient shares these fears and anxieties no one will realize the magnitude of the stress. Such patients receiving a new diagnosis need time to think through their clinical problem and supportive assistance in asking the question which could alleviate some of their perceived stress. The questions and answers need to be provided in a definitive manner. Helberg points out that, "People under stress seem less able to cope with ambiguous or unresolved problems. They feel a need to have things definite, sure and in clear figure, even though this may mean sacrificing accuracy. As a result of 'tunnel vision,' the individual becomes incapable of focusing on the total perceptual field. This results in a drastic reduction in the number of acceptable solutions."[27]

It is interesting to note that the adult or aged patient may distort perception of the stressful event in an attempt to reduce experienced threat. A major surgical operation such as coronary artery by-pass, or reconstructive surgery necessary after severe trauma constitutes a stress situation. These stress situations can be perceived as a catastrophe or disaster in which the patient feels like a victim. In seeing oneself as a victim, the patient faces a combination of three major forms of danger —pain, body-mutilation, and death. Furthermore, the once independent individual is now a dependent patient. The adult or aged patient in the prime of life is found in a clinical setting dominated by a sometimes impersonal health team. The patient perceives the health team as being unable to satisfy needs for pain relief and meaningful stimulation. To the patient ". . . caretakers repeatedly demand submission to painful, dis-

[26]Martin, *op. cit.*, p. 238.

[27]Donald Helberg, "Communicating Under Stress," *Association of Operating Room Nurses Journal*, November 1972, p. 48.

agreeable, and embarrassing manipulation. Needles are jabbed into the patient's arms; probes, swabs, or drainage tubes are poked into sensitive wounds; stomach tubes are inserted through the nose and down into the throat; evil tasting medicine is poured into his mouth; bed pans are shoved under his buttocks and belatedly removed—these and a variety of other disagreeable demands and indignities are imposed upon him at a time when he is already in a state of general malaise, beset by incisional pain, backaches, sore muscles, headaches, distended bowels, constipation, and perhaps a generous spread of angrily itching skin."[28]

Resources

Within the stress framework, resources are assessed according to their external or internal availability. The child may have limited internal resources, while the adult or aged patient may have limited external resources.

Child   The child's external resources consist of the family, friends, and the nurse who becomes a substitute mothering figure. Depending upon the child's age, the mothering figure may be the most significant external resource. The child derives security from the nurse's supportive presence, which reassures the child of protection. The child's age and clinical problem will determine whether or not the mothering figure can remain at bedside or nearby in a family room. Needless to say, the nurse must assess if the mother's presence is a supportive or destructive one. A supportive mother can help to alleviate some of the young patient's stress and thus facilitate recovery.

Friends can be encouraged to send the hospitalized child cards, letters, or drawings. This technique can contribute to the patient's sense of relatedness to home and school. Depending upon the clinical problem, the child becomes a hero to his or her classmates. The last external resource available to the child is the members of the health team, particularly the nurse. As mentioned previously, the nurse becomes a mother substitute, supporting the child through stressful events including intrusive diagnostic or treatment procedures.

The child's age or previous hospital experience may determine internal resources. The older child and adolescent have their own cognitive processes on which to rely for internal strengths. Illness, injury, or disease have thrust the young patient into a world of experience which was not chosen or desired. The clinical problem together with the experience of hospitalization has taught the child things about the self and

---

[28]Janis, *op. cit.*, p. 215.

the ability to adapt to stressful events. For the adolescent it has been a learning experience, in which insight has been gained into one's strength and weakness. Regardless of the child's age, the nurse should assess the patient's internal resources; help the child identify internal strength; and, utilize them in an attempt to minimize the stress experiences and increase stress tolerance.

Adult and aged   The adult and aged patient's internal resources are biological and psychological. Depending upon the severity and duration of the patient's illness, injury, or disease, biological resources may or may not be bountiful. The adult patient may have a greater host of internal biological defenses available than does the aged patient although the opposite can also be true. Illness or disease involves an internal battle between the pathogen and the diseased organ. In most cases the latter defends itself against the catalyst of disease by an adaptive phenomenon. The aged patient may have a weakened or depleted adaptive-protective membrane. Therefore, a particular system or the entire body succumbs to the stress of illness and disease.

An example is the patient with chronic obstructive pulmonary disease or emphysema. The pulmonary system has attempted to adapt to the stress of continued changes in lung tissue and alterations in pulmonary function. For this patient a simple cold is a nightmare because of the potential consequences; pneumonia and/or the additional loss of pulmonary reserve. The patient fears the ultimate will happen; a tracheostomy, dependency on a volume respirator, extensive hospitalization in an expensive respiratory care unit, and inevitable death. As the biological condition worsens, stress is placed upon other biological systems. The patient develops *cor pulmonale* or right sided ventricular failure due to pulmonary hypertension. This may even lead to hepatocongestion. Eventually, the status worsens, every breath becomes a struggle to the point where the patient refuses to eat. In this one example, the pulmonary system tried first to adapt to the biological stress and when it failed to do so, other biological systems were called into action. Eventually healthy organs become weakened due to the continued role they play in adapting to a biological crisis, resulting in decompensation.

Selye has identified three phases in the course of decompensation under excessive stress. "First there is alarm and mobilization, representing a general call to arms of the individual's bodily defenses. Secondly the stage of resistance in which the defensive resources of the body may hold their own against the invading virus or other stress. Lastly there exists the stage of exhaustion and decompensation, in which bodily resources are depleted and the organism can no longer cope with the stress, so that further exposure leads to disintegration and death."[29]

[29]Coleman, *op. cit.*, p. 173.

Stress also has its effect upon the adult and aged patient's psychological reserve. The patient's psychological adaptation to stress can take its toll in different ways. "Under severe stress there is a lowering of adaptive efficiency—a narrowing of the perceptual field and an increased rigidity of cognitive processes so that it becomes difficult for the individual to evaulate the situation or perceive more effective coping responses than the ones he is using."[30] The patient realizes that he or she has adapted to stressful events in the past and therefore, can accomplish the same or similar goals in the future. The patient is then motivated by internal goals, desires, values, and ideas. As a result of stressful events, patients gain confidence in themselves and develop new potentials. In other words, they have confronted a stressful situation and adapted to it.

External resources, as with the child, consist of the patient's family, friends, and members of the health team. The adult patient's family resources may be more or less extensive than those of the aged individual. The latter may have outlived his or her own family. The young adult patient's external family resources consist of a spouse, parents, siblings, and/or children. Each can offer the support necessary to survive the stressful event. The nurse must assess the significance of the family's resources. In other words, the patient's wife may have limited abilities of her own for adapting to a crisis. Therefore, if her reserve becomes depleted, the nurse has two people in need of supportive input. Like the patient, the spouse may demonstrate behavioral responses indicative of reduced stress tolerance. For example, a wife may become angry when her husband's dinner tray arrives without milk. This is a seemingly insignificant omission to the nurse; however, to the wife it becomes an outlet for her own accumulated stresses and anxieties.

Friends become another significant external resource to the patient. This is especially true for the aged patient. If the family support systems are diminished or absent, there is reliance upon friends. Friends should be encouraged to visit the older patient when feasible. They become one of the last contacts with the nonhospital community. They keep the patient informed about social, church, or business events.

Members of the health team can become a source of external support to the patient but they can also become a source of additional stress. The patient may perceive the staff to be the source of stress. Therefore, the patient may direct anger toward them rather than utilizing them as a source of strength. Likewise, the staff may become upset with the patient thus contributing to the stress. Needless to say, the patient's perception needs to be assessed and clarified so that the patient's recovery will be expedited rather than extended.

[30]*Loc. cit.*

NURSING IMPLICATIONS

Nursing interventions focus on the three phases within the stress framework. These include intervening in assessing the degree and duration of stress; the previous experience with stress; and the resources available to alleviate stress.

Degree-duration

The nurse assesses both the psychological and physiological degree-duration of stress as it pertains to the patient's illness, injury, or disease process. Communication is a major factor in lessening the psychological intensity and duration of stress. For example, communication is of significance for the child between ages four and twelve. Such an intervention helps to prevent lasting emotional disturbances long after the young patient is discharged. It may be of benefit to encourage the young patient's manifestation of stress while still hospitalized. In other words, crying may be a way of communicating with the nurse. While the child is crying, the nurse can encourage the child to communicate why he or she is crying. It is at this time that the young patient may express fears of abandonment, intrusive procedures, or needles and illness.

The child may see the parents departure after visiting hours as punishment for the illness, injury, or disease process, thus feeling abandoned. If these feelings are not shared, the child will experience the stressful feelings of insecurity and separation from loved ones. In addition, the child will further perceive injections or other intrusive procedures as punishment. If the child witnesses intrusive diagnostic procedures or treatments done to a roommate, there are fears the same will happen to him or her. All these fears and anxieties need to be communicated thus minimizing stress. Furthermore, the nurse should point out to the young patient that certain behavioral responses are normal.

The adult and aged patients also need to communicate fears and anxieties since illness or disease may have greater significance to them. Prolonged illness may deplete financial reserve thus creating additional stress, which may be more overwhelming than the illness itself. The illness, injury, or disease may cause the patient to lose a job and/or social status. For example, the male patient may have experienced repeated renal infection to the point where he is now dependent upon a hemodialysis machine. His illness and dependency upon the dialysis machine may also lead to role changes. Now his wife must assume the financial responsibilities of the household. Such role changes associated with financial concerns can represent an additional source of stress. Therefore, the nurse needs to assess the degree of stress experienced by the patient prior to behavioral manifestations. The nurse realizes that illness itself causes stress of varying magnitude. Once the nurse assesses what is believed to be the potential source of stress, it is validated with the patient. As mentioned several times, each individual may have a different definition and perception of what is a stressful event. Talking about stressful events gives the nurse insight into the patient's ability to adapt to stress and formulate alternative plans designed to incorporate the stressful event. In addition, it gives the nurse the opportunity to assess the patient's openness for external resources. There are patients who desire total independence in handling their own problems, including biological ones.

Aged patients have their own unique set of problems. Due to their particular illness or debilitating disease, they may be unable to adequately care for themselves. Normally after discharge from the hospital, the patient returns to the security of familiar territory, usually the home. However, the aged patient may, out of necessity, be discharged into a convalescent home. The time spent in the new surroundings recovering from illness or disability is dependent upon the severity of the clinical problem.

The degree and duration of psychological stress can be reduced by assessing the origin of the patient's stress. If feelings of abandonment and separation anxiety are the sources of stress, longer visiting hours may be encouraged between parent and child. If financial concern is the source of stress, a social worker or financial consultant may talk with the patient. The nurse, then, is able to intervene in a variety of different ways, each dependent upon the source of clinical stress.

Alleviating the degree and duration of physiological stress may be a more difficult task for the nurse. Physiological stress as a result of illness, injury, or disease cannot be completely alleviated. In this area, the nurse again assesses the intensity or severity of the physiological problem. The nurse's interventions are designed to help the patient reestablish a physiological balance or stability. The nurse supports the patient through stressful diagnostic tests. Part of the supportive care is to explain the purpose of each test. The patient and the family have a right to know the results of each test beyond the simplistic statement that, "your BUN is slightly elevated." If the patient doesn't understand the meaning of BUN, he or she fails to relate it to a renal function or dysfunction. The nurse also intervenes to teach the patient about a diet, medications, and discharge activities. In this respect the nurse helps to lessen the stress associated with transition from hospital to home. The patient is given a set of realistic guidelines which will hopefully facilitate recovery.

Previous Experience

The patient's previous experience with illness and hospitalization contributes to stress tolerance and perception of stress. The small child's previous experience with the hospital environment, physical illness, and immobilization may be limited. How the child adapts and perceives the new environment will determine the ability to tolerate stress. If the child is afraid of what is seen and what happens to the body, the stress tolerance will be greatly reduced. The child whose life consists of frequent trips to the hospital is familiar with hospital routines. This child knows what is expected of him or her and what to expect from members of the health team. Although the child knows the system in limited capacity, he or she never completely overcomes fears of bodily mutilation through potential surgery or intrusive procedures. In this instance the mere mention of a particular diagnostic procedure will bring a behavioral response of anger or tears from the experienced child. This child knows what to anticipate and how to read the nonverbal language exchange between members of the health team.

If stress is inevitable, the nurse tries to raise the young patient's level of stress tolerance. The nurse intervenes to provide supportive assistance with each diagnostic procedure. If the child is ambulatory, the nurse may treat the patient to a special event such as a walk outside the hospital. This can be done prior to an intrusive procedure such as an IV. During their private time together, the two can talk about the procedure and its implications. Of course such an intervention may not be possible with very young children because of their limited cognitive ability. However, with older children, the intervention is most effective. Together the small patient and nurse set the stage for the procedure. This highly personalized approach demonstrates respect for the child as an individual and more importantly, body integrity is respected. Besides increasing stress tolerance, the nurse also enhances a positive perception of the procedures and hospitals in general.

The adult or aged patient is also in need of a supportive system which will raise stress tolerance and foster a positive perception of bodily changes. Unlike children, the adult or aged patients have many responsibilities. They are responsible for their family, children, and job. Illness, injury, or disease threatens the individual's continued performance in fulfilling these responsibilities. Furthermore, a threat to body integrity also becomes a threat to ego strength. Hopefully both are temporary problems. However, once the illness has stabilized there can be residual emotional effects, such as a lowered self-esteem. This can lead the patient to have reduced stress tolerance to further crisis, such as complications.

As with the younger patient, the nurse assesses the patient's previous experience with illness and hospitalization. In doing so, the nurse assesses how each was tolerated by the patient and family. From this, the nurse learns things about the patient's ability to cope with stress and the patient's likes or dislikes. The nurses primary intervention consists of enhancing the patient's ability to tolerate stress and clarify any misperception regarding care and progress.

Resources

The nurse assesses both internal and external resources available to the patient. Internal resources are of physiological and psychological nature. Physiological resources may be absent, limited, or vast. Psychological resources become the patient's internal strength, values, ideas, and goals. Illness, injury, or disease may temporarily interfere with the patient's life's goals or values. The patient must be encouraged to relinquish these goals simply because of the hospitalization and since the goals, values, and ideas may be in conflict with those providing care. Such conflict needs to be assessed and decreased. If ignored it will only serve to increase the stress experienced by the patient. The patient may not agree that the illness or disease warrants immobilization and/or dependency upon others. The patient feels threatened because there no longer is a sense of security within the body. He or she fears that similar physiological crisis will occur again and won't be noticed. Therefore, the nurse needs to facilitate the patient's sense of security in the external world and internal being. As the physiological problem stabilizes, the patient turns attention toward the future.

External resources can help the patient realize a future. The family can become a tremendous supportive system for the patient. Together they can make realistic plans for the present and future. They need to communicate any stresses regarding potential role changes or financial crisis. If there are children involved, they should be encouraged to communicate with the hospitalized parent. This can be accomplished through telephone calls, drawings, letters, or cards. Friends can be encouraged to communicate in a similar manner. If a telephone is not available in the room, one can be plugged into it. Lastly, the nurse becomes an important external resource, assessing the level of stress, intervening to alleviate or minimize stressful events, and evaluating the effects. The nurse realizes that individuals relate better if they are able to express their own threats, fear, and anxieties to others. The nurse accepts their feelings and encourages expression of stress.

In summary, the nurse assesses the child, adult, or aged patient's stress according to the stress framework. The nurse realizes that illness together with hospitalization constitutes stress for the patient. In assessing the level of stress, the nurse takes into consideration the degree-duration of stress, the previous experience with stressful events, and the resources available to the patient which will alleviate stress.

REFERENCES

Birley, J. L., "Stress and Disease," *Journal of Psychosomatic Research,* 16, 1972, pp. 235–40.

Cameron, Cyril, "Anticipated Disease-A New Concept," *Canad. Med. Assoc. Journal,* 99, August 17, 1968.

Crate, Marjorie, "Nursing Functions in Adaptation to Chronic Illness," *American Journal of Nursing,* October 1965.

Davidhizar, Ruth, "Stress Patient: A New Dimension In Psychiatric Nursing Education," *British Journal Clinical Psychology,* 12, 1973, pp. 130–36.

Dohrenwend, Barbara and Bruce, *Stressful Life Events: Their Nature and Effects,* New York: Wiley, 1974.

Eliot, Robert, *Stress and the Heart,* New York: Futura Publishing Company, 1974.

Foster, Sue, "Behavior Following Acute Myocardial Infarction," *American Journal of Nursing,* November 1970, pp. 2344–48.

Hoffer, Willie, "Notes on the Theory of Defense," *Psychoanalytic Study of the Child,* 23, 1968, pp. 178–88.

Kackett, Thomas, "The Coronary Care Unit: An Appraisal of Its Psychological Hazards," *The New England Journal of Medicine,* 279 December 19, 1968, pp. 1365–70.

Lee, Douglas, "The Role of Attitude in Response to Environmental Stress," *Journal of Social Issues,* 22, 1966, pp. 83–91.

Levine, Seymour, "Stress and Behavior," *Scientific American,* 224, January 1971, pp. 26–31.

Mechanic, David, "Stress, Illness Behavior, and the Sick Role," *American Sociological Review,* pp. 51–58.

Menninger, Karl, "Regulatory Devices of the Ego Under Major Stress, *International Journal of Psycho-Analysis,* 35, 1954, pp. 412–20.

Miller, Stuart, "Ego-Autonomy in Sensory Deprivation, Isolation, and Stress," *International Journal of Psycho-Analysis,* 43, 1962, pp. 1–20.

Peplau, Hildegard, "Interpersonal Relations and the Process of Adaptation," *Nursing Science,* October-November 1963, pp. 272–79.

Rahe, Richard, "Social Stress and Illness Onset," *Journal of Psychosomatic Research*, 8, 1964, pp. 35–43.

Robinson, Lisa, "The Crying Patient," *Nursing '72*, pp. 17–20.

Sczekalla, Rita, "Stress Reaction of CCU Patients to Resuscitation Procedures on Other Patients," *Nursing Research*, January-February 1973, pp. 65–9.

Selye, Hans, "The Physiopathology of Stress," *Postgraduate Medicine*, June 1959, pp. 660–7.

Visotsky, Harold and Others, "Coping Behavior Under Extreme Stress," *Archives of General Psychiatry*, 5, November 1961, pp. 423–47.

Volicer, Beverly, "Patient's Perceptions of Stressful Events Associated With Hospitalization," *Nursing Research*, 23, May-June 1974, pp. 235–38.

Volicer, Beverly, "Perceived Stress Levels of Events Associated with the Experience of Hospitalization," *Nursing Research*, 22, November-December 1973, pp. 491–97.

Weiss, Jay, "Psychological Factors in Stress and Disease," *Scientific American*, 226, June 1972, pp. 104–13.

Wolf, Stewart, "Life Stress and Patterns of Disease," *Psychological Basis of Medical Practice*, 1963, pp. 109–61.

6
Powerlessness

Power is vital to all living things. Rollo May points out that, "Man in particular, cast on this barren crust of earth aeons ago with hope and the requirement that he survive, finds he must use his powers and confront opposing forces at every point in his struggle with the earth and with his fellows. Insecure as he has been through the ages, buffeted by limitations and weakness, laid low by illness and ultimately by death, he nevertheless asserts his powers in creativity."[1]

Modern human beings are essentially alone. Put on their own feet, they are expected to stand by themselves. They can achieve a sense of identity only by developing a unique and particular self to a point where one can truly sense "I and I." This accomplishment is possible only if one develops active powers to such an extent that one can relate to the world without having to draw on it, if one can achieve a productive orientation. An alienated person, however, tries to solve the problem in a different way: by conforming, feeling secure in being as similar as possible to a fellow person. The paramount aim is to be approved of by others; the central fear is disapproval.[2]

Rogers has stated that the basis for incorporating an event into the self may be the person's awareness of a feeling of control over some aspect of the world experience. An individual who has power over objects and persons may make them part of a self-picture. An extension of the self to include objects and persons is accompanied by a feeling of increased self-potency.[3] According to Maslow, "The authentic healthy person may be defined not in his own right, not in his autonomy, not by his own intra-psychic and nonenvironmental law, not as different from

---

[1]Rollo May, *Power and Innocence*, (New York: Norton, 1972), p. 19.

[2]Erich Fromm, *The Sane Society*, (New York: Holt, Rinehart and Winston, 1967), p. 175. Copyright © 1955 by Erich Fromm. Reprinted by permission.

[3]C. R. Rogers, "A Comprehensive Theory of Personality and Behavior," unpublished paper, 1948, cited in David Krech, *Individual in Society*, (New York: McGraw-Hill, 1962), pp. 96–97.

the environment, independent of it or opposed to it, but rather in environment-centered terms, e.g., of ability to master the environment, to be capable, adequate, effective, competent in relation to it, to do a good job, to perceive it well, to be in good relations, to be successful in its terms."[4] Rollo May believes, "Power pushes toward its fulfillment. It is neither good nor evil, ethically speaking: it only is. But it is not neutral. It requires in some way its own expression, although the forms of this expression vary greatly."[5]

Since a generalized expectancy of low personal control is thought to represent a more or less permanent personality trait in adults, it is obvious that one cannot easily or rapidly reduce a high degree of powerlessness. According to Johnson, comparatively little empirical work has been done on the sources of powerlessness, although a link has been established between social structure and alienation.[6] We will examine some of the possible causes of powerlessness, possible behavioral manifestations by patients as they experience powerlessness, and possible ways that the nurse might foster a feeling of powerfulness in various clinical settings. Before discussing the etiology of power and powerlessness, we will define powerlessness and other synonymous concepts.

POWER, POWERLESSNESS, AND
RELATED TERMS DEFINED

Rollo May through his contributions gave new insights to the power concept. In 1959 Seeman pointed out that the term alienation, a pervasive theme in classical sociological theory, appears in a number of ways in the literature. His analysis led him to present research definitions for five basic variants: (1) powerlessness, (2) meaninglessness, (3) normlessness, (4) value isolation, and (5) self-estrangement.[7] We will first define power and then alienation, powerlessness, and meaninglessness. Only the first two terms will be applied in this presentation.

Power

Ancient Greek philosophers defined power as being—that is, there is no being without power. Originally power was a sociological term;

---

[4]Abraham Maslow, *Toward a Psychology of Being,* (New York: Van Nostrand, 1968), p. 168.

[5]May, *op. cit.,* p. 122.

[6]Dorothy Johnson, "Powerlessness: A Significant Determinant in Patient Behavior," *Journal of Nursing Education,* April 1967, p. 42.

[7]*Ibid.,* p. 39, citing Melvin Seeman.

however, people realized that power depends upon emotions, feelings, and motives. Therefore, psychologists began to look more closely at the power concept. "In psychology, power means the ability to affect, to influence, and to change other persons. Each person exists in an interpersonal web, analogous to magnetic fields of force; and each one propels, repels, connects, identifies with others. Thus such considerations as status, authority, and prestige are central to the problem of power."[8]

Alienation

In the last century, Hegel and Marx used the word alienation to refer not to a state of insanity but to a less drastic form of self-estrangement, one that permits a person to act reasonably in practical matters, even though one is marked by one of the most severe socially patterned defects. Marx called alienation the condition of a person in which one's own act becomes an alien power, standing over and against the person, instead of being ruled by that person.[9] Fromm defines alienation as a "mode of experience in which the person experiences himself as an alien. He has become, one might say, estranged from himself. He does not experience himself as the center of his world, as the creation of his own acts—but his acts and their consequences have become his masters whom he obeys."[10] According to Goffman, "the alienated person is out of touch with himself as he is out of touch with any other person. He, like the others, experiences himself as things are experienced, with the senses and with common sense, but he is not related to himself nor to the world outside in a productive manner."[11]

The patient, as an alienated person, feels inferior whenever one suspects himself of not being in line. Since the sense of worth is based on approval as the reward for conformity, one feels naturally threatened in the sense of self and in one's self-esteem by any feeling, thought, or action that one could suspect of being a deviation. The alienated person or patient experiences himself as a thing, an investment, to be manipulated by himself and by others. He or she lacks a sense of self.[12] In this respect, we as humans do not experience ourselves as the active bearers of our own powers and richness, but as an impoverished "thing" dependent on powers outside of ourselves. As Dean has stated, "it may very well be that alienation is not a unitary phenomenon, but a syndrome."[13]

[8]May, *op. cit.*, p. 100.

[9]Fromm, *op. cit.*, pp. 111–12.

[10]*Ibid.*, p. 111.

[11]*Loc. cit.*

[12]*Ibid.*, p. 181.

[13]Dwight Dean, "Alienation: Its Meaning and Measurement," *American Sociological Review*, 26, October 1961, p. 758.

Meaninglessness

According to Seeman, one type of alienation involves the individual's sense of understanding the events in which he or she is engaged. He speaks of high alienation, in the meaninglessness, when the individual is unclear as to what one ought to believe—when the individual's minimal standards for clarity in decision making are not met. The individual cannot predict with confidence the consequences of acting on a given belief.[14]

Powerlessness

Seeman defines powerlessness as the expectancy or the probability held by the individual that his own behavior cannot determine the outcome or reinforcements he seeks.[15] The use of powerlessness as an expectancy is very closely related to the notion of internal versus external control of reinforcements. The latter idea refers to the individual's sense of personal control over the reinforcement situation, as constrasted with the view that the occurrence of reinforcements depends upon external conditions, such as chance, luck, or the manipulation of others.[16] Therefore, powerlessness is a perceived lack of personal or internal control of certain events in certain situations.[17] According to Johnson, powerlessness focuses on the social, psychological aspects of individual personality variables. But in the context of the definition, that is, alienated man in mass society, the term clearly indicates a perceived relationship between the structural feature of social life in modern society and particular aspects of individual psychological structure and functioning.[18]

Johnson further believes that, "powerlessness is equated with the perceived external control of events in the learning variable, expectancy. Operating as this learning variable, it could be expected to influence learning, either in the sense of the acquisition of knowledge or of developing effective, goal-directed behavior. The direction of this influence would be negative since knowledge or goal-directed behavior is simply irrelevant or unnecessary when the individual does not perceive that future events can be controlled by his own actions."[19]

[14]Melvin Seeman, "On the Meaning of Alienation," *American Sociological Review*, 24, December 1959, p. 786.

[15]*Ibid.*, pp. 783–91.

[16]*Ibid.*, p. 785.

[17]Johnson, *op. cit.*, p. 40.

[18]*Ibid.*, p. 39.

[19]*Ibid.*, p. 40.

Each individual, whether well or ill, has a desire for power. This desire is described as *power want*. Krech defines power want as the desire to control other persons or objects, to obtain their obedience, to compel their action, to determine their fate. The concept has enormous significance for the working of a society. Power want may have its origin in self-defense and self-enhancement. The objects that someone incorporates into an extended self are, according to several authors, objects within the control, or power, of that person.[20]

As mentioned previously, everyone wants to maintain an element of power and control over one's being and environment. When illness forces the individual, regardless of age, to relinquish that control to a stranger, one may feel an overwhelming sense of powerlessness. It is safe to state that the more acute the situation or the patient's illness, the less power the patient feels he or she has. Therefore, it is essential to discuss some of the causes of powerlessness in various clinical settings. The concepts alienation and powerlessness will be used interchangeably.

CAUSES OF POWERLESSNESS IN CLINICAL SETTINGS

It is an obligation of the sick person to do everything to get well as soon as possible. On the other hand, the patient is encouraged by the hospital environment to be passive. When a person becomes a hospital patient, others do things to and for that person whether warranted or not. The patient finds a lack of participation, a loss of usual control over his or her environment.

There are essentially two potential causes of powerlessness: loss of control and lack of knowledge. Loss of control implies loss over oneself, one's behavior, and one's environment. Lack of knowledge refers to insufficient knowledge regarding one's illness and the implications it has over one's being, one's family, and one's future.

Loss of Control

Loss of control implies loss of power. Loss of control can be broken down into three large categories and one overall integrating category. The large categories consist of the contributing factors within the psychological, physical, and environmental being of the individual that represent loss of control. The integrating category synthesizes what occurs within the psychological-physical and environmental categories and indicates

[20]Krech, Crutchfield, and Ballachey, *Individual in Society*, pp. 96–97.

how the patient behaviorally manifests loss of control or power. This category contains mechanisms for coping with powerlessness.

   Psychological loss of control   Psychologically Rollo May[21] sees power existing on five different levels. The first level is power to be. This power is seen in the newborn infant who can cry and violently wave the arms as signs of the discomfort within, demanding that hunger or other needs to be met. If these needs are not quickly met, the cries or movements become even more captivating by those attempting to meet these needs. Mothering figures, including nurses, are well aware of the power of control exerted by a crying infant or small child. Such behavior is central to the development of the child even during hospitalization. "Whether we like it or not, power is central in the development in this infant of what we call personality. Every infant becomes an adult in ways that reflect the vicissitudes of power—that is, how he has been able to find his power and use it—indeed, how to be it. It is given in the act of birth, not by the culture as such but by the sheer fact that the infant lives. If the infant is denied the experience that his actions can get a response from those around him—the infant withdraws into a corner of his bed, does not talk or develop in other ways, and literally withers away physiologically and psychologically."[22] The infant's cry or the small child's demand becomes the power to be. Illness coupled with temporary loss of significant others threatens the child's self-esteem. The child may have no other coping resources besides crying or withdrawal-demanding behavior. The nurse understands the comfort a child needs to have and gives the necessary attention. The nurse realizes that, "the power to be is neither good nor evil; it is prior to them. But it is not neutral. It must be lived out or neurosis, psychosis, or violence will result."[23]

   The nurse acknowledges the child's need to develop potentialities. This is particularly significant for infants and small children who are hospitalized frequently or for long periods of time. In either instance, the child feels a loss of psychological control. The child matures potentialities into power to be as he or she talks, crawls, walks, or runs. "The potentiality to explore, to see the world as a person of his age can, will increasingly become an actual power as his neuromuscular structure develops. Everyone who has observed his own development with wonder will be aware that there is both nature and nurture in every step of this actualization of his potentialities."[24]

   The ability to physically explore may be unrealistic for some children

[21]May, *op. cit.*, p. 40.
[22]*Ibid.*, p. 40.
[23]Loc. cit.
[24]*Ibid.*, pp. 121–122.

with multiple fractures, leukemia, or some other equally debilitating illness. The latter two illnesses may keep the child confined to an immediate environment. The child with fractures can at least have the bed moved to the dayroom or nurse's station. The child who is unable to even visually explore the environment may have difficulty with its mastery. The power to be causes the child to experience two developmental or mastery needs. There exists the nutrient side which represents a need to be cared for and loved. On the other hand, there exists the aggressive side which is the need to be assertive, to protest if the situation demands it. Hospitalization has a tendency to create aggressive behavior especially if the child feels that the power to be is threatened.

The adolescent or young adult patient is confronted with the struggle between power and powerlessness. Possibly this is why so many young people experiment with harmful drugs. According to Rollo May, "Drug addiction is another possible effect of powerlessness. The conviction of powerlessness is especially profound with young people, and this is also where drug addiction is most prevalent. Their addiction is a form of violence, first of all, in that the individual violates his own mind—which, indeed, is the purpose of the drug; and there follows later all the petty crime and greater crime that drug addicts get into."[25] The young addict's behavior reflects both weakness and blocked anger. Weakness takes the form of worthlessness, "I can't pass the exam," "I can't get a job," or "My family doesn't care what happens." The anger takes the form of revenge upon the family and the world, becoming the individual's reaction to powerlessness.

The infant, child, or adolescent's capacity to cope with necessities becomes, in the adult, the struggle for self-esteem and for a feeling of worthiness as a human being. This becomes the second level of power: self-affirmation. The individual needs to maintain control over who one is. "Every being has the need not only to be but to affirm his own being. This is especially significant for the human organism, for it is gifted with, or condemned to, self-consciousness."[26]

The adult patient's need for self-affirmation is diminished the moment that patient arrives in the hospital. The patient may be admitted into the hospital system in one of two ways: through the emergency room or directly to a general floor or critical care unit. Those individuals admitted into the emergency room may not have their own personal physician. The physician on call becomes their personal or temporary physician. The patient is powerless over who becomes his or her doctor. Most patients quietly accept the doctor, realizing that they need someone to carry them through the critical stages of the illness. Once successfully through

[25]*Ibid.*, p. 32.
[26]*Ibid.*, p. 41.

the crisis stages, such a patient may feel free to choose another physician. Initially, however, the choice of both doctor and nurse is made by someone else. The patient must quickly submit to these strangers and let them worry about the physical being. The patient may be in such a state of psychological shock that there is a failure to realize the severity of the illness. The feeling of powerlessness, "that is connected with putting oneself in the hands of a doctor or nurse is reinforced when the patient cannot find out what his real worries are. It is not a simple matter to consent psychologically to manipulation or partial destruction of one's own body yet integrate the event as one experience in life among many from which something valuable has been learned."[27]

During the admission and history-taking processes, hospital personnel elicit personal information from the patient, who is again powerless to influence the type of information recorded. This process becomes a "violation of one's informational preserve regarding self. During admission, facts about the patient's social status, history and past behavior are collected and recorded."[28] The patient realizes that to get well, the personal and sometimes tedious questions must be answered. Refusal to answer questions may induce fear that the patient will not receive adequate therapeutic care.

Outside the hospital, the patient could hold objects of self-feeling such as the body, immediate action, thoughts, and some possessions, out of contact with alien and contaminating things. In the hospital, however, the patient soon discovers that hospital circumstances violate the territories of self, invade the boundary placed between the being and the environment, and profane the embodiment of self.[29] The patient has relatively little power over what goes into his or her chart and who reads it. Once in the chart rack, it becomes open territory for one and all. Needless to say, it is understandable that patients begin to feel transparent. Everyone seems to know what is going on with the individual, but the patient may be the least informed as to what is happening. The adult or aged individual questions self esteem and the loss of control over it.

As the patient moves deeper into the admitting web, one may discover that the nursing staff has removed some personal belongings, such as money, valuables, jewelry, or important papers. Personal objects symbolically are a reflection of one's self. More importantly, they represent an identity and provide a sense of recognition. Nurses must realize that with adults or older patients, "the cry for recognition becomes the central cry in the need for self-affirmation. If significance and recognition

---

[27]Hildegard Peplau, *Interpersonal Relations in Nursing*, (New York: G. P. Putnam's Sons, 1967), p. 67.

[28]Erving Goffman, *Asylums*, (New York: Doubleday, 1961), p. 24.

[29]*Ibid.*, p. 23.

are granted as a matter of course in the family, the child simply assumes them and turns his attention to other things."[30]

The third level of power is self-assertion. Like self-affirmation, self-assertion applies to the adult and aged patient. Self-assertion is diminished when the patient feels powerless over controlling decision-making processes. The patient relinquishes the normal ability of deciding and choosing what he or she wants or does not want to do. Now someone else, usually a stranger, makes the decisions and choices. The individual soon discovers that daily activities are tightly scheduled and maintained by other people. All phases of the day's activities are tightly scheduled, "with one activity leading, at a prearranged time into the next, the whole sequence of activities being imposed from above by a system of explicit formal rulings and a body of officials."[31]

Patients may feel that their self-assertion is being threatened through loss of decision-making control. When the individual's self-assertion meets resistance, the patient gives power to one's own stance. That stance may be in conflict with those providing care. The patient with renal failure may choose to increase fluid intake as a demonstration of power. The schizophrenic patient may continue to get involved in stressful situations knowing the consequences. Likewise, the aged individual may choose his or her own treatment plan rather than self-affirmation. It becomes more overt and the behavioral response or defense of attack is universal.

When self-assertion is blocked over a period of time, the individual experiences the fourth aspect of power, aggression. The patient who feels unable to influence the people providing care may become aggressive toward them. Such behavior represents this patient's psychological loss of control. Sullivan believes that the feeling of power in one's interpersonal relations with significant others is vital for the maintenance of self-esteem and for the process of maturity. When this feeling of significance is lost, the individual shifts attention to different, or neurotic, forms of power to get some substitute for significance.[32] The substitute for significance becomes aggressive behavior. This behavior is reinforced if the sense of independence and control falls to other people: a nurse, a doctor, or the family. As a result, a patient may experience anger for having other people, including strangers, assume his or her responsibilities. The patient should be permitted to express aggressive feelings or anger on a verbal level. When such expression is denied, the patient can become violent. Violence becomes the final level on which powerlessness can be perceived.

[30]May, *op. cit.*, p. 41.
[31]Goffman, *op. cit.*, p. 6.
[32]May, *op. cit.*, pp. 35–36.

If the individual is blocked from expression on a verbal level, that individual turns to a physical level of acting out. The physical level may be expressed by hitting or grabbing the nurse, removing various supportive devices, throwing an object, or pulling wires or tubes. The individual may not realize the seriousness of these actions until after it has been done. Acting out or violent behavior is seen most often in the psychiatric setting. It must be remembered that a common characteristic of schizophrenic patients is their feeling of powerlessness.

Powerlessness exists with a constant feeling of anxiety. The patient feels insignificant as a person. It is only through acting out behavior that the patient gains attention and thus a feeling of transitory significance. Nurses working with the more violent schizophrenic patients should understand the meaning of their behavior. "It is important to see that the violence is the end result of repressed anger and rage, combined with constant fear based on the patient's powerlessness. Behind the pseudo-power of the madness we can often find a person struggling for some sense of significance, some way of making a difference and establishing some self-esteem."[33] Psychological feelings of powerlessness are caused by loss of control over admission procedures, the choice of doctor, decision-making ability, schedules, and routines.

Physiological loss of control   Physiological loss of control may not necessarily begin when the individual develops an illness. O'Connor points out that, "Early attitudes toward sickness are important factors in the development of abnormal psychologic reactions associated with injury. The child who discovers at an early age that genuine illness evokes special kindness and attention from the mother may learn to enjoy the role of patient. In some individuals this may predispose to the development of conversion or functional illness for which an organic cause cannot be found."[34] Many adult patients experience physiological loss of control with the onset of illness.

Prior to illness, the patient had what was viewed as power over the body. He or she told the body what to do, where to go, and how to perform. The patient could run, climb, skip, or walk, having control and power over mobility through space and time. The patient may have been the type of individual who took pride in physical accomplishments. However, illness changes the structure of control. The child, adult, or aged patient's physical being is in control.

It is during the initial powerlessness episode that the patient may feel the loss of part of the body. In illness, "It is the fear of loss of the whole

[33]*Ibid.*, p. 26.

[34]Garrett O'Connor, "Psychiatric Changes in the Acutely Injured," *Postgraduate Medicine*, 48, September 1970, p. 210.

or a part of the body that appears to be the focus of psychological concern. While the anxiety is conscious, the idea of loss may not be conscious at all, such an idea may be so grave a threat to the ego that the whole matter is repressed."[35] The patient, regardless of age, may not understand what caused the body to become ill. Physiological loss of control may lead to anxieties over threatened physical integrity. According to Smith, it seems likely that every illness contains some degree of threat to body integrity. Acute illness arouses a fear of loss of function, a loss of ability to understand daily routines, or the sudden awareness of loss of control over one's own physical activities.[36]

Physical illness may totally control the patient's consciousness and render one powerless to do or think anything else. Illness, by its very nature, "tends to preoccupy its victim. Discomfort of pain in the body results in a withdrawal of whatever psychic investments one has made in the outside world."[37] With illness the patient relinquishes physical and psychological control over the body. The adult or aged patient may, on an unconscious level, feel a relinquishing of ego control, which becomes synonymous with relinquishing life. In other words, to give up a type of ownership of the body in illness or injury is to give up the claim to life itself. Therefore, illness or injury causes the patient to physiologically feel loss of control or a sense of powerlessness. It is the powerlessness over the body that brings the patient to the hospital, where a chain of events occur that may further render one environmentally powerless.

Environmental loss of control   Besides psychological and physiological loss of control, the patient also experiences environmental loss of control. Environmental loss of control may be the most threatening to children. A child's environment is not nearly as expansive as that of the adult or aged individual. The child's primary environmental unit is home and more specifically the child's room or bed. Hospitalization removes the child from the familiar and places that child in an unfamiliar setting. To compensate for the loss, the child may bring to the hospital favorite toys, blanket, pillow, games, or stuffed animals. If the personal objects that represent the self and home identity do not lessen the loss, the child may resort to magical powers. Magical powers take the form of fantasies and are not limited to children. They may also be utilized by the schizophrenic patient. Regardless of the situation, the person through fantasies shapes events with the environment by willing them to be. Fortunately, most children's need to lessen environmental loss of control is accomplished with personal objects from home, including the parents.

[35]Sydney Smith, "The Psychology of Illness," *Nursing Forum*, 3, 1964, p. 36.
[36]*Ibid.*, p. 36–37.
[37]*Ibid.*, p. 38.

Most adults choose where they want to live. They take many things into consideration before making the ultimate decision. In a hospital, this is not the case. Environmentally, the patient experiences powerlessness the moment one arrives in the hospital "home." The powerlessness is demonstrated by the patient's inability to explore and choose where one wants to go within the hospital. The patient may not have a choice in terms of the floor; however, once there, the patient should have a voice in choosing a roommate. Many times incompatable patients are placed together. Depending upon the physical problem, the patient's wish may be acknowledged.

The patient may feel powerless within the personal territory. The territory around the patient's bed may be filled with environmental props such as a nightstand, curtain, bedside table, chair, sink, or call light. Other hospital environmental props within the immediate territory may include an IV pole, a Foley bag, chest tubes, a CVP manometer, an oxygen unit, an IPPB, or cardioscope. The patient may desire to have his or her personal environmental props such as watch, glasses, cards, flowers, toys, book, toilet articles, or tissues on the nightstand. Unfortunately the bedside table becomes a place for the nurse to put props, dressings, suction catheters, and bottles.

Behavioral responses   Ideally, whatever emotional changes occur in the patient should be transient and reversible; unfortunately, this is not always the case. The patient is particularly vulnerable from the psychological point of view. Denied the ability to function in a self-help capacity, the patient must accept a position of enforced passivity and reluctant dependency. Most often those responsible for care are strangers, yet the patient must place hopes for survival in their hands. Finding himself in strange surroundings and plagued with various worries about the future, the patient is prone to psychological complications.[38]

As the patient reaches a limit of physical, psychological, and environmental loss of control, he or she may experience the frustration of powerlessness. The patient was powerless to choose a doctor, a location in the hospital, how props will be organized around the bed, what diagnostic work and treatments will be done, or how the days tightly scheduled routine will be accomplished. The individual may be frustrated, "as a consequence of the discrepancy between the control he may expect and the degree of control that he desires—that is, it takes no direct account of the value of control to the person."[39] A patient's experience in the hospital is controlled by other people; the patient becomes another person's experience. This may eventually become alarming to the patient.

[38]O'Connor, *op. cit.,* p. 200.
[39]Seeman, *op. cit.,* p. 784.

As Fromm said, "the sense of self stems from the experience of myself as the subject of my experience, my thought, my feeling, my decision, my judgment, my actions. It presupposes that my experience is my own, and not an alienated one. Things have no self and men who have become things have no self."[40] The patient, regardless of age or clinical problem, must relinquish the "my" aspect.

Physical illness and the resulting immobility creates an emotional intolerance that may complicate the patient's recovery. The patient may no longer be able to tolerate not having choices or decision-making responsibilities. The patient no longer has the power to guide and direct daily activities. It is no wonder that the patient may have nothing to do but, "concentrate upon his own misery to the exclusion of whatever is happening around him. Most illness and its accompanying pain are likely to be transitory, but for the period of time an illness dominates its victim's consciousness, there is a shift of psychic energies to the self that results in an enlarged egocentricity."[41]

As the patient reaches the intolerance of powerlessness, he or she may exhibit a temporary behavioral response. Patients can express themselves in a variety of ways such as anger, hostility, withdrawal, or depression. When the patient reaches an intolerance of powerlessness, that patient may not be able to recognize that people in the environment are concerned with his or her well-being and restoration of power.

Lack of Knowledge

Just as loss of control creates feelings of alienation and powerlessness, lack of knowledge can have same or similar effects. We keep the child, adult, or aged patient powerless if we do not provide knowledge about what is happening within and around the patient. This is quite unintentional on the part of the nurse or physician. The clinical situation may dictate actions that do not necessarily include exploration and teaching. Such input has low priority. Hopefully, it will be only postponed until a more opportune time.

Many children or adult patients have never been ill, nor have they experienced the powerlessness of illness. Therefore, they feel frightened when placed in the hospital in one of its specialized areas; pediatrics, psychiatry, or critical care. If the patient does not understand what is happening, that patient may choose to deny the seriousness of the entire event. As discussed earlier, children or schizophrenic patients may temporarily turn to a world of fantasies if their world of reality is threatening

[40]Fromm, *op. cit.*, p. 130.
[41]Smith, *op. cit.*, p. 38.

or meaningless. The fantasies give them temporary control of the situation until such time as other coping mechanisms can be identified and successfully executed. Denial is common to many patients, whereby their illness and/or environment has no meaning. The patient can understand nothing except the fact that he or she is ill, anxious, or separated from significant others. Therefore, some knowledge input is imperative and it need take only a few minutes or seconds to begin the process.

It is natural that the patient, who has answered questions about a previous illness and/or current symptoms, may want some simple explanations in return, excluding the usual medical technology or professional jargon. If the patient receives only highly technical explanations of a current illness, that patient will still be without knowledge. The patient does not understand the complicated language that may have become second nature to the medical-nursing team. Not wanting to look stupid before the staff, the patient may fail to seek further explanations of professional jargon. Therefore, the patient remains essentially less informed and more confused or frightened.

The health team may believe the child to be incapable of understanding physical problems or treatments, and may withhold information. As with the adult, the child remains ignorant. According to Smith, when one leaves the patient in ignorance about what is going to happen, one provides a fertile field for the activation of fantasy. All kinds of distortions, many of a fearful nature, may creep into the patient's thinking.[42]

A patient's sense of powerlessness or lack of personal control influences the learning about his or her illness; the higher the level of alienation, the less the learning. Seeman pointed out that greater alienation accompanies limited knowledge, for in an important sense, knowledge acquisition is irrevelant to those who believe that fate, chance, luck, or external forces control what happens.[43]

The patient seeks knowledge about illness as it relates to care, treatments, family, and future prognosis. The child who is to experience an invasive diagnostic study or treatment needs a meaningful explanation. Likewise, the adult or aged patient who is to receive an AV shunt or permanent pacemaker implant, a chest tube insertion, peritoneal dialysis infusion, or skin grafts obviously needs explanations and time to assimilate the explanations adequately. Even the simplest of procedures should be explained, since "what the health team views as simple may be complex to the child, adult, or aged individual. If the patient's, "emotions are properly dealt with . . . that is, if in preparation for a treatment he is given some understanding of, and help in coping with his feelings

---

[42]*Ibid.*, p. 37.

[43]Melvin Seeman, "Alienation and Learning in a Hospital Setting," *American Sociological Reivew*, 6, December 1962, p. 773.

. . . much can be done to reduce the emotional complications of illness."[44] Each time the nurse performs a treatment, its significance should be explained so that the patient sees meaning in the actions. The patient may see members of the health team as taking knowledge from his or her biological systems, but relatively little information is being put back into it. If patients are able to derive meaning from their nurse's actions, then they can realize that these interventions are purposeful or goal-directed.

A patient who lacks knowledge about an illness may not realize how it will affect a role in the family. The patient may not realize that a role shift or alternation may be necessary. The family may be informed, but often the patient is not. This is not intentional on the part of nurses or physicians; they, with the family, may believe they are protecting the patient. This is particularly true for the child or adult who has newly diagnosed terminal illness. The family or health team does not realize that the patient may be fantasizing various unrealistic complications and limitations. In such clinical situations, the patient experiences intellectual powerlessness. The adult patient may need to know how much the family knows and what the prognosis will be so that patient can make both short and long term plans, primarily financial ones.

When the nurse, in any clinical setting, provides the patient with knowledge, the nurse is actually facilitating progress through the stages of illness. One must remember that there are times when the nurse must be sensitive to the degree, type, and readiness of the patient for knowledge. If the patient has knowledge about oneself, the patient is able to ask the physician or nurse additional questions that will further expand this knowledge. The end result of this process is a reestablishment of the patient's intellectual power.

ENCOURAGEMENT OF POWERFULNESS

The patient's experience with nursing care may discourage one from taking any initiative in one's own care or progress. The patient's contacts with nurses may have been nurse-active, patient-passive, nurse-guided, or patient-obedient. In certain clinical settings, the nurse may unintentionally carry activities beyond the necessary point. The nurse may do things for the patient when he or she is quite capable of doing them, with guidance, for themselves. As the patient's physiological or psychological problem stabilizes, the nurse returns the power. Nurses accomplish this

[44]Smith, *op. cit.*, p. 43.

goal in two basic ways: restoring control to the patient, and reinforcing new knowledge.

Restoration of Control

The nurse may restore psychological, physiological, and environmental control to the child, adult, or aged patient. By restoring control, the nurse may alleviate unnecessary or debilitating behavioral responses.

Psychological control   The nurse's interventions involve restoration of psychological control by encouraging the patient to express feelings, to participate in self-care, and to make choices and decisions. The nurse who permits the patient to express feelings assists that patient in viewing the illness as an experience. In this respect, the individual, regardless of age, feels significant. When one feels significant, one can also experience a sense of power. "Power and the sense of significance are intertwined. One is the objective form and the other the subjective form of the same expression. While power is typically extrovert, significance may not be extrovert at all but may be shown (and achieved) by meditation or other introvert, subjective methods. It is nevertheless experienced by the person as a sense of power in that it helps him integrate himself and subsequently makes him more effective in his relations with others."[45] Given the opportunity to express feelings of frustration, anger, hostility, anxiety, or fear, the patient has a sense of power. He knows that messages will be received by a listening and understanding nurse. The seemingly simplistic intervention of listening gives power through a building up of the patient's own self-affirmation.

Instead of telling the patient to rest and not to talk, the nurse encourages verbal participation. The nurse realizes that by giving patients the opportunity to verbalize concerns, needs, or desires, it restores control and participation in the patient's own care. The nurse further realizes that approaching a patient as a responsible person, having the power to accept or reject care, actually enhances the effectiveness of that care. Furthermore, both patient and health team are satisfied with the result. The nurse should actively listen to her patient's concerns regarding his family, job, finances, and future. Active listening implies that the nurse permits the patient to talk without interruption. The nurse carefully listens for themes in the conversation which can actually be concerns the patient has for the illness and its possible outcome. As the nurse actively listens the patient believes that he or she is a significant person within the hospital setting. The nurse assesses the level on which the patient is able

[45]May, *op. cit.*, p. 35.

to participate. Initially, the patient's participation may be only on a verbal level. Of course, this depends upon the severity and stability of the patient's condition. Once it has been assessed that the patient is able to progress to a more active involvement, this should be encouraged.

The nurse may unintentionally continue in an active role rather than reassess the appropriateness of an intervention. It is essential that the nurse reassess any actions before continuing on an active level. It is easier and faster for the nurse to actively perform than it is for the patient. The patient's illness or injury may have reduced mobility. This does not negate the nurse's encouraging slow participation. Most patients, especially children and older people, need to become involved in directing and planning their own care. The participating patient assumes some responsibility for care in terms of its outcome or effectiveness. As a participant, the patient is able to utilize members of the health team. Furthermore, participation increases the patient's knowledge of the suggested course of therapy and enables him or her to express feelings regarding the care.

As the patient begins to participate in self-care, he or she obtains the power to choose or decide how the nurse should participate. This implies that both participants are sensitive to each other's need. We know that, "if one is to have satisfactory interpersonal relationships, he must be senstive to the feelings and attitude of the people in his environment. The more one distorts, or misperceives the personalities of those around him, the less likely he is to make a good adjustment to his surroundings."[46] Hopefully, both people have gotten to know each other. It is important to involve all patients, especially children. Inclusion can be done on a simple level. For example, the child who has had surgery can, in time, help the nurse with dressing changes. In this respect, the patient actually sees what is under the dressings rather than fantasizing. Furthermore, the child with a cardiac problem may be encouraged to listen to the heart beat.

With children or adults, the nurse must know the patient before assessing one's readiness to assume decision-making responsibilities. If the patient is ready, the nurse begins the process on a lower significant level. For example, the nurse may give a patient power to decide when and how that patient would like certain treatments to be performed. The patient may choose to sleep before an IPPB treatment. If the lungs are clear and blood gases are adequate, the nurse can approve this decision. Of course, this implies that the nurse had already collected the data before giving the patient a choice. Little by little, the patient's decision-making powerfulness is increased.

[46]Anthony Davids, "Alienation, Social Apperception and Ego Structure," *Journal of Consulting Psychology*, 19, 1955, pp. 24–25.

The nurse can foster decision-making powerfulness when allowing the patient to make a choice. Rollo May believes that, "Man becomes a self only as he participates in his development and throws his weight behind this or that tendency, no matter how limited this choice may be. The self never develops automatically; man becomes a self only to the extent that he can know it, affirm it, assert it."[47] The nurse permits the patient to choose which personal environmental props will go in the closet, remain in the luggage, go into the nightstand drawer, or be placed on top of the bedside table. These personal environmental props may be the only daily contact the patient has with home or family. Pictures of animals, children or grandchildren become important to the patient. Furthermore, patients like their cards displayed on their table. This serves to remind them that they are significant to friends.

Instead of collecting the patient's props and placing them "out of the way," the nurse should leave the patient's toys, stuffed animals, games, watch, glasses, pictures, or books within easy reach. The nurse also helps the patient achieve a type of environmental powerfulness by keeping the bedside table within reach. This may seem like an obvious intervention, but it is frequently overlooked. If the patient has received a diuretic and does not have a Foley catheter or bathroom privileges, the nurse should attempt to keep a urinal empty and within reach. The patient who is encouraged to cough should have a tissue within reach. Last, the patient who is told to force fluids needs a full water pitcher close at hand.

Physiological control   As mentioned earlier, a patient sees an illness or injury as a threat to security. The insecurity that results relates to feelings of death. Physiologically, the fear can become a reality. No matter what the precipitating crisis may have been (MI, leukemia, pulmonary edema, third-degree burns, diabetic coma, cystic fibrosis, open heart surgery, overdose, or bilateral nephrectomy), the patient's physiological systems go through adaptive changes in response to the insult. These changes may necessitate temporary disequilibrium and reorganization on the part of certain bodily systems.

It is during such reorganizations or adaptive processes that additional complications can occur. As the nurse carries out an assessment of the patient, he or she will note that the patient's fears are either intensified or reduced. Regardless of what the patient's primary problem was, there are needs for reassurance as to how the physiological systems are regaining control and, hopefully, reaching stability. The nurse can point out to the MI patient, for example, that an EKG pattern shows less S-T elevation or an absence of arrhythmias, or that serum enzymes may be decreasing from their previous high levels. The child or adult patient with

[47]May, *op. cit.*, p. 141.

kidney problems will be reassured upon learning that the kidneys are diuresing and the BUN and/or creatinine levels are decreasing. Of course, the nurse must assess the child's readiness to receive teaching input and evaluate his or her comprehension. This basic principle applies to all patients but particularly to the child. The burn patient feels less insecure when beginning to see a skin graft take control. The pulmonary patient feels hopeful when learning that the blood gases are stable and that he or she is being successfully weaned off the volume respirator.

To point out that the body is regaining control means that the nurse must know the expected physiological changes that accompany an insult. The nurse must be able to differentiate expected responses from the positive changes in a patient's condition. As the positive changes occur, the patient will feel a sense of physiological powerfulness. This feeling can occur only when the physician and nurse inform the patient of the body's daily restoration of control. One must keep in mind, however, that there will be patients whose condition vacillates and may never reach total control.

For example, some patients may not regain normal physiological control as quickly as desired. It may become more difficult for the nurse to identify areas in which power can be returned to such patients. The nurse's most important intervention, in this instance, is to point out to the patient that progress has reached a slow stage of physiological adaptation. A positive factor is that the condition is not regressing. In other words, a physiological plateau is more desirable than physiological regression. In this respect, the nurse maintains what power has previously been given the patient before reaching a plateau.

Environmental control   The nurse can insure environmental powerfulness by seeing that a patient's environment is organized and contains the elements of his or her personality. All too frequently a patient's environment becomes congested or cluttered with various pieces of supportive devices. Such devices should be kept, when possible, to a minimum. In addition it is important that the child, adult, or aged individual maintain communication with members of the health team. Such communication may only be possible by means of a call light or intercomm. The nurse should see that the light is securely fastened in an accessible area of the patient's bed. Frequently, older patients prefer to hold their light or have it pinned to their gown. The call light is an important communication device for the tracheostomy patient. Such a patient may also need a magic slate board near the bed to use as a way of writing notes to the nurse so the patient's needs will be better understood. This gives the patient a feeling of control within the environment.

If the nurse strives to foster psychological, physiological, or environmental powerfulness, he or she may alleviate negative behavioral responses. According to Peplau, "Feelings of crying or anger for the benefit of the nurse may be expressed in order to get attention. If sustained assistance or self-enhancement is not provided in other ways, patients often do use these forms of behavior to express the powerfulness that they feel."[48] Therefore, these feelings can be reduced if the patient can identify with a nurse who helps the patient to feel less threatened and more in control or powerful. As the patient, young or old, is able to identify with the nurse, that patient is ready to learn.

Reinforcement of Learning and Knowledge

When the nurse reinforces or promotes learning, the nurse must assess a patient's readiness to learn. The infant or child may be too young for teaching input. The adult or aged patient may feel anxious about acquisition of new knowledge and may subscribe to the philosophy that, "what you don't know won't hurt you." But lack of knowledge can be harmful to the future of the patient. During the initial crisis, the nurse must take extreme care in talking with the patient. The patient in crisis may be in a highly suggestible condition, and most insignificant remarks by the health team can make a lasting impression on the patient. Therefore, early explanations should be brief and simple.

As the patient progresses in care, he or she will be exposed to certain treatments and procedures. Nurses working with children can develop creative teaching strategies through play therapy, role playing, or games. For example, a doll can become a substitute for the child. On a psychological level the doll can say what the child is feeling. Therefore, the nurse gains knowledge regarding the patient's anxieties. On a physical level, the nurse can simulate various diagnostic or treatment procedures on the doll. A small vial and tubing can represent an IV or small dressing and bandage can represent surgical dressing similar to the child's. The child who is to experience an amputation can remove the altered body part (leg) from the doll. Obviously such a teaching approach must be actively supported on a verbal level by the health team and family.

The nurse should remember that while various procedures and treatments are routine to him or her, they may be new to the patient. Before the nurse decides on the type and extent of explanation required, the patient should have an opportunity to express views on the forthcoming event. The patient's description may be grossly inaccurate, weird, or fanciful, but if communication does not start with recognition of the perception of the situation, the most careful explanation may fail to assure

[48]Peplau, *op. cit.*, p. 31.

the patient.[49] After providing the original explanation, the nurse must evaluate its impact by assessing whether the messages were necessary, internalized, and returned by way of a demonstration. It is at this time that the nurse evaluates the need for reexplanation or clarification.

The nurse may choose to give a patient learning input on a one-to-one basis. The nurse may spend time teaching one day and follow it with a return demonstration. This enables the nurse to see how much the patient actually retains from the original learning session. Furthermore, it gives the patient time to assimilate new knowledge so questions can be asked if necessary. The nurse continues to reiterate certain pertinent points in order to reinforce the patient's learning. Once the patient seems to have a grasp of the illness, and its causes and prognosis, the nurse can bring the family into the teaching input sessions. The nurse may even have the patient teach his or her own family. The nurse may simply be an observer, participating only when specific questions arise from the family. By teaching both the family and patient, the nurse provides them with equal knowledge, knowing that what one forgets, the other might remember. In any respect, knowledge does give the individual a feeling of powerfulness.

Being a patient is an unfamiliar experience. The child, adult, or aged patient takes cues from those around him. When the patient is encouraged to ask questions, to express feelings, and to participate in planning for care, that patient will know what behavior is expected. If one is discouraged from self-expressing and from taking part in care, that patient may well assume that the power role is passive, and will not be able to take responsibility when warranted. The patient can only experience powerfulness as the nurse is able to restore certain controls and reinforce new knowledge.

REFERENCES

Aiken, M, "Organization Alienation: A Comparative Analysis," *Am. Social Review*, 31, 1966, pp. 497–507.

Allardt, E., "Types of Pretest and Alienation," *Alienation and Social System*, (Ed: A. W. Finifler), New York: Wiley, 1972, pp. 289–305.

Bullough, B. L., "Poverty, Ethnic Identity and Preventive Health Care," *Journal of Health and Human Behavior*, 13, 1972, pp. 347–59.

[49]Margaret Aasterud, "Explanation to the Patient," *Social Interaction and Patient Care*, (Ed: Skipper and Leonard), (Philadelphia: Lippincott, 1965), p. 83.

Coleman, J. S., "Loss of Power," *Am. Sociol. Rev.*, 38, 1973, pp. 1–17.

Crawford, T. J., "Relative Deprivation, Powerlessness and Military: The Psychology of Social Protest," *Psychiatry*, 33, 1970, pp. 208–23.

Gamson, W. A., *Power and Discontent*, Illinois: Dorsey, 1968.

Geyer, R. F., "Alienation and General Systems Theory," *Sociol. Neer.*, 10, 1974, pp. 13–41.

Johnson, F., *Alienation: Concept, Term and Meanings*, New York: Seminar, 1973.

Kaufman, A. S., "On Alienation," *Inquiry*, 8, 1965, pp. 141–65.

Lystad, M. H., "Social Alienation: A Review of Current Literature," *Sociol. Quart.*, 13, 1972, pp. 90–113.

Murchland, R., *The Age of Alienation*, New York: Random House, 1971.

Netter, G., "A Measure of Alienation," *Am. Sociol. Rev.*, 22, 1957, pp. 670–77.

Pearlin, L., "Alienation From Work: A Study of Nursing Personnel," *Am. Sociol. Rev.*, 27, 1962, pp. 314–26.

Ransford, H. E., "Isolation, Powerlessness and Violence," *Am. Jour. Sociol.*, 73, 1968, pp. 581–91.

Schacht, R., *Alienation*, New York: Doubleday, 1970.

Seeman, M., "Powerlessness and Knowledge: A Comparative Study of Alienation and Learning," *Sociometry*, 30, 1967, 105–23.

Simpson, M. E., "Social Mobility, Normlessness and Powerlessness in Two Cultural Contexts," *Am. Sociol. Rev.*, 35, 1970, pp. 1002–13.

7
Loss

It is ironic that as we live in an age devoted to youth and life, death, in its various forms, is all around us. Through our advanced nuclear technology, each individual is only minutes away from nuclear death. In addition, our communication system makes us cognizant of senseless bombings, killings, and accidents. Shneidman points out that, "Life has become both more dear and more cheap. And if it can be taken by others, it can also be thrown away by oneself. Senseless killing and the wanton destruction of one's own mind reflect the same debasement of man's basic chain: life itself. In the Western world we are probably more death-oriented today than we have been since the days of the Black Plague in the 14th century."[1]

Man realizes that death is inevitable. It is a phenomenon associated with life itself. What one doesn't know is when or how one's own death will occur. Many individuals intellectualize death as it pertains to another death, not their own. This is because man is basically future oriented, planning the future as if one will live forever. While one is free of illness and the threat of a limited future, such behavior is normal. It does not imply denial. However, as loss moves beyond the boundaries of loss in function or part, death and denial sometimes become fused together. Denial for many individuals is a copying mechanism, one that enables them to guard against threat of death or dying.

Loss involves loss of function, part or whole. It can also take the form of death and dying. The purpose of focusing on loss in any one of its forms is to help those who must cope with their own loss. In addition, it provides help for members of the health team who care for the dying. The goal of the latter is to help the individual attain what Weisman refers to as *significant survival*. This implies achieving a purposeful death. "Significant survival is a quality of life that means much more than simply not to die. Purposeful death also means more than dying; it includes a measure

[1]Edwin Shneidman, "The Enemy," *Psychology Today*, August 1970, p. 37.

of fulfillment, quiescence, resolution, and even traces of personal development."[2]

Many people die each year of terminal illness. A growing awareness of the dying process had led various professional people to identify behavioral stages of the dying process. Even though there is a growing body of literature on the patient's behavioral reaction to the dying process, many agencies fail to utilize the various theories.

DEFINITION OF LOSS AND ITS STAGES

Loss includes both biological and psychological loss. Biological loss includes loss of function, part, and/or whole. Illness necessitating hospitalization causes biological changes ranging from temporary alteration of a system's function to complete removal or loss of that system. Take for example the patient who develops a renal infection. The inflammatory process leads to chronic renal failure and ultimate loss of both kidneys. Similarly such loss can involve the myocardial, pulmonary, endocrine and neurological systems. Losses within these biological systems can cause further impairment of mobility, speech, and/or hearing. Psychosocial losses are equally as significant. They can occur simultaneously with biological loss or as independent problems. Such losses involve loss of employment, family member, or status. Some losses are externally visible whereas others are known only to the individual. Regardless of the degree of loss or its implication, the individual involved can experience grief and mourning.

The component of loss to be defined involves death, dying, grief, and mourning. The latter two are behavioral responses to death and dying, encompassing the overall stages of death and dying.

Components of Loss

For many, the dying process only pertains to the aged and terminally ill. Terminal illness does not only apply to those individuals dying from various forms of cancer. It also applies to noncancerous patients whose biological system progressively deteriorates toward total failure. The dying process is longer for some patients than for others. Nevertheless, "Dying becomes an important, noticeable process insofar as it serves to provide others, as well as the patient, with a way to orient to the future,

---

[2]Avery Weisman, *On Dying and Denying*, (New York: Behavioral Publications, 1972), pp. 33–34.

to organize activities around the expectability of death, to prepare for it. The notion of dying appears to be a distinctly social one, for its central relevance is provided for by the fact that it establishes a way of attending a person."[3]

Just as the dying process makes the individual cognizant of a limited future, it also has the similar effect upon those providing care as well as family members. The dying process seems to serve the function of putting into perspective roles, values, and expectations of each of these involved. Thus, the dying process, as previously mentioned, becomes social. Some family members temporarily abandon their own personal needs and attend to the immediate needs of the dying individual. Likewise, the health team can attend to more than the physical needs of the dying patient. In selected settings in which dying is the anticipated outcome, the staff may be better equipped emotionally to handle its behavior by offering both patient and family the emotional support needed to eventually orient themselves to the expectation of death. Needless to say, this process does not take place immediately but occurs in various stages. The individual at each stage will present certain behaviors. The behavior may range from initial fear and panic to quiet withdrawal. Weisman states that, "Fear of dying is a state of episodic alarm, panic, and turmoil. It is associated with excessive autonomic symptoms, and usually conveys a preemptive conviction that collapse is at hand. When the fear of dying is intense, reality testing abandons the hopeless victim."[4]

Death usually represents finality, the end of one's biological being, while for others it represents a spiritual beginning. At some point in time the patient's fear of dying evolves into fear of death. "Fear of death is not an immediate event, but rather a reflection about man's helplessness. . . . As a rule, fears about death are much stronger than the evidence produced by actual disease and invalidism."[5] Those who remain after the patient has died go through the process of mourning. Those remaining are usually the members of the family and health team. Each has become involved with the dying patient in varying degrees. Similar to the dying process, the mourning process can be painful.

Mourning takes place when those who remain realize the loss of a loved one. According to Bowlby, mourning, "Refers to the psychological processes that follow a loss of a significant or valued object, or that follow the realization that such a loss may occur. These processes usually lead to giving up the lost object."[6]

---

[3]David Sudnow, *Passing On The Social Organization of Dying*, (Englewood Cliffs, N.J.: Prentice-Hall, 1967), p. 68.

[4]Weisman, *op. cit.*, p. 14.

[5]*Ibid.*, p. 15.

[6]John Bowlby, "Processes of Mourning," *International Journal Psychoanalysis*, 42, 1961, pp. 317–40.

Not only does the dying individual mourn a loss whether it is physical, psychological, or social, one also grieves the potential loss, which involves anticipatory grief. "The anticipatory grief of the dying patient is a total response to the realization of future total loss, it is characterized by absolute finality. It is felt before the actual fact of loss and yet may never be experienced since, in a philosophic sense, death presumes the end of all experience."[7] Anticipatory grief implies the internal changes experienced by the significant others who must watch the dying patient. It occurs prior to the actual grief process which occurs when loss is associated with death. Therefore, actual grief occurs after the real loss whereas anticipatory grief is associated with potential loss.

Torpie further states that, "Anticipatory grief must be compared, interpreted, and magnified by the patient's sense of past loss and grief and past premonition of threat of loss. This anticipation, therefore, consists of elements of fantasy which have a realistic basis, but which also may be colored quite unrealistically by weakness, fear, isolation, feelings of inadequacy, and loss of control."[8] Grief, whether it is anticipatory or normal, consists of a culmination of behavioral responses. Some of the behavioral responses are hopelessness, loneliness, powerlessness, depression, anger, hostility, and guilt. The various behavioral responses can be found within the different stages of the grief and mourning process.

Stages of Loss

Engel and Ross have delineated various stages through which the dying patient and remaining significant others progress as they cope with death and dying. Engel's stages involve shock, disbelief, awareness of loss, and restitution. Kubler-Ross, on the other hand, has identified five phases of dying: denial and isolation, anger, bargaining, depression, and acceptance. Therefore, when the nurse assesses a particular behavioral response in a patient, it may represent a particular phase or stage in the grieving process. Yet Lipowski has identified four categories through which an individual may progress. He refers to the four categories as having subjective meaning for symptoms and disability of the patient. They consist of threat, loss, gain (relief), and insignificance. Because the latter categories are unfamiliar to many, they will be explained.

According to Lipowski, "The process of evaluation resulting in meaning begins with the first perception of a pathological process or

---

[7]Richard Torpie, "The Patient and Prolonged Terminal Malignant Disease: Experience From A Radiation Therapy Center," *Anticipatory Grief*, (New York: Columbia University Press, 1974), p. 120.

[8]*Ibid*.

injury and continues unabated throughout the course of illness and its sequelae. . . . The meaning is the core of the person's psychological response to his disease. It is of crucial importance for his emotional and behavioral response."[9]

We will discuss the first category, threat. Threat implies anticipation of an event over which the individual may feel there is no control. If the event leads to personal physical or emotional suffering, it becomes all the more threatening. Anticipation of a threatening event may result from perception of bodily changes that signal potential loss or disability. Again the loss may be loss of physiological function or social status. Loss need not always be associated with dying and death. Even the slightest biological change (toothache) can be threatening with the perceived threat ranging from a simple filling to complete removal of the tooth. Threat then causes anxiety. Anxiety in turn causes behavioral responses designed to avoid, reduce, or work with the anticipated threat. All of which help the patient to eliminate the unpleasant experience of anxiety. The dying patient utilizes defense mechanisms which help him cope with the future.

Loss is the second category. As previously discussed, loss encompasses many facets ranging from simple loss of a fingernail to the more complex loss associated with death and dying. Lipowski says loss, "refers not just to body parts and functions actually lost but also to deprivations of personally significant needs and values. The latter are related chiefly to self-esteem, security, and satisfaction. The emotional response to each anticipated loss, whether concrete or symbolic, takes the form of a grief reaction."[10]

Some patients' loss represents gains. The patient who has sustained a myocardial infarction involving loss of myocardial tissue and temporary loss of social mobility, may have certain unconscious dependency needs fulfilled. In this respect, illness has a secondary gain. Through the illness, the sick individual is able to control others either directly or indirectly. The patient can control family members or staff directly by giving orders and indirectly by inflicting guilt feelings. "On the whole, when subjective gains derived from illness, disability, and so forth, outweigh the losses the patient is likely to cling to his sickness and develop an emotional disturbance when recovery occurs."[11]

The last category is insignificance. The patient who is dying should be permitted to approach death with dignity. Even though the individual has sustained or is in the process of sustaining a biopsychosocial loss, that

[9]Z. J. Lipowski, "Psychosocial Aspects of Disease," *Annals of Internal Medicine*, 71, December 1969, p. 1198.

[10]*Ibid.*, p. 1199.

[11]*Ibid.*, p. 1200.

patient needs to feel significant. However, there are times when the loss makes the patient feel insignificant as a human being. Insignificance associated with loss has two meanings for the patient. First the patient, attaches insignificance to the illness, injury, or impending loss. Initially, the loss may be perceived as insignificant if the patient denies any threat. The second implication of insignificance involves other's perception of the individual. There are times when the chronically disabled or terminally ill patients are made to feel less significant than the more healthy patients around them. Possibly the patient experiencing loss perceives that more time is spend caring for patients with less complicated and disabling problems. The dying patients make the health team cognizant of their own vulnerability and inevitable death. This is particularly true of younger patients. In addition, death or dying implies failure to alter a potentially fatal process. It must be kept in mind that loss, no matter what the cause or degree of severity, need not be perceived as a failure. Instead the loss can be approached in a more positive manner. Even though the patient is unable to reestablish a previous level of mobility, that patient can still be a significant member of the family unit. To further this feeling, the health team needs to maintain a sense of hopefulness in the patient's emotional contributions.

Regardless of the stages or phases, each patient who experiences a loss manifests a unique behavioral response. Loss has a different meaning for each patient. Furthermore, it is possible that one patient may bypass a particular stage or phase as one adapts to the immediate or impending loss.

APPLICATION OF LOSS AND STAGES
OF MOURNING

It must be remembered that regardless of the cause, severity, or duration, illness implies a loss. The loss involved can range from temporary loss of function to loss of life. Regardless of the duration or severity, loss has significance for all involved, including the patient, family, and members of the health team. Loss occurs in all age groups. It can affect the lives of many people irrespective of age or clinical setting. Each individual due to a placement in the growth and development continuum reacts differently to the loss experience. Depending upon the age of the patient, the nurse is confronted with different behavioral manifestations of inner feelings.

According to Shusterman, "Some persons withdraw from the threat of death into a life pattern of hopelessness and lose personal control; others regress in their behavior to an immature level of self-centeredness, psychosomatic complaints, and bitterness at being dependent on others. Awareness of impending death may also be minimized or eliminated by such defense mechanisms as repression, rationalization, devaluation, or obsessive-compulsive ritual."[12] Needless to say, more complex losses such as those associated with complete dysfunction of a biological system or impending loss of life are the most difficult with which to cope. Each individual from childhood to old age has a unique way of coping with loss. Loss has different significance for the child than the aged patient. Hopefully, the way each patient copes will not be maladaptive.

Child

Nagy[13] has identified three childhood developmental stages associated with loss, specifically death and dying. In stage one, the child until age five has no concept of death. The child likens everything external to himself or herself according to a self-image. Lifeless objects are thought to be living. Usually the child's first encounter with loss may be through the death of a favorite pet. The child learns that even though the pet died it is quickly replaced with another one. This child may even give the new pet the same name as the dead pet. Therefore, death implies life. The lost object will be replaced. The exception is loss of human life involving a grandparent, parent, brother, sister, or friend. Within stage one, the small child does not comprehend death in the same manner as an adult.

Nagy points out that stage one involves two components. The first component revolves around loss as a departure. The child considers the dead individual to be simply asleep or gone away to another place. Therefore, when anyone goes away the child considers that person to be dead. The child sees death as a temporary departure. The individual is still alive but under a different set of conditions. When death occurs to a favorite person (grandparent, parent, or sibling), a change may not occur within the child since death is equated with life. The child's life together with those of the remaining significant others changes because the dead person no longer lives with them. Even though the dead person is viewed as departed, the child has numerous questions usually involving where the lost one has gone, how he got there, and why he had to leave. Within the second component, death is viewed as gradual or temporary. The child is able to acknowledge physical death; however, it cannot be divorced from life itself. This applies to children between age five and six.

[12]Lisa Roseman Shusterman, "Death and Dying: A Critical Review of the Literature," *Nursing Outlook*, 21, June 1973, p. 366.

[13]Marcia Nagy, "The Child's View of Death," *The Meaning of Death*, (Ed: Herman Feifel), (New York: McGraw-Hill, 1965), pp. 80–81.

The child is still unable to accept an abstract idea that death or dying is an absolute negation or definitive fact. As with departure, the child thinks of loss as temporary or gradual.

Stage two deals with the personification of death for children between ages five and nine. Nagy believes that personification of death takes place in two ways. First, death is fantasized as a separate person. Some children within this age group view death as a distinct personality. "Either they believe in the reality of the skeleton-man, or individually create their own idea of a death-man. The death-man is invisible for them. This means two things: (a) it is invisible in itself, as it is a being without a body; (b) we do not see him because he goes about in secret, mostly at night."[14] At this point in the developmental continuum, the child accepts the fact that death does exist. In accepting its existence, the child accepts its absolute definiteness and seeks ways to avoid it. When going to bed at night, small children will tell their parents "see you in the morning." They are seeking to reassure themselves that both parents will in fact be present when they awaken. Second, death is identified with the dead. Some children view death as a person. Their concept of death may have been influenced through the many television programs they watch. Regardless of its origin, children in this age group attempt to keep death or dying at a distance. The distance sometimes takes the form of anger. If the child is frequently hospitalized for an illness, the loss experienced is parental.

Friedman discovered in his research of children with leukemia that the young child openly rejected parents. Such rejection was evident through statements such as "I hate you." The parents experienced guilt thinking they had failed their child. "This pattern of behavior appeared most commonly after the children had been ill for some time, and seemed in part related to the patient's inability to prevent painful procedures and prolonged hospitalization with consequent damage to the usual childhood faith in parental omnipotence."[15] In addition to separation from significant others, the child with leukemia experiences physical alterations in the self-concept or body image. The illness itself together with the various treatment procedures causes weight changes, disfigurements, and possible hair loss. The child must cope with the various physical losses or changes associated with the disease process, treatment procedures, or anticipation of death. As the disease process progresses, the child experiences additional losses.

Besides separation from the family, the child is separated from school, friends, pets, and eventually the home. With each subsequent

[14]*Ibid.*, p. 95.

[15]Stanford Friedman, "Behavioral Observations on Parents Anticipating The Death of a Child," *Pediatrics*, October 1963, p. 615. Copyright 1963, American Academy of Pediatrics.

hospitalization, the losses are replaced with more diagnostic procedures, treatments, tubes or wires, physical changes, and pain. It is no wonder that the child manifests certain behavioral responses. The nurse assesses that a young patient behaviorally copes through crying, anger, hostility, depression, or intellectualization. Even though the child is surrounded by a caring health team and supportive family, he or she must experience the loss and/or eventual death alone. According to Langer, "Dying is difficult to do alone, and yet in so many ways it cannot be shared. If anyone is aware of this, it is the dying child. He knows and observes the restrictions against speaking about death. If he tries to break taboos, he rarely does so directly and then, perhaps, only in a highly symbolic manner."[16]

The last developmental stage occurs at age nine or later. At this time, the child acknowledges death as a process which eventually happens to all individuals, the difference being that it occurs at different times and under different circumstances. Beginning at about age nine, the child realizes that death means the actual termination or cessation of all bodily functions. Furthermore, the child realizes that death or dying is a process which occurs within the individual and that it has implications for all, not only the very old. It is at this time the child realizes that illness necessitating frequent hospitalization has the potential of loss. The older child or adolescent acknowledges an illness. In his research Friedman discovered that, "some acknowledgment of the illness is often helpful especially in the older child, in preventing the child from feeling isolated, believing that others are not aware of what he is experiencing, or feeling that his disease is too awful to talk about."[17]

The adolescent is in a difficult position, experiencing everything in the here and now. The immediate world is an intense one. It is surrounded by everything that is significant or valuable. Unlike the adult patient, the adolescent views the future as immediate. The adolescent sees life as just beginning and moving toward meaningful events. Needless to say, illness resulting in various losses is not a part of that future. Illness which takes the adolescent away from family and friends has little value. Kastenbaum states that, "The adolescent occupies a pivotal position. His maturing outlooks on life and death are strongly influenced by the existing cultural matrix, and the resultant configuration of personal beliefs will strongly influence his future experiences. But it would be a mistake to suppose that the individual is passively shaped by the external forces which operate upon him."[18]

[16]Myra Langner-Bluebond, "I Know, Do You? A Study of Awareness, Communication, and Coping in Terminally Ill Children," *Anticipatory Grief*, p. 180.

[17]Friedman, *op. cit.*, p. 615.

[18]Robert Kastenbaum, "Time and Death in Adolescence," *The Meaning of Death*, (Ed: Feifel), (New York: McGraw-Hill, 1959), p. 104.

The nurse attempts to support both the young patient and the family as they cope with their immediate and/or future losses. Like the child, the parents need continual reassurances. In particular, the parents need reassurance that they are, in fact, good parents. As mentioned previously, parents verbally or nonverbally express feelings of guilt. More specifically, parents have questions regarding how much their child knows about the illness or disease process. The parents seek support as to whether the young patient should be told what is happening to his or her body. Initially, as a way of protecting themselves, they refrain from telling the child. However, as time progresses and the child's frustrations increase, the parents realize that he or she must be informed. Throughout this time, the nurse can alleviate the families anxieties regarding their decision.

This is particularly difficult for the parents of a terminally ill child. Friedman found that parents of children with leukemia, "eagerly look forward to the time that their child would go into remission and be discharged from the hospital, but their pleasurable anticipation of this event was frequently tempered by considerable concern regarding the necessity of again assuming the major responsibility for the child's care."[19]

The nurse together with other members of the health team have a responsibility to assist the child and parents as they adapt to various losses associated with the illness or disease process. Furthermore, they need to help both make the necessary transition between hospital and home. This is particularly true for the child whose leukemia is in remission or whose disease process has stabilized. The adult and aged patients also cope in their own unique way to loss.

Adult and Aged

Loss or the threat of loss can be a new experience for the adult or aged patient. The loss can be the result of acute illness, chronic disability, or terminal process. Regardless of the cause, the patient may be unable to fulfill psychological or physiological needs. Illness is an inconvenience for the adult or aged patient who must temporarily submit ownership of the body to others. The patient depends upon the nurse to feed, bathe, turn, or assist one to the bathroom. As the illness or disease process increases in severity or chronicity, the patient may be totally dependent upon others. "For most people, sickness is uncomfortable, inconvenient, temporary, but rarely a menace. Then, if sickness persists, enduring beyond the healing effects of treatment and time, the personal dimensions of being

---

[19]Friedman, *op. cit.*, p. 616.

sick gradually become more conspicuous."[20] In discussing the adult or aged patient, two factors are of significance. First is the concern for biological survival. Second is the competent behavior utilized as each copes or adapts to their biological threat.

Acute or prolonged illness involves primary loss in bodily functions or organs. Myocardial infarction, chronic obstructive pulmonary disease, or renal failure causes loss in function, part or whole, of a particular system. The patient with acute renal failure is threatened by the possibility of total loss in renal function resulting in ultimate dependency upon hemodialysis. When a biological crisis occurs, the individual is removed from the familiar territory and rushed to a nearby hospital. While the sirens scream, the individual has thoughts of final separation from family and life itself. These feelings intensify as the patient becomes quickly absorbed into a rapidly changing environment. In all probability these fears will continue throughout the initial days of biological crisis. The fears and anxieties may be even more intense if the patient is hospitalized several times for the same problems.

Each patient in biological crisis seeks the same goal of biological survival. Depending upon the patient's particular problem, biological survival has different meanings. For the patient with a myocardial infarction it means surviving the initial crisis and threat of death. To the patient with chronic emphysema or renal failure, biological survival means pain relief, decrease in suffering, physical stability, and adaptation to reduced stamina. A diagnosis such as myocardial infarction or renal insufficiency is not as threatening as that of cancer. Although patients can survive any of the above biological problems, cancer is still synonymous with death. In addition cancer is associated with extended illness and hospitalization. "The meaning of illness becomes more pertinent when sickness is extended and involves helplessness and the threat of death. Survival itself may be uncertain. Effective performance within a familiar orbit of activity is drastically, and perhaps permanently compromised. The affected patient must, therefore, assess his place in the world. He asks himself what has happened, where he is going, what he can expect, and what it all means."[21]

Loss resulting in threats of death does not limit itself to patients with biological alteration. The adult schizophrenic patient with schizophrenia also experiences fantasies about death and dying. Feifel says that, "Death themes and fantasies are prominent in psychopathology. . . . There is the stupor of the catatonic patient, sometimes likened to a death state and the delusions of immortality in certain schizophrenics. It may well be that the schizophrenic denial of reality functions, in some way, as a magical

[20]Weisman, *op. cit.*, p. 52.

[21]*Ibid.*, pp. 95–96.

holding back, if not undoing, of the possibility of death."[22] The schizo-phrenic is not sure of his or her own body. The schizophrenic sometimes has difficulty realizing body boundaries let alone the boundaries of the future. In many instances, the schizophrenic has grown up feeling inept with his or her physical being, having little or no sense of relatedness with the self and the surrounding outer world. The emotionally stable or secure individual experiences a dread of death and an overwhelming amazement of life. The schizophrenic feels this more than anyone else because of an inability to build a positive self-concept or self-confidence necessary to permit this temporary denial. Becker states that, "The schizophrenic's misfortune is that he has been burdened with extra anxieties, extra guilt, extra helplessness, an even more unpredictable and unsupportive environment."[23]

Regardless of the biological or psychological problem, the adult patient desires to live. Likewise, the aged patient may have different or similar desires. The nurse must recognize that there are aged patients who, because of chronic debilitating illnesses, enter the hospital without the desire, will, or motivation to live. The nurse may hear the patient say, "Please let me die in peace." Oftentimes nurses will attempt to instill the desire to live, even though the patient has already willed the self to death. Positive peripheral factors such as spouse, a family to give the desire to live, or social activities may not be operating in this group. On the other hand, there are times when it seems that medical technology is more concerned with prolonging death than life. The aged patient is almost inevitably confronted with the issue of prolongation of life.

This is particularly applicable to aged patients in critical care units. It must be pointed out that there are many aged patients with acute or chronic biological problems who maintain an active desire and motivation to live as long as possible. They are usually people who have been relatively healthy all their lives and for whom illness is simply an incon-venience or waste of valuable time. Such patients are eager to return to their homes, families, social activities, and pets. There are several posi-tive peripheral factors in their lives which motivate them to return to a level of health. One may be the fact that they have been free from repeated, debilitating illness. Another significant factor may be that the aged patient realizes that a spouse is home waiting for his or her return. Because such aged patients in acute and chronic care facilities have a strong motivation to live, their wishes should be acknowledged and respected. Both the adult and aged patient's desire to live causes each to behave in certain ways. The way utilized becomes a factor; competent behavior.

[22]Herman Feifel, "Attitudes Toward Death in Some Normal and Mentally Ill Popula-tions," *The Meaning of Death,* (New York: McGraw-Hill, 1959), p. 115.

[23]Ernest Becker, *The Denial of Death,* (New York: McMillan, 1973), p. 63.

Competent behavior signifies that an individual who is ill can choose the manner in which to solve or cope with biopsychosocial losses. The way chosen will depend upon the direct or potential loss involved and how it interferes with life goals. A patient may choose to deny the loss of existence or severity; to bargain with significant others for the loss's removal; to develop an awareness of the loss's relatedness to physical being; and, to resolve or accept the loss.

The adult or aged patient uses negation as a process through which the individual responds to something perceived to be a threat. Negation behaviorally manifested as denial is a defense behind which the patient, family member, or nurse can retreat. If one denies the loss, then its meaning or future implication cannot be emotionally assessed. Sometimes it is difficult for the nurse to assess whether or not the patient is denying. The nurse may falsely assume that since the patient does not discuss the loss, it has been both assimilated and accepted. Therefore, denying and denial are missed. The nurse's assessment should include how and when denial seems to occur. Keeping this in mind, Weisman has identified three degrees or orders of denial which he relates to death. His orders can also be applied to patient's experiencing loss of which death is one example. Weisman's labels these orders as first order denial, second order denial, and third order denial.[24]

First order denial deals with the period of time in which an individual realizes that something is wrong. This period of time involves two phases. The first is the initial impact of a biological crisis such as myocardial infarction, respiratory failure, or sudden abdominal pain. The symptoms tell the individual a potential problem exists. The person may choose to acknowledge the pain's or symptom's presense and seek professional help. On the other hand, one may intellectualize the problem's magnitude or etiology through self-diagnosis and self-treatment. Take for example the hard driving young male executive who experiences chest pain while conducting a business meeting. He has experienced a similar pain on previous occasions. With each new occurrence, he rationalizes or intellectualizes its significance and origin. He attributes the pain to indigestion and prescribes antacids. Therefore, through self-diagnosis and self-treatment, he denies the threat of a biological crisis. He continues to deny until the time when the symptoms can no longer be hidden behind denial. Unfortunately, for some this time of awareness is at death.

The second phase begins when the individual's problem is professionally labeled or diagnosed. At this point fears are confirmed. Denial begins at either phase and it is interesting to note that the patient does not realize the denial. Besides sheltering the patient from reality, denial also allows the patient to maintain and present a positive self-image. Ameri-

[24]Weisman, *op. cit.*, p. 67.

can society places great emphasis upon youth and life. Therefore, one who is experiencing several biological losses resulting in a premature dependency, disability, or death becomes life's mistake. Obviously, this should not and is not always the case. To avoid such feelings of worthlessness, the patient will attempt to deny the seriousness of the biological loss or potential death. According to Weisman, "Patients who deny a great deal seem to do so in order to preserve a high level of self esteem. For this reason, they need to preserve contact and stabilize their relationship with someone essential to self esteem. Even when there seems to be no one in particular who threatens or could be threatened by a patient's illness, deterioration, or death, the patient himself may deny because he wants to maintain the status quo of already existing relationships."[25]

The adult or aged patient is expected to present courageous behavior even when death approaches. Such notions require that the patient maintain relative composure and cheerfulness or, at the very least, that death should be faced with dignity. The patient should not cut himself or herself off from the world, nor turn the back on the living; if one has a family, one should continue to be a good family member. The patient should "be nice" to other patients as well and should cooperate with the staff members who provide care, and avoid distressing them.

In critical care units, nurses frequently hear family members say, particularly to aged patients, "Now, Papa, be nice to the little nurse. Do what she says and don't complain." It may be, however, that complaining or arguing with the nurse is the only control he feels he has over the situation; he may be physically too weak to fight, so his control takes the form of verbal abuse. The nurse may be controlling him through a pacemaker, dialysis machine, or intravenous therapy; he is controlling his nurse through yelling, or pushing his light frequently. Critical care units in any hospital, with their atmosphere of heroic recovery, are geared toward prolonging life at almost any cost. Equipment is clustered near every bed, so that prolonging may be just a matter of leaning over and "hooking the patient up." The atmosphere in such units counters staff's attempts to make the patient comfortable to let him die. As Fletcher has beautifully said, "It is the living that fear death, not the dying."[26]

Just as the patient or the family experiences first order denial, the health team may not realize that they also deny the reality of a serious or terminal illness. Some doctors feel that a patient's death puts their professional competence, rather than the state of medical knowledge, generally in question, and as a consequence they will not relinquish the recovery

---

[25]*Ibid.*, p. 64.

[26]Joseph Fletcher, "The Patient's Right to Die," *Harpers Magazine*, October 1960, p. 139.

goal until they feel assured that their own skills are not at issue. A favorite rationale of the doctor who persists in the ideal of indefinitly prolonging life is the assertion that he or she is simply an instrument of society. The doctor feels that society has vested in him or her the duty of sustaining life, and that the doctor is therefore obligated to abdicate personal responsibility for judging the advisability of whether a particular life should or should not be prolonged.[27]

With first order denial, the patient attempts to minimize the illness or disease. Minimization may continue even when the illness reoccurs. When pain is involved, the patient is unable to deny its existence, and may instead deny its significance. A tumor that is cancerous and malignant may be emotionally treated as though it is benign. Such behavior indicates second order denial.

Biologically, second order denial refers to the phase of more extensive losses associated with illness or disease. During this phase, the patient emotionally may or may not see the extension and overall implications of the illness or disease. It will be remembered that first order denial revolves around the patient's first reaction to the diagnosis. However, once the patient accepts the fact that one is ill, there is an inability to comprehend the implications and severity of the loss.

For example, the patient with acute renal failure may deny the probability of the illness evolving into chronic renal failure. The latter's extensiveness would indicate dependency upon a supportive device such as hemodialysis. The cardiac patient experiencing a second myocardial infarction associated with congestive heart failure in six months may choose to deny the severity of the loss. For this patient the loss may be temporary. The nurse realizes that the loss is more extensive even to the point of death. Likewise, the patient with a malignant disease may deny the extensiveness of the illness. Such behavior represents the patient's coping mechanism. The nurse may assess that the patient, at this phase, is only able to take in and assimilate small aspects of the illness.

In second order denial, "Denial of implications often takes place when a patient fractionates his illness and persistent symptoms into many, minor complaints, each of which can then be handled separately. As a result, the total illness cannot amount to much."[28] These become the patients who refuse to adhere to an overall restrictive treatment program. Each may follow one aspect yet refuse to follow an equally significant aspect. The patient with myocardinal infarction may refuse to remain in bed even after having been instructed of the dangers of early mobilization. The patient with renal failure may fail to follow a proper diet, eating

[27]Barney Glaser and Anselm Strauss, *Awareness of Dying,* (Chicago: Aldine Publishing Co., 1965), p. 202.

[28]Weisman, *op. cit.,* p. 71.

food high in protein and potassium content. The patient with schizophrenia might refuse to participate in individual or group therapy. Likewise, the patient with pulmonary edema who refuses to restrict fluid intake only contributes to the biological crisis. Regardless of the biological or psychological problem, each patient has a unique reason for refusing to adhere to a particular treatment procedure. The adult or aged patient, through assimilation, finally reaches the transitional stage in which one becomes aware of one's possible extinction. The nurse assesses that such behavior is reflective of third order denial.

Third order denial deals with the patient's acceptance of loss, various hazards, or complications. However, the patient may still resist associating a terminal illness with death itself, since it represents finality and extinction. Naturally, not all patients are unable to face their own finality. However, some younger adult patients are unable to imagine their own terminal illness and eventual death, thinking that death is reserved for the very old. Loss affects all age groups. Loss can be painful for the young adult patient because it implies separation from those one loves. The young adult must temporarily or permanently leave the work one enjoys and the family one loves. On the other hand, loss for the aged patient may or may not be a painful experience. There are many older people who feel that they have made their contribution and lived long enough.

The nurse should realize that it is possible for the patient to acknowledge his or her own loss and its finality sooner than either the nurse or health team. Some family members request heroic measures even when the patient's losses are so extensive that only death will be prolonged, not life itself. The nursing and medical staff may need to go along with the family until the family can understand that such measures may not be the wisest choice. If the patient is being kept alive by equipment, the doctors have greater control over life than in the case of natural prolonging of life. The doctor also has more time to plan, to calculate risks, and to negotiate with the family and nurses.

Although the medical ideal of prolonging life at all costs and with all possible facilities conflicts with the awareness that prolonging life may be useless and unduly expensive; the ideal often wins out. According to Glaser and Strauss, one physician stated, "There are too many instances . . . in which patients in such a situation are kept alive indefinitely by means of tubes inserted into their stomachs, or into their veins, or into their bladder, or into their rectums—and the whole sad scene thus created is encompassed with a cocoon of oxygen which is the next thing to a shroud."[29]

Denial, with its three orders, is one component of competent be-

---

[29]Glaser and Strauss, *op. cit.,* p. 202.

havior experienced by the patient. Other competent behavior associated with loss includes hopelessness, depression, fear, and finally an awareness of the loss. The severity of a patient's loss influences the degree of depression and hopelessness. A more serious biological illness, possibly resulting in death, causes the patient to feel less hopeful about the future. Instead of looking forward to an expansive future, the patient becomes depressed thinking of a constricting one. Verwoerdt believes that, "Loss of hopeful prospects in fatally ill patients is associated with a turning away from the future. A certain amount of satisfaction with the past is associated with a more hopeful outlook and with looking forward into the more distant future. The degree of disability for current life activities shows a significant relationship to loss of hope and to constriction of future."[30]

Normally an individual looks forward to the future, anticipating positive accomplishments. One dreams of how leisure time will be spent in the pursuit of yet unmet goals. The individual, together with the family, plans for the future because there is hope in its existence. Hope is a future-oriented concept. Loss resulting in a contricting future removes the patient's sense of hope and replaces it with the feeling of hopelessness and depression. To protect oneself from the hopeless feelings of one's finality, the patient may avoid any reference to the future. The family or nurse attempts to offer the patient a sense of hope by focusing upon positive aspects of the present and future. Such an approach may eventually have a positive effect upon patients with biological losses leading to disability rather than immediate or impending death. The chronic pulmonary or dialysis patients need an element of hope in order to cope with their constricting future. Their attention may only focus upon the present state of biological loss. Each patient needs to find hope in the present so that, in case of survival, a future, no matter how limited, still exists. The terminally ill patient's focus is upon the past and present because the future is too painful. Therefore, the patient recoils into events of the past that represent pleasure.

Feelings of hopelessness and depression are normal adaptive behavioral responses to a loss. Maladaptive behavior occurs when the patient, whose loss only means temporary obstruction to future goals, continues to feel hopeless and depressed. The nurse may assess that the loss was a greater threat to emotional integrity than anticipated or realized. The biological crisis may reach stability; however, the patient's emotional equilibrium may remain unstable. Free from diagnostic studies and treatments, the patient has time to think about the loss. It may be at this point in the hospitalization that the patient requires a greater degree

[30]Adriaan Verwoerdt, "Psychological Reactions in Fatal Illness, The Prospect of Impending Death," *Journal of the American Geriatrics Society*, 15, 1967, p. 16.

of attention from the nurse. Unfortunately, the health team shifts their attention to someone else in biological crisis. As a result, the patient is left alone with unresolved conflicts and unanswered questions; consequently, fears remain and sometimes become intensified.

Initially, with a biological loss, the patient experiences fear of dying or death. It is natural that fears are dependent upon the nature and severity of the loss. The biological insult may not be as threatening as the diagnosis itself. For example, a 34 year-old woman had recently passed her yearly physical examination with flying colors. Two months later she begins complaining of nonspecific symptoms such as generalized aches and tiredness. Shortly thereafter she develops some rectal bleeding. Still unconcerned about her symptoms, she nevertheless enters the hospital for diagnostic studies. To everyone's amazement the studies reveal what was not anticipated, leukemia. What was two months earlier assumed as perfect health and an expanding future was later diagnosed as leukemia and a very constricting future (three to twelve months). For this patient and others like her the fear of dying and death become a reality. The fears of dying and death may be experienced during the early stages of a terminal illness. As the disease progresses, the patient, more so than the family, becomes more accepting of the losses. Consequently, as death approaches its growing fears may be subsiding. Instead, the awareness of one's own biological finality has made the patient more accepting of it. The nurse should keep in mind that the absence of fears does not always imply denial. It may imply that the awareness has led the patient into the last stage of mourning; acceptance.

The patient whose loss results in denying and death, becomes aware of a limited future sooner than the family or sometimes the health team. After all, the adult or aged patient is living within the body that is experiencing a biological or emotional loss. Elmore points out that, "To the extent that the individual perceives and interprets the nature of the internal messages and is consequently able to plot the rate of decline, and to extend this declining curve from the present into the future to a terminal point—to this extent we can speak of a premonition of death."[31] The internal messages received by the patient are constant. They keep the patient continuously informed about biological stability or decline. No matter how hard a patient may try to deny, he or she cannot avoid the close monitoring of biological events with the body. Therefore, the internal messages contribute to awareness. As the messages become more intense, the patient begins to accept the reality of one's death.

Not all patients respond to a loss in the same manner. A patient's response may be dependent upon age, previous experiences with loss, or

[31]James Elmore, "Psychological Reactions to Impending Death," *Hospital Topics,* November 1967, p. 36.

severity of the loss. Nevertheless, there are stages, previously mentioned, through which each individual moves. The nurse assesses the patient's behavioral response in an attempt to assist in coping with the loss. In addition, the nurse simultaneously helps the patient's family cope with their feelings. The nurse keeps in mind that each individual, family, or patient is unique and that some move toward acceptance faster than others. To effectively assist the patient, the nurse assesses and utilizes various influencing factors or variables as they specifically apply to the individual.

NURSING IMPLICATIONS

The nurse needs to assist the patient in adapting to the loss. The nurse realizes that the loss can imply a threatening fatal disease and a diminishing self-worth. Weisman states that, "The healing effect of treatment and time are not his. Therefore, as his illness progresses, he is forced to settle for less and less, to compromise his expectations, and to become less than what he had been or might be. Finally, survival becomes an end in itself."[32] To accomplish his or her goals, the nurse assesses both internal and external influencing factors or variables. Once assessed, the nurse intervenes to either alter, maintain, or strengthen the variables.

Internal Variables

Internal variables are concerned with the pathological and psychological processes. The nurse assesses the loss according to its nature, extent, rate of progression, degree, and reversibility of the reduced function. These become the biological variables through which the nurse and other members of the health team intervene. Take for example Mr. J., an aggressive 39 year-old who maintained his own construction business. He was married and the father of three children. His job involved both physical and emotional pressures. Throughout his life he has enjoyed relatively good health. However, one morning while jogging, he experienced severe chest pain. He was quickly admitted to a nearby coronary care unit. A social history revealed that he smoked 2-3 packs of cigarettes per day, drank, and maintained late hours. An emergency cardiac catheterization revealed 95 percent occlusion of both his right and left coronary arteries. The patient's cardiologists felt surgery was mandatory; otherwise his preinfarction status could lead to severe myocardial damage or death. Mr. J. submitted himself to the surgery.

[32]Weisman, *op. cit.*, p. 57.

Needless to say, his family was quite concerned. Because Mr. J's symptoms, diagnostic evaluation, and surgery all took place in the same day, he had difficulty relating to his own loss. Postoperatively he minimized the entire event as if it had never happened. He felt that in a few weeks he would resume his previous life style. The surgery saved his life; however, Mr. J. never completely internalized that his life was in danger. Mr. J's image of himself was that of "one of the group at the construction site." He wanted to continue his active life, including smoking, drinking, and keeping long difficult hours. Any discussion to the contrary was avoided by the patient. He denied that any change in his future life style was necessary.

In the above situation, the nurse and health team intervened to alter events that led to the biological crisis; maintained those factors which reduce its extension or achieve stability; and, strengthened already stabilized processes. When the patient, like Mr. J., denies events contributing to his illness, it becomes difficult for his nurse to alter those events. The nurse can allow the patient to deny a loss; however, the nurse does not support him in his denial. The patient's denial is important in attempting to continue presenting a positive image. The nurse keeps in mind that regardless of the patient or the loss, "The greater the value and psychodynamic significance the body part or function affected by disease has for the patient, the more intense this psychological reaction is likely to be."[33]

Recognizing the patient's need to present a positive physical body image, the nurse helps the patient realize that there are other aspects of the physical being and personality which permit the patient to continue a positive self-image. In other words, the patient need not depend upon what he thinks are the behaviors of "the construction gang," such as drinking, smoking, and physical labor. Once the illness has stabilized and the loss realized, the patient can be helped to look at contributing factors which led to the biological crisis. These events can then be altered. All treatments or activities designed to stabilize the biological loss should be maintained. Last, those factors which strengthen the patient's adaptation to the loss and eventual recovery should be encouraged.

Regardless of the biological loss, it is important to remember that patients who set a high value on their physical well-being, including the ability to physically move through their environment, are threatened when faced with an illness or pathological process. Different parts of the body have different significance for each individual. Therefore, this becomes an important variable. According to Lipowski, "Different organs and functions may have different value and psychological significance for different persons. These values often have little to do with biological factors related to survival. An injury to the nose or amputation of a breast

[33]Lipowski, *op. cit.*, p. 1201.

may have greater psychological impact on a person than, for example, hepatic disease directly threatening his life."[34] Pathological processes can and do lead to psychological changes, which become the second internal variable.

The psychological changes experienced by the patient, regardless of age, are directly related to the loss. The nurse realizes that certain behavioral responses such as anxiety, depression, anger, avoidance, or denial are normal. The same behaviors become abnormal if the patient remains depressed, anxious, angry, or fails to seek and follow medical advice. Regardless of the specific behavioral response, it begins the moment an individual perceives a change in the body. The patient is the first to realize that a biological change is taking place. For example, the hypertensive patient complains of severe headaches. The cardiac patient complains of tiredness and minor chest pain which is attributed to indigestion. The patient's perception is then confirmed by a physician in the form of a diagnostic study, laboratory tests, and finally a diagnosis.

Many times the patient is cognitive of a potential problem prior to its confirmation by a professional. Likewise, the same individual remains aware of the body's altered state throughout the illness or disease process. It is because of the patient's body perceptions that he or she is able to assess the seriousness of the illness or disease. This is a significant variable for the nurse to utilize when intervening to assist the patient and family through a difficult time.

There are times when the family requests that the patient not be informed of the seriousness of an illness or disease. The patient realizes the illness or disease is serious; however, the patient wants to protect the family from the pain of potential or eventual death. Therefore, the loss is avoided through jovial behavior. As previously pointed out, the patient wants to maintain a positive self-image. Likewise, the family, thinking it is protecting the patient, avoids discussion of the loss and threat of further loss. Both are aware of the loss, but each avoids open discussion. Each thinks it is protecting the other. The nurse assesses each's readiness to begin sharing its support with the other. The nurse encourages the patient and the family to openly acknowledge the loss and its implications. Together they can begin resolving it.

Within the resolving phase of an individual's loss, one may manifest behavior previously referred to as anxiety, depression, anger, avoidance, or denial. Such responses are considered coping behaviors. The nurse intervenes to channel the patient's behavior in an adaptive direction by aiding behavior recognition. However, there are times when this becomes a difficult task. With a serious loss leading to eventual death, the nurse assesses that the adult or aged patient seems to withdraw. The

[34]*Ibid.*, p. 1202.

patient pulls away from surrounding significant others. The avoidance may be wrongly assessed as preoccupation with oneself, when it is really self-preservation. The adult patient withdraws internally in an attempt to hold together. This usually occurs as death approaches. According to Lieberman, "Many observers have commented on the psychological withdrawal of the dying patient and have suggested that the withdrawal is functional in that it protects the individual from intense separation anxiety. On the other hand withdrawal represents an attempt to cope with the experience of inner disintegration. The disintegration probably precedes the reduced emotional investment in others."[35]

The behavioral response of anger and withdrawal may be seen more frequently with the young adult patient who becomes angry, frustrated, and anxious about a constricting future. The young married patient worries about his or her family. The patient becomes anxious upon realizing that he or she can only enjoy the family's existence to a certain point. The aged patient, on the other hand, becomes less anxious and depressed over a loss since there may no longer be family responsibilities, therefore the concern focuses on self. The nurse remembers that the psychological variable which leads to behavioral changes is a result of the patient's inability to cope with the loss. This is particularly significant for the dying patient. "The psychological changes preceding death are best viewed in terms of the individual's lessened ability to cope adequately with environmental demands, particularly because of a lowered ability to organize and to integrate stimuli in his environment. Perhaps the aged individual, approaching his own death, experiences upheaval because of currently active disorganizing mental processes, rather than because he fears his approaching death."[36]

The nurse assesses the pathological variable in terms of the degree of temporary or permanent loss and the meaning it has for the individual. The nurse realizes that its meaning relates to its attachment to the patient's ego. The second internal variable (psychological) is assessed in terms of the patient's behavioral response to the illness. The behavioral response can take many forms such as anxiety, depression, denial, avoidance, and anger. Each behavior becomes a component within the grieving process. Once the nurse assesses internal variables, she then assesses external variables influencing the patient.

External Variables

External variables or influencing factors involve the patient's previous experience with hospitalization, social value or situation, and available support systems such as family, health team, or friends.

---

[35]Lieberman, *op. cit.*, p. 189.
[36]*Ibid.*, p. 189.

Illness or disease resulting in loss may be a new or recurring experience for the individual. As a new experience, the patient may not know how to respond to it. Hospitalization means loss in the form of separation from parents to the child. Besides being separated from a familiar home, bed, toys, family, or dog, the child is confronted with threatening and sometimes intrusive diagnostic procedures. The entire experience can be threatening unless the nurse is aware of the young patient's fears and anxieties.

Hospitalization can also be a new experience for the adult or aged patient. The adult who has maintained total control over the being becomes threatened when faced with forced dependence upon strangers in a sometimes highly technical world. Depending upon the patient's biological problem, the environment in which he or she is hospitalized can be emotionally threatening. Take the patient who enters the hospital's emergency room complaining of chest pain. Even though the patient realizes that the biological crisis is serious, it is rationalized as indigestion. The patient soon finds himself hospitalized in a critical care unit. The patient next relinquishes the body to various pieces of supportive equipment and strangers who poke, probe, and percuss. The patient does not know what to expect nor what is expected of him. The nurse intervenes to create a nonthreatening environment. This goal is accomplished by explaining the various supportive devices as they relate to a particular problem. In this respect the patient knows what is expected of him or her.

Illness or disease as a recurring problem can be even more threatening to the patient. Due to previous experience, there is knowledge of the hospital's environment, intrusive diagnostic procedures, and various supportive devices. The patient also has knowledge of his or her own biological frailty. The patient realizes that with each subsequent hospitalization one experiences greater loss. The nurse recognizes that the patient, alone, perceives biological changes which could result in further disability or even death. Therefore, depending upon the biological loss, each hospitalization brings one closer to the thing feared: death. Since hospitalization is not a new experience, the patient needs less environmental support and more emotional support. Instead of discussing external environmental events, the nurse focuses on the patient's external feelings. The nurse encourages expression of internal feelings and supports the patient with fears.

The second external variable or influencing factor is the patient's social values or situation. An individual's social value is assessed according to age, wealth, education, profession, and appearance. Patients with the highest social value seem to receive the greatest degree of attention. A patient with high social status in the community may receive special care in addition to administrative concern. A room is quickly made available.

This patient receives diagnostic studies and laboratory tests at the prescribed time and may even receive special privileges given only to high status people. On the other hand, another patient may lose certain privileges because of a low social status. Regardless of their position in the community, each should receive the same degree of concern and attention. This means that the nurse will assess the patient's social status as it relates to education, occupation, and previous illness experience. These social variables become significant to the nurse as he or she formulates a teaching plan designed to raise the patient's level of understanding. Furthermore, it enables the nurse to more fully understand the potential for coping with a crisis situation.

The nurse realizes that age is a significant social variable. A younger patient may receive greater attention and heroic measures than an aged patient. Our society has become extremely youth-centered. An individual will try to deceive himself and others by remaining as young as possible. The health team responds with greater sorrow when learning of a loss affecting a younger patient. The same loss can affect an aged patient, however, it would be looked upon as expected for the age. This is particularly true when the loss involves death. According to Weisman, "The death of a child is always a tragedy. It is unforgettable and futile, because so much of a child's worth depends upon unrealized potential and its capacity to evoke tenderness. In contrast, the death of the very aged fits into an acceptable order of nature and we find reasons to explain why it is right and proper for an old patient to die when he does."[37]

Illness or disease resulting in loss has no age boundaries. It affects each individual at some point in life. Regardless of the age involved, the nurse recognizes that for the patient and the family the loss is significant. The various social values of age, occupation, education, or wealth all become variables to be utilized by the nurse.

Finally, the support systems available to the patient can assist one through the loss experience. The support systems consist of family, health team, and friends. A patient's family can be a supportive asset throughout the illness or disease process. The patient can draw upon the family's strength. In this respect, they can help the patient cope with a difficult situation. The nurse realizes that, "The response of the family and other meaningful people to the patient's illness or disability, to his communications of distress, and to his mobility to perform the usual social roles may spell the difference between optimal recovery or psychological invalidism."[38] However, the nurse should remember that the family can become emotionally depleted. Therefore, it becomes important to offer the family as much assistance as offered to the patient.

---

[37]Weisman, *op. cit.*, p. 144.
[38]Lipowski, *op. cit.*, p. 1200.

The family needs to be continually appraised of the patient's biological status. If not appropriately appraised, the family develops unrealistic expectations that the patient's loss is not serious but temporary. In the latter instance, the family may request heroic measures even when they will not alter the disease process. The family fails to realize that they are only prolonging the dying rather than the living process.

When everyone, especially the family, is aware that there is "nothing more to do," the goal of recovery has, in effect, been changed to a goal of comfort. This seems to be the ideal time for ceasing to prolong the dying patient's life. Of course, in critical care the means by which the patient is allowed to die depends on whether life is being prolonged naturally or by equipment. When families request unrealistic heroics, the health team has a tremendous responsibility to aid the family in understanding the hopelessness of the situation. The nurse can convey to the family how the terminally ill person is progressing. By keeping family or significant others continually informed of the acuteness of the situation, the nurse also psychologically prepares the family for the eventual death of the child, adult, or aged patient.

It is at this time that the nurse can be an attentive listener to the family member. Many times a member of the family will want to share with the nurse memories of their loved one. Allowing the family to discuss pleasant memories, to reminisce, will help the family accept termination with the dying patient. This is part of facilitating their awareness of the patient's potential death; it initiates some of the grief work and perhaps makes it easier when the time comes to cease heroic measures.

The family often seeks reassurance that everything that can be done is currently being done for the aged patient. The nurse can reinforce their feelings that, yes, everything is or has been done. Such feedback assists the family not to request heroics based on their own guilt feelings. Families who react, instead of act, because of feelings of having not done more for a parent often drain their financial resources. Hospitalization in intensive care is expensive enough and the expense of various pieces of equipment used to prolong death can be astronomical. In some instances families may incur tremendous financial burden for having tried to assuage guilt.

The family may put the nurse on the defensive by asking if an aged parent is, or will get better. Many times, if it is hard for the nurse to respond honestly, he or she will resort to trite cliches such as, "You never know about these things," or "Why don't you ask your doctor?" Unfortunately the family rarely sees the physician, because the physician may have given up on the patient, realizing that the prognosis is terminal.

The family may be caught in a double bind of wanting to do what is best, but not realizing what is best for the patient. As the family begins to understand that their loved one is being kept alive by equipment, they may ask the staff to stop treatments which result in the usless prolonging of life. When the family or doctors decide to turn off the pacemaker or respirators, the family should be present either in the waiting room or patient's room. If the family is at home when the doctors make their decision to turn off life-prolonging equipment, the family may have guilt feelings about a loved one dying alone, surrounded by unyielding pieces of equipment.

There is a need for ministers, physicians, and nurses to discuss the concept of loss and the issue of prolonging versus nonprolonging death. As openness toward the once-taboo topic of loss including death increases, nurses, physicians, and ministers may be able to decide under what conditions termination of life-prolonging techniques and procedures is appropriate for the child, adult, or aged patient, and they may also feel better about the decisions they shared in and carried out.

REFERENCES

Agate, John, "Ethical Questions in Geriatric Care," *Nursing Mirror*, 19, November 1971, pp. 40–41.

Aquilera, Donna, *Crisis Intervention: Theory and Methodology*, St. Louis: Mosby, 1970.

Barrell, Lorna, "Crisis Intervention Partnership in Problem Solving," *Nursing Clinics of North America*, 9, March 1974.

Bowlby, John, "Childhood Mourning and Its Implications for Psychiatry," *American Journal of Psychiatry*, December 1961, pp. 481–97.

Burnside, Irene, "Loss: A Constant Theme in Group Work with the Aged," *Hospital and Community Psychiatry*, 21, June 1970, pp. 173–77.

———, "Multiple Losses in the Aged: Implications for Nursing Care," *The Gerontologists*, 13, Summer 1973, pp. 157–62.

———, "You Will Cope, of Course," *American Journal of Nursing*, December 1971, pp. 2354–57.

Carlson, Carolyn, "Grief and Mourning," *Behavioral Concepts and Nursing Interventions*, (Ed: Carlson), Philadelphia: Lippincott, 1970.

Dayan, Yael, *Death Had Two Sons*, New York: McGraw-Hill, 1967.

DiFabio, Susan, "Crisis: A Complex Process," *NCNA*, March 1974.

Engel, George, "Is Grief A Disease?" *Psychosomatic Medicine*, XXIII, 1961.

Gramlich, Edwin, "Recognition and Management of Grief in Elderly Patients," *Geriatrics*, July 1968, pp. 87–92.

Guther, John, *Death Be Not Proud: A Memoir*, New York: Harper and Row, 1949.

Hinton, John, *Dying*, Penguin Books, 1967.

Janken, Janice, "The Nurse in Crisis," *NCNA*, March 1974.

Kendig, Isabelle, "The Denial of Illness," *British Journal Medical Psychology*, 36, 1963, pp. 37–48.

Kübler-Ross, Elisabeth, *Death: The Final Stage of Growth*, Englewood Cliffs, N.J.: Prentice-Hall, 1975.

Maguine, Daniel, *Death By Choice*, New York: Doubleday, 1974.

Martin, Harry, "The Stages of Illness-Psychosocial Approach," *Nursing Outlook*, March 1962, pp. 168–71.

Parad, Howard, *Crisis Intervention*, New York: Family Service Association of America, 1965.

Parkes, Colin, *Bereavement: Studies of Grief in Adult Life*, New York: International Universities Press, 1972.

Popoff, David, "What Are Your Feelings About Death and Dying," *Nursing '75*, August, pp. 15–24; September, pp. 55–62.

Quint, Jeanne, *The Nurse and the Dying Patient*, New York: MacMillan Company, 1967.

———, "Awareness of Death and the Nurse's Composure," *Nursing Research*, Winter 1966, pp. 49–55.

Rochlin, Gregory, *Griefs and Discontents: The Forces of Change*, Boston: Little Brown and Company, 1965.

———, "Dying with Dignity," *Canadian Nurse*, October 1971, pp. 31–35.

Schoenberg, Bernard, Psychosocial Aspects of Terminal Care, New York: Columbia University Press, 1972.

Schulz, Richard, "Clinical Research and the Stages of Dying," *Omega*, 5, 1974, pp. 137–43.

Strickler, Martin, "The Concept of Loss in Crisis Intervention," *Mental Hygiene*, 54, April 1970.

8
Hopelessness

Much has been written about love and faith. However, little has been written about hope and hopelessness. Until recently, hope seemed to have had negative connotations. To say a person has hope usually implies that one has nothing else and that one is standing close to the brink of despair. This thought could not be further from the truth. "Hope comes close to being the very heart and center of a human being. It is the best resource of man, always there on the inside, making everything possible when he is in action, or waiting to be illuminated when he is ill. It is his most inward possession and is rightly thought of, according to the Pandora story as still there when everything else has gone."[1]

People realize that no matter how hopeless things may be, they still maintain an element of internal hope. This is probably the most motivating force behind prisoners of war and their families. Each has hope that the other exists. The prisoners have hope that the war will end and that they will be returned to their families. Each family has hope that their loved one is still alive. In spite of the great physical separation and the dismal condition of prison camps, hope still prevails. But hope cannot be achieved alone. Hope must be an act of the community, an organization, or two people struggling together. People develop hope in each other, hope that they will receive help from the other.

Hope relates to things outside of us. If we did not know that hope is related to the outside world and to help, we would all become despondent. People in good health hope for a response from the world, whether they are breathing, working, or in love. Trouble starts when the response is not there. The ill have fewer relationships, and there is more fear for lack of help or response when it occurs. Hope must rediscover the other half of itself, the outside world and the idea of help.[2] While people have hope, they also wish. They hope for a response; this may involve wish-

---

[1]William Lynch, *Images of Hope*, (Baltimore: Helicon Press, 1965), p. 31.
[2]*Ibid.*, p. 32.

ing. The two go hand in hand. If we do not wish for something, then we have no hope in the thing we want. We are then playing games with ourselves, and at times we become apathetic about achieving the thing we originally hoped for. This is particularly true of mental illness.

More has been written about mental illness and its relationship to hopelessness than any other illness, except perhaps for the hopeless feelings of a patient's experiences while dying. Death and dying have gained prominence in nursing literature throughout the last several years. Ross noted in her studies of dying patients that hope was the only thing that persisted throughout the stages of dying. Hope provided these people with strength at a time when they desperately needed it.[3] Nursing should look at other clinical situations and take note of the void regarding the explanation of their feelings of hopelessness.

Little has been written about the hopeless and helpless feelings of the hospitalized patient, regardless of age. When the body becomes ill, one experiences the frustration of hopelessness and helplessness. Both frustrations do not necessarily go hand in hand; they can occur separately. The hospitalized patient can feel helpless about an illness, but may not lose hope in the body's ability to restore itself. There are times when the patient does feel helpless, because a physical or emotional condition may seem so very hopeless. It then becomes the nurse's role to foster a realistic sense of hopefulness. The nurse should try to make the patient responsible for his or her own care.

It is ironic that even with modern technology our bodies still become sick. The only saving factor is that technology allows us to live longer. We now face a dilemma; with all our technology, will we increasingly prolong death rather than life? Regardless of the outcome, we have hope because we know science has progressed and is progressing to unmeasurable limits. We realize that we can accomplish virtually anything we choose. If this is true, then why does the patient still experience hopelessness? What causes the feeling of hopelessness? These are a few of the issues that should be examined from the viewpoint of the patient.

HOPE: HOPELESSNESS AND HELPLESSNESS DEFINED

The greatest hope of the sick is that there is nothing wrong with them that is not wrong with all humans. This becomes the individual's hope, and one might suffocate it while building a too high psychological wall between the well and the ill. The more people push illness out of their

---

[3]Elisabeth Kübler-Ross, *On Death and Dying*, (New York: MacMillan, 1971).

minds, the greater the distance to hope. The individual is subjected to one's own sense of hopelessness. Hope is a sense of the possible, and hopelessness is ruled by a sense of the impossible.

Hope

Lynch defines hope as the fundamental knowledge and feeling that there is a way out of difficulty, and that things can work out. It implies that we as humans can accommodate internal and external reality. Furthermore, Lynch's definition indicates that there are solutions in the most ordinary biological and psychological senses of that word; that, above all, there are ways out of one's illness.[4] Hope gives the individual a sense of security in the knowledge that there are solutions to life's various problems. Sometimes it may seem that the solutions are long overdue, but the patient with hope feels that a solution is possible. The doctors may be deciding which drug or treatment would be of greatest benefit in altering an illness, and many patients trust that their physicians will pick the best one. If the individual did not feel this way about himself and others, that patient would have nothing; no energy.

Wishing and hoping generate a degree of energy. This energy is channeled into desire or motivation to achieve a particular goal or set of goals. The goal for a patient may be simple (to dangle, stand, or sit beside another person) or more complex (to ambulate, run, or communicate with another). Regardless, the individual young or old, has hope that the goal will be accomplished. Absence of energy greatly reduces the patient's sense of motivation. The patient is dominated by feelings of the impossible. The patient has no direction. "Hope, therefore, is energized by belief in the possibility of getting somewhere, in the possibility of reaching goals, the somewhere, the goals, can be as many as the wishes and things we propose to ourselves."[5]

Each of us moves into the future as long as we have hope. For example, we would not brush our teeth after eating unless we had hope of avoiding tooth decay. Apparently hope is something, halfway between knowing and willing, for none of us can know the future or know what will happen if we do not participate in that future. We know from past experience that brushing our teeth limits tooth decay. Our action rests upon our knowledge of the past. Hope is opposed to despair. The individual who despairs essentially gives up, separating from the selfness and peers.

[4]Lynch, *op. cit.*, p. 32.
[5]*Ibid.*, p. 34.

The individual who hopes can transcend the situation, having the inner strength to overcome the difficulty, thus being liberated from the darkness. The sense of hope is that there is a way out. On the other hand, the individual who has a sense of hopelessness believes there is no way out. According to Lynch, "Hope is truly on the inside of us, but hope is an interior sense that there is help on the outside of us . . . the act of taking help from the outside is an inward act, an inward appropriation, which in no way depersonalizes the taker or makes him feel less a man."[6] Hope and help are closely related. There are times when we realize that our own internal resources or strengths are not sufficient to handle or cope with the situation. These strengths must be supplemented from the outside. This need for help is a continuing fact for every human being. Many difficulties make us increasingly more aware of it.

Helplessness

Helplessness is, "the conviction that everything that can be done has been done, which results in an ability to mobilize energy and effort for intervening in illness."[7] Each of us has experienced a moment when we have had a helpless feeling. There may have been a time when we have watched a child run, trip, and fall. Maybe we were only an arm's length away but were helpless to break the child's fall. When an individual becomes ill, he or she feels helpless. The body has lost control and can no longer rely on its own physiological adaptation or homeostatic mechanisms. The body needs external help. Nurses also experience helpless feelings, especially when they watch a patient die and realize that they have done everything possible to make the patient comfortable.

An ill person realizes that there is an inability to help oneself. The person is confronted, at a critical moment, with a medical problem that cries out for help. Although one may be able to help oneself, serious illness or injury obliges the seeking of external help. Sometimes individuals feel both a sense of helplessness and hopelessness; the individual accepts the fact that the disease process or emotional instability is progressive and irreversible and that all efforts to intervene are of no use to either the people in the helping relationship or to the patient. Hopelessness, more so than helplessness, is one of the most difficult areas in which the nurse works, for he or she must try to feel hopeful, no matter how grave the situation.

[6]*Ibid.*, pp. 31–32.

[7]Frank Shea, "Hopelessness and Helplessness," *Perspectives in Psychiatric Nursing*, 2, 1970, p. 32.

Hopelessness

Hopelessness is always appearing in our lives. It will always be with us, to be used in a positive or negative way. If allowed to take over, it becomes an immobilizing monster that incapacitates the individual. In all probability, hopelessness occurs when an individual has experienced emotional or physical suffering for a long period of time. Feelings of hopelessness become manifested at certain times in our lives. At these times, we learn about ourselves and try to channel hopelessness toward a positive end. If not channeled in a positive manner, hopelessness can block any effort to change a situation constructively.

Lynch says, "Hopelessness is rooted in structure of thought, feeling, and action that are rigid and inflexible. They are absolutized and repetitious structures that have become so many traps. If, therefore, one of the central qualities of the hopeless is the feeling of entrapment, a central quality of hope is freedom."[8] Hopelessness involves a number of powerful human feelings. It arouses a sense of the impossible; what a person wants to do or accomplish is beyond reach. One comes to a wall that cannot be climbed. The individual may also experience the feeling of futility. Hope allows the individual to believe in a future. Hopelessness, on the other hand, lacks this central vision, or image, of what could be.

Therefore, "Hopelessness does not imagine and it does not wish. Hope does, but hopelessness does not. It is characteristic of the latter that it does not have the energy for either imaginary or wishing. It is deeply passive, not in any of the good senses of the word, but in its most unhappy sense. Its only fundamental wish is the wish to give up. In a particular situation it cannot imagine anything that can be done or that is worth doing. It does not imagine beyond the limits of what is presently happening."[9]

There are times in life when everything seems to collapse on us at once. Many crises may happen to an individual or family in a limited time. After multiple crises, the individual will say, "I feel like just giving up," or "What's the use, nothing seems to go right anymore." Most persons have enough inner strength to handle each crisis, or crises, even when they occur simultaneously. They maintain a sense of hopefulness that the storm will pass. The hopeless individual not only feels like "giving up," but sometimes actually does. He or she decides that even if one has resources and even if help is available, there is no use, no good, no sense in action or in life. The feeling of hopelessness is a major concern of a nurse. The nurse needs to foster hopefulness, but before doing this must

[8]Lynch, *op. cit.*, p. 63.
[9]*Ibid.*, p. 50.

be aware of how the patient, regardless of age, comes to feel hopelessness in the first instance.

HOPELESSNESS AND ITS CLINICAL APPLICATION

Human beings respond to stimuli from many sources; emotions, physiological state, attitudes, beliefs, perception of others, and environment. Illness itself can be a stimulus. "The hopeless individual is devoid of hope, i.e., he does not strive to solve problems, or cope with difficulties of life, because he does not really believe that any change can be effected. This type of individual usually does not envisage choice or alternatives which are available to him; those individuals who do perceive choice at their disposal usually lack the initiative, or the motivating power, which would enable them to become involved actively in changing their life."[10] The factors influencing the patient's hopelessness fall into two categories. First, there are factors threatening the internal resources of the patient; the illness and the ability to cope accordingly. Second, are the perceptions of the external resources such as the environment and persons within that environment who can help him.

Threats to Internal Resources

Threats to the patient's internal resources involve threats to the sense of autonomy, self-esteem, independence, strength, and integrity. The patient may feel an internal hopelessness if the ability to function is impaired, if the goal of existence is frustrated, or if separated from those one loves. Developmentally, the child, adult, or aged individual each clinically experiences hope and hopelessness in different ways.

The child   The child, since infancy, has been equipped to handle the problem of hopelessness and separation. Separation as an experience takes place initially through physical separation from the mothering figure. Subsequently, separation takes place through play activities with such games as peek-a-boo or hide and seek. The child learns that if one hides, usually in a not too difficult location, one will be sought and found. There is a sense of hopefulness in the outcome. Eventually, the child crawls through the environment away from the mothering figure. He or she is increasing territorial distance away from dependency. However, if

[10]Joyce Travelbee, "Concept: Hope," *Interpersonal Aspects of Nursing,* (Philadelphia: F. A. Davis Company, 1971), p. 81.

the child becomes frightened with this new found independence, he or she copes by crying or demanding behavior. The child has learned that when uncomfortable or frightened in the past, such behavior brought mother to the rescue. Therefore, if separated, the child has hope of a reunion.

Such behavior begins in infancy where need for help is the core of being. "First of all, there is the charm of babyhood, which naturally attracts help. Secondly, children are skilled in demanding. They are indeed demanding in their relationship to help. After all, they have a right to be; they have a right to help, and a right to be angry when its substance is refused. Their hope is a demand, demanding is their way of solving a crucial problem."[11] Therefore, the child's hope is acknowledged and responded to with help. All the child need do is cry and the need is fulfilled. As Lynch said, "His complete helplessness is solved by his complete omnipotence: he concludes that it is only necessary to say an inarticulate word and the world moves about him."[12] As the child continues to grow and develop, he or she learns many things about the self. Hopelessness helps in this self-discovery. Through experimentation with hope and hopelessness, the child learns more about his or her own power and limitations.

Limitations are learned when the child realizes that not all crying or demanding behavior will be acknowledged by a mothering figure, whether a parent or nurse. Illness makes the child aware of certain physical limitations. Crying may not restore a broken bone, lost limb, or diseased body part. Rather, it gains the immediate supportive attention necessary to emotionally cope with the crisis. In time the nurse assesses the patient's behavior for its appropriateness in relationship to the physical-emotional problems. The child may cry because the problem seems hopeless.

Illness necessitating hospitalization may be a new experience for the child. Therefore, the child has no previous experience on which to test internal resources for hoping in the present or future. The only previous experience may have been a cold, flu, or measles. In each instance, the child remained at home, in his or her own bed, and surrounded by the family. Acute illness or injury forces the child to be separated from this home and family. A child with a physical disability, on the other hand, may have spent much time in hospitals rather than at home. The latter child's hope in the future is based upon any present success in the physical being no matter how small it may seem.

A study done by Wright[13] on children with physical disability de-

[11]Lynch, *op. cit.*, p. 59.

[12]*Ibid.*

[13]Beatrice A. Wright and Franklin C. Shontz, "Process and Tasks in Hoping," *Rehabilitation Literature*, 29, November 1968, pp. 322–31.

monstrated their future orientation when answering the question, "What do you hope to be like when you are grown up?" The responses were, "I would like to be a policeman," "a nurse," or "a bachelor." Needless to say some hopeful goals in the future are not realistic. The child's disability (cerebral palsy, crystic fibrosis, or muscular dystrophy) may be too limiting.

Small children without a disability are primarily present oriented. To the child, the future is not necessarily available to be acted in. As a result the child can express hope in future things (when I grow up) because he or she is not concerned with the probable outcome or consequences. The future is too far away and it will be handled through actions of adults. Therefore, the nurse must refer to events in the present framework. Such a child cannot wait until next week for needs to be met. Instead, the child demands that they be met in the here and now. If not, the child becomes temporarily frustrated and hopeless. This becomes significant for nurses working with small children. Lynch points out that, "Frustration of any immediate hope, on the other hand, can throw him into an omnipotent rage, driving him to use still more omnipotent means. He is so absorbed in his own problem, whatever it be, that he cannot be expected, temporary god that he is, to be aware of any reality to save himself."[14]

Children are not always reality oriented as documented by Wright's study. Unlike the adult, the child may have difficulty hoping in the self because "self" is not fully developed. However, as the child grows older these hopes change. Wright believes that, "when the hopes of an older child are challenged by an outsider, reality thoughts are only tenuously forced, for at best the child remains content simply to acknowledge that his hopes may not come true. However, when the young person begins to take charge of his future, then one can expect a more substantive surveying of reality and a launching of the adult hope structure."[15] Adults are more reality based and future oriented whether or not the future is certain.

The adult   The adult might despair when a function is impaired or lost. One may feel that he or she will never be whole again. The adult fears being forced to give up those things vital to the internal being. The adult loses hope in the self and in his or her own internal resources. Normally, the patient who hopes refuses to give up before the inevitable. The patient accepts the situation, and realizes the inability to rise above and beyond it by self-will, knowing that assistance will be coming and that he or she will be helped according to his or her own hope. On the other hand, the patient who despairs will submit to the imminent loss of

[14]Lynch, *op. cit.*, p. 59.
[15]Wright, *op. cit.*, p. 324.

integrity and being. Hope is both future and reality oriented for the adult. Those who hope in the future are somewhat dissatisfied with the present. The ill individual is no different. He or she has the now of the present moment. The task is to use the now as a foundation on which to structure the future. Hopefully this will provide what is desired even though it involves change.

Regarding the adult patient's reality orientation, Wright believes that, "Upon reality surveillance hinges many further complexities of the hoping process. The person surveys reality because he realizes that hopes must have a realistic base if they are to come true. Not only is the person threatened by the prospect of false, but he also recognizes that the actualization of his hopes requires action on his part, action that must be coordinated with reality during the time intervening between the present and the future."[16] The internal biological or emotional resources may be so altered or damaged that action is not immediately possible. Therefore, the future seems dubious.

Take for example those patients entering critical care for various clinical reasons. The cardiac patient who is hospitalized for the third myocardial infarction certainly despairs. The planned future may no longer be realistic or obtainable. The patient who develops acute renal failure necessitating hemodialysis or the individual burned over 50 percent of the body both experience an element of despair in their own way. Furthermore, if complications occur, the patient may lose a sense of hope and quickly submit to hopelessness. The critically-ill patient is not unique in these feelings or behaviors. Other patients with different clinical problems manifest hopelessness.

The nurse must learn to assess the patient's behavior for signs of hopelessness. Such signs may be difficult to recognize or validate because the patient is not always cognizant of his or her own despair and hopelessness. According to Isani, "The manifestations of hopelessness include action, thoughts and feelings in the following categories: actions characterized by a lack of paralysis of intellectual and gross behavioral efforts towards the attainment of a goal, thoughts about the inability to achieve the desired improvements, and feelings of powerlessness to achieve the desired improvements."[17]

An example of this is a study done by Schmale.[18] He studied forty women who on repeated examination discovered they had possible cervical cancer. The presence or absence of cancer was predicted on the basis

[16]*Ibid.*, p. 325.

[17]Rebecca Isani, "From Hopelessness to Hope," *Perspectives in Psychiatric Care,* March-April 1963, p. 16.

[18]Arthur Schmale, "The Affect of Hopelessness and the Development of Cancer," *Psychosomatic Medicine,* XXVIII, 1966, p. 714.

of interview criteria defined as high hopelessness potential and/or recently experienced feelings of hopelessness. Those interviewed expressed feelings of "doom," "the end," or "failure." The study found that their feelings were ". . . experienced in connection with a loss of gratification for which the individual assumes responsibility. There is the associated thought that nothing can be done to overcome or reclaim the lost gratification. Furthermore, since the individual assumes primary responsibility for the loss, there is no expectation that anyone else can provide a solution."[19] In his study, Schmale made thirty-one correct predictions and nine incorrect predictions. Hopelessness need not only be the result of illness but it can also be the cause of illness.

Hopelessness is frequently observed in the schizophrenic patient. Everyone including the schizophrenic lives by hope. Our action in life is based on the hope that by doing something we will get somewhere. We do not always knows where that "somewhere" will be. Even the individual who is hopeless finds hope. The schizophrenic who commits suicide has hope that actions will solve problems. Hope is flexible and does not confine itself to only internal resources. This description of hope makes life tolerable for the patient, "But it would be an intolerable burden for the well or mentally ill if hope turned out to be a rigidly and exclusively interior thing. The sick, who have reached the limit of their interior resources, are often told to hold onto this completely inward kind of romantic hope."[20] The schizophrenic patient assumes that he or she has no internal resources in crisis. The hopelessness revolves around the idea that if internal resources or external help were available, it would be of no assistance. The schizophrenic, therefore, sees no action in life, which becomes the ultimate despair, death. He or she just wishes to give up. One may need to discover the origin of this hopelessness. Lynch believes that ". . . one of the major causes of this interior hopelessness and futility is the inability or the refusal to face all the forms of actual hopelessness as they occur in real life. The hopelessness of the sick comes largely from an overextension of hope, an absolutizing of its range."[21]

The schizophrenic patient is really helpless, functioning within a self-imposed closed system. The system permits the patient to fantasize what he or she wants to see and believe. Therefore there is an inability to imagine what is on the outside of this closed system. "One way of describing schizophrenia is this: a few rigid and absolute categories are set up in the mind to describe and handle reality; when reality is widened, when life introduces some new element, the schizophrenic is unable to reconstruct his managing concepts to the point of adjustments; the result-

[19]*Ibid.*, p. 715.
[20]Lynch, *op. cit.*, p. 31.
[21]*Ibid.*, p. 53.

ing confusions will be proportionate to the amount of unassimilated material from the world and people that thus accumulate."[22] The individual remains in a closed system choosing not to communicate with the surrounding world. The schizophrenic's hopelessness even encompasses communication itself.

Nurses who work in psychiatry frequently observe verbally noncommunicative patients. Such individuals do not see hope in language, in talk or discussion, or in the use of words. They find themselves helpless at putting words or thoughts together to express how they feel. The patient who feels this way withdraws further into this self-imposed closed system. The hopelessness forces the patient to see surrounding events as overwhelming. People in the environment may take an unusual shape and size thus making the patient feel more threatened. Oftentimes, the distorted individuals represent authority figures. If the patient becomes too threatened, he or she withdraws.

Hopefully, the patient can be reached from this feeling of hopelessness before it forces withdrawal. Stotland said that, "Once the individual begins to withdraw, to hallucinate, to communicate poorly with others, to have delusions, there are additional consequences. He perceives that there are difficulties, "sick" behavior, either in himself or in the world about him. He tends to develop schemes of less hopefulness about an improvement in his life situation."[23] The schizophrenic becomes motivated to avoid a hopeless situation. In doing so, the patient creates for himself or herself an autistic world, whereby the significance of surrounding things are reduced. Their reduction leads to a lessening of internal anxieties.

Regardless of the adult patient's clinical problem, there is a time when internal resources become threatened or even totally drained. It is during this traumatic time of realizing one's own emptiness and a need for seeking external help that the patient may experience the most overwhelming period of hopelessness. Illness may evoke within the patient a life-long dread of the vulnerability of the body. The patient may feel that the wholeness is destroyed. The body is in essence quite vulnerable and helpless. In order to feel any hopefulness at all the patient needs to understand the origin of the illness. "The individual's degree of hopefulness about overcoming his difficulties may also be influenced by the way he understands the causes of his illness. He may feel hopeless and despondent if he regards his illness as something that has burst upon him, as a terrible calamity that has been imposed on him by a cruel fate. His perception of his illness in these terms may be derived from a variety of culturally learned sources."[24] Naturally, the patient despairs, realizing

---

[22]*Ibid.*, p. 86.
[23]Ezra Stotland, *The Psychology of Hope*, (San Francisco: Josey-Bass, 1969), p. 153.
[24]*Ibid.*, p. 162.

the vulnerability of the body. But the patient submits to desperation, and loses an important internal resource: motivation.

Motivation plays a significant role in the recovery process. According to Stotland, "Motivation is a positive function of the perceived probability of goal attainment and of the importance of the goal. Motivation is indicated by the organism's acting, either overtly or cognitively, toward the attainment of goals. These actions include attending to and thinking about those aspects of the environment that are perceived as relevant to goal attainment."[25] The patient's goal is a major determinant of motivation. The patient must believe that actions will bring about a result. The patient's goal may be good health, although he or she is realistic enough to know that due to the particular illness, there can never be a restoration to the same previous level of wellness. In this instance, future orientation is reality based. Good health at any level becomes the goal. The patient might be highly motivated to achieve a goal with low expectation of actually achieving it. The goal still has great significance.

As long as the patient's biological illness remains essentially stable, motivation continues. Likewise, the nurse helps the schizophrenic patient achieve a degree of emotional stability. This may include a reduction in the frequency of regressive behavior. As with other adult patients, the nurse helps the individual formulate realistic and attainable goals. Nurses instill within their patients a sense of hope. The hope for goal attainment becomes an internal resource. The goal becomes increasingly more realistic with each positive day or experience. The patient is more receptive to things within the environment that will facilitate attainment of the goal. The patient may become preoccupied with how to obtain the goal of wellness. The individual has a sense of hopefulness in attaining this goal. There are, however, other patients who do not have this same internal positive motivation. Their illness pushes them into the darkened world of hopelessness. Hopelessness becomes most apparent in the aged patient.

The aged   Unlike the child or adult patient, an aged individual lives within the future on a daily basis. An aged patient's future is no longer looked upon in terms of years, but rather days. Therefore, goal attainment is not necessarily getting somewhere but rather remaining somewhere. Depending upon the clinical problem, the aged patient's hope rests in the maintenance or restoration of biological being. Hospitalization with its sometimes threatening diagnostic tests and treatments causes emotional instability.

Nurses frequently see their aged patients become disoriented and confused. Confusion that is unrelated to a biological change becomes possibly the most painful manifestation of hopelessness for the individual. "Confusion is a necessary part of the human but when it passes

[25]*Ibid.*, p. 14.

beyond a certain degree, it tends toward panic and hopelessness. The essence of this confusion in the ill is that people, feelings, and things which should have their own absolute identities, limits, boundaries, begin to dissolve and lose themselves in each other. Instead of helping to create and liberate each other their movement is toward blaming and destroying each other."[26] Confusion serves to make the aged patient's future seem fleeting. The patient knows not where he or she exists either in the past, present, or future. Such behavior further reinforces other feelings of hopelessness; a sense of impossibility.

The aged patient can experience hopelessness as a manifestation of certain power feelings. The internal coping resource although good in the past may be exhausted for future use. Thus, one senses the impossible. What one wants to do can be no longer accomplished. Such goals must remain the responsibility of the young. The patient also realizes that no matter how the biological systems attempt to adapt they will reach a plateau. It is no wonder that the individual feels trapped and hopeless. In addition, the aged individual may be confronted with feelings of "too muchness."

The biological or emotional crisis is too much to handle, especially alone. On occasion, nurses see patients in their 70's or 80's who have attempted suicide. This, then, becomes the epitome of despair and hopelessness. Eventually, if the aged individual's feelings of hopelessness over biological instability or future limitations continue unchecked, this person will submit to futility. Futility is probably the most difficult of all feelings to counteract. It essentially signifies a lack of feeling in general.

Some aged individuals have hope even though they may or may not realize its futility. Take for example the terminally or chronically ill individual who hopes for a cure or recovery. "In such an instance one can say the process of hope is operative; however, the goals of the individual are, barring a miracle, unrealistic and probably unobtainable. The individual who lacks hope perceives no prospect of change or improvement in his life, neither does he perceive a solution to problems or a way out of his difficulties."[27] If the treatment fails, the individual moves into the world of futility. The futility is manifested through statements such as, "Why should I follow the doctor's orders, it won't do any good now," or "It's too late for such treatment." The patient assumes the attitude of what's the use. For this individual, there is no goal or reason to hope in an uncertain future. Therefore, he or she turns the energies toward the present.

[26]Lynch, *op. cit.*, p. 81.
[27]Travelbee, *op. cit.*, p. 77.

Perception of External Resources

External resources are the environment and other people. The people are those who guide and plan the patient's care; the nurse and physician, and the family members or friends. The patient's perception of external resources may be as he or she wants to perceive them. According to Hadley, "Human beings are creatures of hope and are not genetically designed to resign themselves. This characteristic of man stems from the characteristic just described: that man is always likely to be dissatisfied and never fully 'adapts' to his environment. Man seems continually to hope that the world he encounters will correspond more and more to his vision of it as he acts within it to carry out his purposes, while the vision itself continually unfolds in an irreversible direction."[28] Children, adults, and aged individuals may each, in varying degrees, perceive their environments to be threatening.

The child   The hospital environment, although new, different, and sometimes exciting during the day, becomes frightening at night when those most significant to the child leave. The child does not know the strangers within the environment and perceives them in a nontrusting manner. Nurses working with patients of all age groups realize that establishment of trust is the very foundation for meaningful interaction. The child who can trust finds hope in the one trusted. According to Erikson, hope emanates from a favorable ratio of trust to mistrust. The individual learns to hope provided his environment is suitable to the development of this virtue.[29]

The child learns to trust things and people in the environment through the mothering figure. The mothering figure can be either parent and later those who become significant to the child. Eventually the nurse becomes a substitute mothering figure. The child learns basic trust in knowing that help is available as needed. The child has come to learn this through early testing of the parents. The child has knowledge of the trust with them but does not have the same assurance with strangers. Therefore, he or she tests them to see if help outside the "self" is available in time of need and distress. As the nurse passes the "trust examination," the child learns to transfer previous knowledge of trusting from the mothering figure to the substitute, the nurse.

[28]Hadley, "The Human Design," *Journal of Individual Psychology*, 20, November 1964, p. 132.

[29]Richard Evans, *Dialogue with Erik Erikson*, Dialogues with Notable Contributors to Personality Theory Vol. III (New York: Harper and Row, 1967), pp. 12–18.

Hopefully, the child realizes a need for external help. Lynch says, "The child needs external help. He is helpless but not altogether. He has devices by which he calls for help. Let us imagine the statistically normal situation in which to the usual call there is the usual response. A growing sense of the mutual interaction between call and response is part of the growth of hope. If I ask I shall receive."[30] This same framework applies in the clinical setting.

As discussed earlier, the child hopes in the here and now therefore trusting that needs or discomforts will be taken care of now by the one in whom he or she hopes. The nurse realizes that some expectations cannot always be met. The time spent with mother is ideal and those ideal moments are not always found in the hospital setting. Consequently, the child becomes frustrated when desires or wishes are not immediately fulfilled. For example, "Some things and moments begin to produce deep frustration. The child cannot reach the toy, or cannot reach it immediately; but he must, or so he thinks, and at once, so he thinks, but it is impossible, so it seems."[31] Many individuals have experienced the anger that can develop out of this example of hopelessness. Hospitalized adults frequently fall victim to their feelings of frustration.

The adult   The adult patient, depending upon the need for hospitalization, can find the immediate environment to be threatening. The environment around the critically ill patient is noisy and busy. The patient must lie in bed connected to various pieces of equipment such as IV's, a chest tube, an oxygen mask, or cardioscope leads. The patient realizes that each piece of equipment serves a special purpose. Some of the equipment, such as the cardioscope, reassures the patient of being observed, but most of the equipment serves to make the patient aware of how really helpless he or she has become. It also forces one to realize how vulnerable the body is. Now the patient depends upon objects to record, monitor, or maintain body function. Each new piece of equipment makes the patient feel even more helpless and hopeless. The patient feels that death must be the next alternative.

Patients normally assimilate the original treatments or pieces of equipment into being because of perceiving it to be part of the recovery process. The IV's, oxygen mask, Foley, CVP, or cardioscope leads all gain acceptance. The patient hopes these things will be disconnected when the condition stabilizes; at least this is what the people in the environment convey. But if additional pieces of equipment are added while none are removed, the patient may despair at this situation. The patient believes that the body is steadily losing control, necessitating more external en-

[30]Lynch, *op. cit.*, p. 42.
[31]*Ibid.*, p. 58.

vironmental help. He or she realizes that the hospital is the place for help and that if recovery is possible it can only be found there. The schizophrenic, on the other hand, may see the hospital environment as depressing or impoverished, fearing prolonged hospitalization for therapy. If the schizophrenic sees the immediate environment as impoverished, he or she will feel hopeless.

The hopelessness of the schizophrenic within the environment contributes to behavioral changes seen by the nurse. The schizophrenic tends to withdraw from any anxiety-producing situation. This behavior is seen in the seemingly low self-evaluation, poor performance in doing tasks, and in lack of internal ambition to overcome failure. The schizophrenic has a tendency to withdraw from other people. The schizophrenic has been hurt by people in the past and seeks to avoid such pain in the future by withdrawing into his or her own internal world. This withdrawal behavior reinforces the feelings of hopelessness. He alone is incapable of solving the problems. The internal resources for coping are no longer helpful and there are fears of help from outside. Such patients are caught in their own double bind. They want help but are afraid of it. In addition, they fail to recognize meaningful external help because they may not have experienced it in the past. External environmental help for patients in various clinical settings is more than assistance from equipment. It also involves people.

External environmental help comes from both pieces of equipment and people, as supportive devices. Patients in various clinical settings realize that their own inward resources are not always sufficient and that they must be supported from outside. Unfortunately, it is only during crisis that we become acutely aware of this external need. The act of taking help from the many supportive people within one's environment is an inward act. Taking supportive help when available should not make the individual feel less of a significant being. The patient's perception of the nurse and other members of the health team can reinforce or negate this feeling. The health team plays a vital role in determining a patient's hope—or hopelessness. Obviously, there are times when it becomes difficult for the nurse to be anything else but hopeless. The terminally ill, chronically disabled, chronic schizophrenic, or sometimes the critically ill all can contribute to the nurse's feelings of hopelessness. Nurses, like patients, need to see improvement in order to be encouraged in their efforts.

The nurse conveys a personal attitude to the patient and the family. The nurse must remember that, "when the patient becomes the object of the hopeless and helpless feelings of the staff, his hopelessness and helpless feelings about himself become intensified."[32] The hopelessness

---

[32]Shea, *op. cit.*, p. 33.

of the patient's illness or injury may render the nurse helpless. There will be times when the terminally ill, chronically disabled, or schizophrenic patient's condition does seem hopeless. The nurse may feel justified about internal feelings of hopelessness; but if such feelings are communicated, the patient may reach a premature level of emotional standstill. The patient would succumb to a sense of hopelessness in biological integrity, underscored by a perception of hopelessness in the health team guiding therapy. The patient views events internal and external to the being as, "waste of time." If the health team seems hopeful, the patient will also feel hopeful. If the patient has hope in the biological-psychological integrity, the nurse must be careful not to express, verbally or nonverbally, feelings of hopelessness, so that the patient will continue to emotionally strive for a higher level of wellness.

According to Shea, "The fusion of helplessness and hopelessness into an entity results from the fact that when staff members feel helpless about intervening in a patient's illness, they utilize hopelessness as a defense for protecting them from feelings of failure. This response is frequently rationalized by the use of stereotype and diagnostic labels that enable the staff to feel comfortable about ceasing to interact effectively with the patient."[33] Therefore, the nurse could use the feelings of hopelessness as a defense. The nurse assumes that the critically-ill patient with multiple complications will die or the chronic schizophrenic will never change adaptive behavior. The hopeless defense serves to protect the nurse from becoming too emotionally involved with the patient. This is a normal expression of feelings. The nurse may fear that investing too much energy in the patient's care or becoming too close will leave the nurse a void feeling if the patient dies or regresses.

The nurse may need help in channeling energy toward both the patient and the family. The nurse should keep in mind that along with other members of the health team, they are making the patient as comfortable, relaxed, or reality oriented as possible. There are times when the patient's illness reaches stability; however, the mechanical devices decorating the immediate environment or group behavior give the impression of instability. Various supportive equipment or the patient's acting out behavior can discourage the nurse from making personal close contacts on a frequent basis.

The aged   Like critical care patients, the aged realize their need for external help, although they may not acknowledge it until a crisis occurs. Even though society views older individuals as wise, independent, and autonomous, they nevertheless need help. There are times when it is

[33]*Ibid.*, p. 32.

difficult for the aged to seek and accept help. Dependence on others is interpreted as a threat to autonomy and self-esteem. It may be difficult for the aged patient to seek help from an available family member, not wanting to become a burden. The patient therefore turns to members of the health team for support and assistance.

Modern technology takes away some of the nurse's technical responsibility. This may only serve to make the aged patient feel more helpless; after all, the equipment and machines cannot provide motivation and give hope for continuing. These cannot talk to the patient, listen to concerns, answer the many questions, give positive reinforcement, laugh or cry with the patient, or tell of the patient's progress. The aged patient may finally put hope in the machines. The nurse must help the patient seek other ways of maintaining hope, or hope that comes from within and is reinforced by people who help from the outside. The nurse's goal is to instill a sense of hopefulness in the patient, no matter how small it may be.

ENCOURAGEMENT OF HOPE AND HOPEFULNESS

Following the initial crisis of illness, injury, or emotional breakdown, the patient should begin to feel hope and hopefulness in encounters with people around him. These encounters have two dimensions: they involve other patients in the environment and members of the health team.

Pediatrics as an organized unit could be an example for all patient groups. Pediatrics is usually organized according to age groups as well as types of illness. In this respect children or adolescents can each enjoy the other's company because they share commonalities. Other clinical settings are not organized according to age but rather disease or treatments. Critical care categorizes illness according to which part of the body has been altered. No matter where the patient is hospitalized, he or she, in many instances, becomes concerned with fellow patients. Quite frequently, a patient will say to the nurse, "How is Mr. J. today? You know he had surgery the same time I did." Besides demonstrating concern, the patient may be seeking information about himself or herself. The other patient becomes a reference point. The patient is indirectly asking the nurse, "Am I doing as well or better?" In some critical care units, such as burn or hemodialysis units, patients seem to develop an early realization that there are other people experiencing the same kind of injury. When the burn patient sees visual evidence of another patient's progress, a sense of hopelessness or hopefulness increases.

Terminally ill or schizophrenic patients may not always benefit from contact with other patients. The nurse must assess a patient's readiness for other-patient environment. The terminally ill patient who has accepted an uncertain future may support another cancer patient. Likewise, the surgically altered cancer patient can give supportive care to someone anticipating the same or similar surgery. The schizophrenic patient, because of a lack of hope in others and language, may not want to communicate in group therapy. The schizophrenic may feel anxious about failing in the eyes of others, seeking to avoid group activity.

Whenever realistic, involvement with other patients should be encouraged. Another approach in utilizing patient-peer contact is to involve a postoperative patient in the teaching of a preoperative patient. The nurse can certainly instruct the patient from a theoretical level, but it is the other patient who has actually experienced the surgery. This can be a useful technique for open heart surgery patients. Naturally, the one helping must have had a positive experience. Patients can help and support each other on a very practical level.

The nurse can serve as a tremendous motivating force in the patient's environment. Patients in crisis are able to perceive the attitude of hopelessness or helplessness of those providing their care. The patient begins to believe that the nurse has power and ability to help. The patient derives comfort in knowing that the nurse must want to help. He or she has trust in this stranger who is steadily becoming a very important friend. This is particularly significant for the hospitalized child who seeks a mother substitue in the nurse.

The patient, regardless of age, reaches out beyond the self, hoping in others. The patient is the individual who hopes, but he or she must hope in external others, since the internal reserve may have become depleted. Before the patient can truly hope in the nurse, he or she must sense that the nurse hopes that interventions will be effective and that the crisis will be resolved. The patient can then transcend the crisis. Unfortunately, and too often, nurses have a tendency to give up prematurely on a particular patient. We prematurely reach a level of hopelessness when not all avenues of care have been explored. We give up because we feel that the situation is hopeless. Then the patient quite miraculously responds to therapy and gets well, much to our amazement.

All patients need to be encouraged. A frequent source of discouragement becomes the patient's own diagnosis or clinical location. Besides the diagnosis, one is further categorized according to degree of severity: acute or chronic. Depending upon the latter classification, the patient is placed in a critical care unit or general floor. The patient placed on a general floor feels more encouraged than the one placed in critical care. This patient feels hopeful that once diagnostic tests or surgical intervention are completed, he or she will return home. Initially, the critically-ill patient does not have this assurance. Instead, he or she succumbs to feelings of hopelessness if multiple complications occur. The nurse's realistic encouragement is an important aspect of the recovery process.

Patients, particularly the schizophrenic, need encouragement from an authority figure. As an authority figure, the nurse realizes the need to motivate the patient. The nurse accomplishes this by channeling internal energies towards a goal the patient can attain; one that is realistic for the level of biological or emotional illness. The nurse motivates by influencing the internal and external resources.

Motivation refers to action, to doing something rather than doing nothing. That something can be overt or covert; it can entail skeletal, perceptual, or cognitive behavior. Moreover, "motivation refers to the directed quality of the action taken; the organism will choose acts that seem more likely to lead to goal attainment over acts that seem less likely to do so, and it will attend to those aspects of the environment that are relevant either in an instrumental or in a consummatory way."[34] The nurse attempts to reduce the threats the patient feels against internal resources. The nurse simultaneously reinforces the realistic perceptions the patient has of the environment and the people in it. The nurse accomplishes this by becoming a catalyst. He or she attempts to mobilize the patient's positive attributes toward a higher level. In this respect, the patient becomes encouraged to take the first, sometimes unsteady, step toward a goal.

The key word in helping all patients overcome their feeling of hopelessness is goal. The nurse might devise a plan involving degrees of goal attainment from simple to increasing complexity. The nurse realizes that a patient could be highly motivated for a goal of minor significance but of high probable attainment. For example, within two days after a myocardial infarction the patient may be allowed to brush his teeth and wash his face. These are relatively simple tasks that are taken for granted until they are restricted. When the responsibility for such tasks returns to the patient, one senses improvement and feels hopeful. The next day the patient might be given another goal: shaving with an electric razor.

The schizophrenic patient should also be given simple success-oriented tasks. Possibly the most important task lies in the area of interpersonal relationships. If the patient feels a sense of comfort and accomplishment with the nurse-therapist, the process can be transferred to other people. The first goal may be to quietly sit beside another patient and not become anxious. Next the patient may be encouraged to participate in a small group activity (games). The last goal would be to participate in group therapy, first nonverbally and then verbally. The latter goal will not be accomplished quickly but through step by step encouragement if it is

---

[34]Stotland, *op. cit.*, p. 8.

possible. With success-oriented tasks accomplished, the individual's achievement level increases. The nurse should start on a safe level, one that he or she knows the patient can attain. After evaluating the positive or negative effects of the activity, the nurse can create another goal. The nurse realizes that, "hope of attaining a goal and the importance of that goal also influence the organism's affective state. The higher an organism's perceived probability of attaining a goal and the greater the importance of that goal, the greater will be the positive effect experienced by the organism."[35]

As the patient moves closer toward a goal, he or she becomes increasingly motivated. If the patient feels too may goals are to be accomplished before achieving the big one, motivation will diminish. Therefore, nurses should establish goals. An initial goal should be close to the patient's starting point, and it should have a high probability of attainment. As the patient moves toward the goal, the nurse evaluates the positive or negative outcome. If the patient's movement is in a positive direction, then the nurse's intervention has been successful. Then the patient may be ready for more complex goals. Most significant of all, the nurse must follow up on a patient's progress toward goal attainment. For example, the schizophrenic or chronically disabled individual may fluctuate between periods of hope and hopelessness. Either patient needs to be supported and encouraged; however, the decision for continued goal attainment always rests with the patient.

Hopefully the patient has a choice in his or her future. We know that hope is related to choice. The hoping individual, regardless of age, believes in the availability of choices. As the patient hopes, he or she perceives some alteration to the clinical confronting problem. In other words, choices provide the patient with avenues of escape. Even though the choice may not be realistic, the individual has freedom to choose and make a unique decision. The nurse has a tremendous responsibility in helping the patient make the correct choice and decision. The nurse allows the patient to make choices regarding care whenever possible. The patient's biological problem may dictate what choices are available, but the patient might prefer one treatment procedure or measure rather than another.

A sense of hopefulness is maintained through encouragement, motivation, and establishment of a number of small goal-directed interventions. As the patient becomes more hopeful about internal resources, the original feelings of threat will lessen. The patient realizes that the internal resources can be stimulated toward execution of a plan. The nurse creates an atmosphere conducive for goal attainment and goal

[35]Judy Monaco, "Motivation By Whom and Towards What?" *American Journal of Nursing*, 69, August 1969, p. 1719.

satisfaction. The goal must have a high probability of attainment, have meaning to the patient, and should build upon attainment of more complex goals. The nurse can accomplish such a plan only by maintaining the proper personal attitude.

The nurse should maintain an attitude of hopefulness with each patient and family, no matter what the clinical situation may be. Hopefulness is a necessary condition for action, for without this positive attitude, very little can be accomplished. The hopeful nurse is enthusiastic, active, and energetic about the care he or she provides. The patient draws upon this energy in an attempt to replenish the curative outcome; the nurse becomes more involved with the patient.

As mentioned previously, hopelessness can be a defense utilized by the critical care nurse to avoid closeness or involvement. The hopeful nurse enters the situation with this awareness, but will usually believe that it is far better to have actively touched another's life in an attempt to meet needs than to turn away from the patient in a fatalistic manner. The latter approach only fosters guilt feelings and perpetuates a sense of failure. If the patient should go into crisis or die, the nurse feels guilty. Frequently, the nurse might say, "I wonder if I could have done more?"

The activist approach fulfills the nurse, the patient, and the family. The nurse should continue to work in a positive manner. This does not imply that the nurse denies a possible outcome of further crisis or death in a patient; such a concern is constantly present in the nurse's mind. It does imply that the nurse realizes the alternatives and chooses to work in an affirmative direction.

A nurse should trust a patient's will to live. The nurse mobilizes those internal and external resources which will strengthen a patient's will to live. In most clinical situations, the nurse helps the patient look forward to some worthwhile life goal. The patient who hopes does not stop at the momentary crisis. Instead, the patient extends and reaches out to being. In reaching out, the patient must reach toward someone. That someone must share a similar hope. When the patient finds this hope shared by nurses, he or she can be restored to being.

REFERENCES

Fromm, Erich, "Hope," *The Revolution of Hope*, (Chapter 2), New York: Harper and Row, 1968.

Menninger, Karl, "Hope," *The American Journal of Psychiatry*, 1959, pp. 481–91.

Novak, Michael, *The Experience of Nothingness,* New York: Harper and Row, 1971.

Schmale, Arthur, "A Genetic View of Affects with Special Reference to the Genesis of Helplessness and Hopelessness," *Psychoanalytic Study of the Child,* 19, 1964, pp. 287–310.

Travelbee, Joyce, "To Find Meaning in Illness," *Nursing '72,* December, pp. 6–8.

Vaillot, Clemence Madeline Sister, "Hope: The Restoration of Being," *American Journal of Nursing,* February 1970, pp. 268–73.

9
Hostility and Anger

From childhood to adulthood, we find constructive ways of handling anger or hostility. The child uses play to display accumulated anger. Play enables the child to channel energy toward another child in a game like dodge ball or in fantasies like cops and robbers or cowboys and Indians. These activities involve, "great hostility ranging from primitive games in which one is penalized either by being sent back or being estranged or actively physically punished, to the make-believe games such as cowboys and Indians where one may get 'shot' and 'killed.' All these games are acceptable as long as no one is seriously injured."[1]

We have all watched a small child constructing a building out of blocks. Once finished, the child takes tremendous pleasure in its destruction. After deliberately destroying the building by kicking the blocks, the child jumps up and down with great excitement and enthusiasm. The excitement diminishes and the child, once again, gathers the scattered blocks and begins a new building, repeating the cycle several times until tired or bored. To the adult observing this phenomenon, the entire episode seems strange. To the child, the experience has been an acceptable way of displaying anger.

If an adult were to enter into play activity with the child, he or she might discourage the child from destroying the creation. Adults want to preserve their energetic and creative endeavors. An adult's gratification comes from construction, whereas the child's gratification comes from destruction. If a child holds gratification in control, he or she becomes further angered or frustrated. The frustration may be directed toward the adult who unintentionally interrupted normal play activity. The child may hit the adult construction partner, beginning a battle that might end with an angry adult and crying child. The whole incident seems ridiculous, since both people entered the game with different goals and needs.

In adulthood, sports become an acceptable outlet through which

[1]Lee Madow, *Anger*, (New York: Schribner's, 1972), p. 37.

one channels energies. Anger should be converted into something useful or acceptable. The individual who has difficulty finding an acceptable way of directing energies becomes more angry and frustrated. Eventually, a person reaches limits and explodes. Anger leads to violent behavior when the individual becomes blinded by one's own rage. All reason is momentarily lost in a violent act such as rape or murder. According to Madow, "Man is an extremely complex emotional organism. His greatest pleasures in life come from the realistic fulfillment of his emotional drives. If his emotions are mishandled, however, this not only can lead to unhappiness but also may actually interfere with the normal healthy functioning of his body. One of the emotions that can cause the greatest harm is anger."[2]

The hospitalized patient is not immune to these emotions. Like any other person, he or she also becomes angry. The patient resents being sick, limited, disabled, or disfigured. The illness has prevented the patient from doing all the things he or she wants to do. The patient, regardless of age or clinical situation, experiences anger in two ways: first, one expresses anger at the illness; second, the illness creates additional hostile or angry feelings within the individual. The individual may cope with these feelings in one of two ways. The patient may turn the anger and hostility inward or he or she may externalize it by displacing it onto agents within the environment.

DEFINITIONS OF HOSTILITY AND ANGER

Humans are complex emotional creatures. We can experience love and hate for the same object at the same time. Children quite frequently enter into the love-hate emotions with their parents. These emotions continue into adulthood and are transferred from parents to spouse. For example a man may love his wife dearly, but he dislikes it when she tells him, "Pick up your shoes!" The adult realizes that he responds negatively to his wife's behavior, not her personally. Any emotions can be considered potentially destructive. The significance lies in the degree of emotional response. The concepts, hostility and anger, will be defined and then developmentally applied.

Hostility

Horney defines hostility, "as a response to subjectively experienced humiliation. A person finds or thinks that another person does not have

---

[2]*Ibid.*, p. 71.

the expected respect for him. Rather than feel anxiety, he feels and/or expresses hostility."[3] In reality, it is the person who is unable to look within to find respect. Therefore, the patient projects or displaces the blame onto someone in the environment. The patient feels that another individual has become the harmful agent that produced feelings of lowered self-esteem or respect. The outsider, or "harmful agent", becomes the object of the hostility. Hostility can be viewed as the tendency of an individual to harm others or even oneself. Aggression is not always hostile, for it can be constructive. Likewise, hostility is not always aggressively expressed; rather, it can be passively expressed. Kiening states that hostility is an antagonistic feeling; the individual wishes to hurt or humiliate others. The result may be a feeling of inadequacy or self-rejection due to loss of self-esteem.[4]

In many instances, individuals do not realize that they are hostile or angry. The behavior of one individual may initiate hostility or anger feelings in another person. The individual initiating the feeling may be totally unaware of his or her own behavior. This is because each individual displays hostility in a unique way. One person may say, "I am upset," whereas another may react more intently by saying, "I am so mad I could kick down the door." The first individual may be controlling hostility, minimizing the expression of feeling to a simple statement. The latter individual expresses more intensity by putting the hostility into action terms. Both people may be experiencing a similar level of hostility, but each expresses it differently.

Behaviorally it is difficult to assess the degree of hostility present within an individual. It is known that behavioral responses vary from individual to individual. Circumstances evoking hostility in one individual may not do the same for another. An individual who has always enjoyed good health experiences tremendous stress when confronted with illness, especially illness that leads to separation from significant others, limitation, disability, or disfigurement.

There are several factors which lead to feelings of hostility. These include frustration, loss of self-esteem, or unfulfilled needs of status and prestige. The patient's illness, with its forced hospitalization and restriction, causes one to feel frustrated. Self-esteem becomes threatened as the patient is thrust into a forced dependency role. If the patient was a socially prestigous individual who enjoyed self-achievement, there is difficulty accepting dependent relationships with the doctor and nurse. The adult or child of a prestigious family may continually inform members of the health team of his or her social significance and may become hostile when the health team does not respond with awe.

[3]Dorothea Hays, "Anger: A Clinical Problem," *Some Clinical Approaches to Psychiatric Nursing*, (New York: Macmillan, 1963), p. 112.

[4]Sister Mary Kiening, "Hostility," *Behavioral Concepts and Nursing Interventions*, (Ed: Carlson), (Philadelphia: Lippincott, 1970), p. 188.

Anger

Anger can be viewed as a derivative of anxiety. Incorporated in the feeling of anxiety is a sense of powerlessness. Thomas identifies how anger follows a social order of events beginning with anxiety. First, one perceives the anxiety-producing situation as something that can or should be managed through overpowering thoughts and/or actions such as fighting, conquering, or subtly opposing. Next, one blunts or avoids it by transforming the energy created by anxiety into thoughts and/or actions designed to control or disguise one's own feelings and/or to overpower a situation or another person. Last, the degree to which one perceives thoughts and/or actions as being successful influences the degree to which one feels personal security.[5]

Similar to avoidance and denial, hostility and anger can be viewed as normal behaviors within the adaptive process. The hospitalized individual, young or old, moves from shock and disbelief to developing awareness. It is within the developing awareness phase that the patient realizes what has happened. Furthermore, all the anxiety accumulated prior to this time converts to energy. The amount of energy accumulated depends on the degree of anxiety experienced by the patient in the initial crisis. It also depends on the amount of energy output permitted by the patient. In other words, if one actively denied an illness for fear of confronting the threat, he or she may not have realized energy was accumulating. Individuals under stress situations can accumulate only so much energy before it must be channeled constructively or destructively. The excess energy can take the form of hostility or anger.

Anger has advantages and disadvantages. Anger that is turned inward can force the patient into depression. This may impede the patient's movement, temporarily, toward resolving the loss phase of adaptation. Anger that is turned outward may serve to motivate the child, schizophrenic, chronically or critically ill adult, or aged patient. It is as if the patient maintains the idea, "I'll get better in spite of you." Both anger and hostility, within limits, are normal human responses. The fundamental dynamic force behind hostility is frustration. Likewise, anger reveals a sense of frustration in attempting to achieve a goal that has been osbtructed. But the hostile or angry person is too preoccupied worrying about the obstructed goal to think of alternative ways for achieving it. The hospitalized patient, regardless of developmental age, is no exception. The patient daily experiences similar frustration, which leads to hostility and anger.

[5]Mary Thomas, "Anger: A Tool for Developing Self-Awareness," *American Journal of Nursing*, 70, December 1970, p. 2587.

Hostility and anger can affect us physically and mentally. As a form of energy it must manifest itself in some manner. Even repressed hostility and anger will eventually be manifested. It is important to remember that accumulated anger can influence us physically to the point of illness and emotionally to the point of acting out such behaviors as rage or violence.

HOSTILITY AND ANGER CLINICALLY APPLIED

We can view hostility and anger as psychological defense mechanisms. They involve, "an unconscious process employed by an individual in order to obtain relief from the anxiety produced by a sense of danger."[6] Both types of behavior can be found within the developing awareness or accepting illness phase of adaptation. This is the time when an individual who has been defined as ill assumes the sick role. In all probability, the patient has relinquished attempts at avoidance or denial, and recognizes the dependency role. The dependency role arouses feelings of regression and powerlessness that create, sometimes unconsciously, additional feelings of hostility and anger. Besides dependency and powerlessness, the patient is aware of the reality of loss. The degree of loss, whether biological, emotional, or social, may determine the degree of hostility or anger. The patient may have the feeling of losing something of tremendous value.

The loss in terms of illness, disability, or disfigurement creates anxiety within the individual. The patient experiencing illness for the first time is subjected to anxieties associated with the unknown. He or she may not understand what is expected sick-role behavior. Patients whose illness dictates frequent hospitalization experience anxieties of their own. Such a patient may be predisposed toward tension and worry. This patient may have a need for acceptable channels for dependence on others. The repeated illnesses leave the patient confused and uncertain about himself in relation to other people and to life goals. Unfortunately, the patient may interpret the frequency of admissions as diminishing the chance of ever getting well.

Whether hospitalization is a new or frequent occurrence, the patient will feel hostility and anger at some point. This is likely to occur because the patient's integrity has been threatened. Hostility and anger are psychological defense mechanisms that serve to mask the vagueness and powerlessness of anxiety. It is imperative that the nurse identify when the child, adult, or aged parent is experiencing some degree of anger. This

---

[6]N. B. Levy, "The Psychology and care of the Maintenance Hemodialysis Patient," *Heart and Lung*, 2, May–June 1972, p. 401.

behavior may be difficult to recognize. The patient may make verbal and nonverbal attempts to control, attack, or even injure himself. The adult, through childhood experiences, may have learned ways of coping that camouflage true feelings of anger.

Used constructively, anger can provide mental and physical strength. An individual should not be overwhelmed by internal anger. Such anger will immobilize him or her. In addition, the individual should not fear anger. Feared anger leads to its unhealthy expression. Individuals, including patients, should be permitted to express their anger in socially acceptable ways. Hostility and anger can be observed as on a continuum. Behavioral manifestations range from polite behavior to the more extreme form externalized as rage, violence, or murder. Anger which is internalized may be behaviorally manifested as depression or even suicide.

We will discuss hostility and anger as they apply to the child, adult, or aged patient in two ways: inhibited and open expression. A patient who inhibits anger internalizes it, and may express it by indirect means. Open expression of anger appears as an externalized outburst or acting out behavior.

Anger and Hostility Expression
Inhibited: Internalized

There are two general characteristics of inhibited anger and hostility expression. The first characteristic is perception of a threat, and the second is location of the agent of harm.

Perceived Threat

The threat perceived consists of a blow to the individual's view of self. A blow to the self-view takes the form of illness, disability, disfigurement, or removal from significant others. The patient, including the child, may perceive the crisis to be more or less threatening than it really is. "A person's perception of a situation directly determines his response to that situation. If the situation is perceived as threatening, anxiety will result. When personal security is disrupted through anxiety, energy is created and transformed into various types of behavior. Manifestations of anger may be the resultant behavior if the person perceives the anxiety-producing threat as one that can or should be managed through overpowering actions or thoughts."[7]

[7]Thomas, *op. cit.*, p. 2586.

The child   For the infant life begins as a state of bliss. All needs are anticipated and met before the infant has a chance to make them known, via limited means of communication. The infant has only to smile, cuddle, or coo to obtain satisfaction. He or she is totally dependent upon the mothering figure. The infant's goals are satisfaction or comfort. Any discomfort such as wet diapers, hunger, or pain, is communicated through crying. As the small child grows, he or she is forced to become more independent. The child must now feed himself even though the act is sometimes frustrating. Continued growth brings about limitations on immediate satisfaction of needs. The child must learn to satisfy certain needs him- or herself or put them off until a later time. Depending upon the need, this can cause frustration. The child fears that the expression of anger in the form of crying will displease the mothering figure. Therefore, the only threat initially perceived is loss of mother's love or presence.

The latter is significant for the child who must be hospitalized due to illness or injury. If hospitalization occurred from injury such as being hit by a car while riding a tricycle, bicycle, skate board, or motorcycle, the child fears that the mothering figure will be angry. The child may repress feelings of fear and anxiety. The child may be angry over losses; immobility due to fractures and a broken bicycle. However, he or she is discouraged from expressing anger toward the person who created the loss. Discussion of events leading to the crisis displeases the mother. She reacts according to her own fear of what might have happened. The child is forced to repress anger at himself or herself and the driver of the car. Repressed anger leads to anxiety and guilt. The child perceives the threat as a blow to self and integrity. These early experiences with frustration affect coping behaviors in later life.

The adult   Like children, adults who internalize the anger and hostility are turning this excess energy inward. Each has discovered through past and present situations that externalization or expressed anger is socially unacceptable. Both create indirect means of coping with anger and hostility. If such defense or adaptive mechanisms are unacceptable to the adult, that individual may react by escaping. The adult avoids self-feelings, and withdraws. According to Kiening, illness and the circumstances surrounding it are sufficient to cause intense anxiety and/or hostility. The patient is in a position comparable to childhood. In other words, the individual is weak and inadequate in an environment of powerful people upon whom the patient depends. The individual is acutely aware of this dependency and the threat to self-identity posed by the impersonal world of the hospital.[8]

The critically ill patient resents being ill. The patient is prevented

[8]Kiening, *op. cit.*, p. 193.

from doing what he or she wants. Most critically ill patients perceive a threat of loss. The threat involves loss of biological, psychological, and social integrity. Loss of biological integrity affects those alterations in the homeostatic process that result from illness, irreversible pathology, or trauma. In addition, the patient may perceive that he or she is an inconvenience to the family. This causes a threat to psychological integrity. Such threats revolve around loss of independence and self-respect. Patients who make statements such as "I doubt if the treatment will do any good," or "My career is finished," are indirectly expressing feelings of bitterness, hostility, anger, hopelessness, and powerlessness. Threats to psychological integrity suddenly become overwhelming; the patient becomes angry.

The adult who is chronically ill also experiences anger. According to Madow, "The chronically ill may build up anger because they are outside the mainstream and no longer able to get their share of the world's pleasures. They feel they do not matter any more and are of no value either to themselves or society. In addition, they can develop hostility because of the resentment of well people at the burden of the chronically ill."[9] This is particularly true of the chronic schizophrenic who is frequently hospitalized for varying periods of time. Due to feelings of resentment, he or she may not seek help until an overwhelming crisis occurs.

The individual who is exposed to a forced illness, injury, or disability experiences feelings of anger and hostility. Hostility may arise from either anxiety about the illness or the patient's dependency feelings which accompany acceptance of the illness. The basis for hostility varies according to individual mechanisms for handling stressful situations.

Patients such as the critically or terminally ill, chronically disabled, or schizophrenic, experience unfulfilled or obstructed goals. An obstructed goal, whether it be career mobility, watching one's children grow, making a business deal, or planning a vacation, can lead to frustration. Many independent adults with goals and dreams become frustrated when unable to attain them. A goal takes on value when the individual has time and energy invested in it or when it is shared by significant others. The goal's value to the patient relates to the intensity of behavioral response when the plan is interrupted. Consequently, the patient reacts against an obstructed goal, enforced illness, and dependence.

Exposure to a threat of physical-emotional illness or body damage resulting from injury, disfigurement, or mutilating surgery, "tends to sensitize the individual to unacceptable hostile and destructive tendencies in his own aggressive behavior, so that even relatively minor aggressive actions, which are normally tolerated without affective involvement,

[9]Madow, *op. cit.*, p. 26.

are consciously or unconsciously felt to be violations of inner superego standards."[10] Patients who say "My career is finished," "Group therapy will not help me," or "I am going to die anyway so why take the medication," are each unaware that such expressions represent repressed anger. Furthermore, a patient may not realize that anger at being sick.

Madow believes that, "Emotions are repressed because they are unacceptable. Anger may be denied because we feel too guilty about it or are afraid of it. The conflict between the anger and the guilt may be completely unconscious. If we try to bring out those feelings, they may be held in tighter than ever, because they were unacceptable in the first place, and trying to reveal them openly will only increase the resistance to their expression."[11] Repressed or internalized anger can produce physical symptoms such as headaches, backaches, or diarrhea. Furthermore, it is believed that arthritis, skin disorders, hypertension, and coronary artery disease, to mention a few, can be outward manifestations of internalized anger. Anger is also capable of aggravating already existing physical illness. The hospitalized patient becomes angry at being physically ill or disabled, being unable to work, or having insufficient financial help. The patient may feel that it is not masculine to express his anger therefore it becomes internalized.

Anger that is turned inward to the patient's self leads to other behavioral problems. These have significance to patients hospitalized in any clinical setting but are of greater concern to the chronically disabled, terminally ill, or schizophrenic patient. Accumulated anger leads to the clinical problem labeled depression. Depression is sometimes disguised as insomnia, poor appetite, and feelings of hopelessness. The individual may describe himself as worthless, blaming himself for everything that seems to go wrong. The terminally-ill patient becomes depressed realizing that life and therefore goals are coming to a close sooner than ever anticipated. The severely disabled arthritic or neurological patient is depressed over loss of mobility and/or bodily changes. The schizophrenic patient's depression may be his or her only means of coping. Psychologically the patient pulls within, even though wanting help from outside. The patient fears the threat of rejection or failure by others if feelings should be shared.

Repressed anger can become a serious clinical problem; suicide. "Suicide is, in reality, hostility turned inward, an attempt to destroy something within one's self."[12] Therefore, the nurse's goal is to help the patient find acceptable ways in which he or she can act out or externalize anger. The severely depressed patient, regardless of physical or emo-

[10]Irving Janis, *Psychological Stress*, (New York: Academic Press, 1974), p. 54.

[11]Madow, *op. cit.*, p. 108.

[12]Gertrude Flynn, *Perspectives in Psychiatric Care*, 7, 1969, p. 155.

tional problem, who externalizes anger verbally will not destroy himself. Besides repression, regression is also a clinical problem.

It must be remembered that during an illness the patient seems to regress. Regression can be directly related to the meaning and length of the illness. As previously mentioned, illness is a threat to psychological integrity. In certain areas of the hospital (critical care) illness is sometimes magnified. The patient is unaware of the threats to physical integrity. Regression, "in itself is neither good nor bad; in illness it is simply inevitable. It often serves a useful function, but at times it can become an obstacle to recovery. If a busy executive has a heart attack and must go to bed, it should be obvious that he cannot, for the time being, carry on at his previous position. This circumstance is beneficial; it allows for rest and the process of healing."[13] While it may be physically beneficial to the patient, he or she may not, in time, continue to accept the forced dependency. The patient eventually expresses anger or hostility in a verbal or nonverbal manner.

The nurse can facilitate expression of a patient's feelings by helping one to realize that they are normal. Anger serves the purpose of giving the patient a sense of power. This type of power serves to enhance lowered self-esteem. Furthermore, anger stimulates the individual to fight against the obstacle standing between himself and the goal. Whatever the reason, the normalcy of anger should be looked at by the nurse and the patient. The patient needs to know it is normal to feel angry or hostile, particularly when it seems than an illness is not progressing as desired. By helping the patient to see a behavior as normal, the nurse also helps that patient to see it as acceptable.

The nurse should allow the patient to react to a situation even if the reaction is directed toward the only person in the immediate environment, the nurse. Once expressed, the patient must not feel guilty or embarrassed. There are three ways in which the nurse can facilitate expression: allowing the patient to feel as he or she does, explaining behavior in terms of its normalcy, and alleviating any feelings of guilt. The hospitalized patient, either on a specialized unit, such as critical care or psychiatric, or on a general floor, experience relief in knowing that the nurse is aware of how he or she feels and actually encourages communication.

The aged   The aged individual becomes fearful of the future and all the unknown elements it contains. It is as if the aged has become a forgotten member of a youth-oriented society. At the peak of a productive life when one has accumulated great knowledge and possibly status, one is told to retire. Naturally, there are many individuals who look forward

[13]Harry Martin, "The Stages of Illness-Psychological Approach," *Nursing Outlook*, 10, March 1962, p. 168.

to this day. For others, retirement reinforces a growing sense of uselessness, worthlessness, powerlessness, and lowered self-esteem. When one retires one either continues to live in a present location or seeks the companionship of similar others in retirement communities. Some aged individual's physical stamina may not permit mobility. They find themselves alone and unable to care for themselves. Consequently, if not hospitalized, they find themselves in a convalescent home.

The aged individual perceives threats to physical integrity and a sense of worthlessness or lowered self-esteem. If the latter feeling is repressed because one has no one in whom to confide or one senses that no one cares, repressed anger turns to depression. As with the adult, the aged individual's depression can become manifested in the act of suicide. Unfortunately, the suicide attempt may be attributed to confusion or senility, overlooking the real reason for the behavior. The nurse keeps in mind that suicide is not solely a problem for youth or adulthood. It also confronts the aged members of our society.

Agent of Harm Located

The patient may locate what is believed to be the harmful agent; the patient may, in fact, believe that he or she is the harmful agent. Such awareness is enhanced when looking into the eyes of loved ones. The child feels that he or she will lose the love of the mothering figure. The adult or aged individual fears there will be a financial or physical burden for the family.

The child The infant is unable to sufficiently identify objects as being separate from himself. This is validated when one watches an infant play with a soft toy. The first goal is to incorporate it into the mouth as was done with the hand. To the infant the object is merely an extension of the self. In time the infant differentiates between those objects which communicate pleasure instead of pain. The infant learns to turn away from the threatening stimulus or attempts to push it away with the hand. As the infant's coordination develops, he or she is able to physically move away from the threatening stimuli.

With continued growth and development, the child learns what pleases the mothering figure on whom the infant is dependent. Kiening points out that a three-year-old has learned to anticipate punishment from an adult; to protect oneself, the child retreats to a safe area. The child feels weak encountering an authority figure and is discouraged from expressing hostile feelings. The child's unmet needs can lead to hostility in adulthood.[14]

[14]Kiening, *op. cit.*, p. 189.

The growing child learns that the mothering figure insists he do things, once taken for granted, for himself. This leads to restriction of the total freedom which was once enjoyed. The feeling of restriction leads to further feelings of frustration. The resulting anger cannot be fully expressed and as a result it accumulates. Expressed anger displeases those significant to the child. Therefore, for fear of losing the thing valued most, the mother's love and security, the child internalizes anger.

The child who is hospitalized transfers this coping process. The child fears that expressed anger will create feelings of displeasure in the new mothering figure, the nurse. In both instances, home or hospital, the child learns that by creating displeasure in the mother or nurse, he or she has become the harmful agent. Such a realization can be frightening to the child who already may feel a sense of alarm, especially when hospitalized. The child should be encouraged to express frustration before becoming angry or hostile. How the child copes with anger and hostility can determine how one copes with similar feelings as an adult.

The adult and aged   As with the child or adolescent, the adult's self-perception is that of a harmful agent. As mentioned previously, the adult dislikes being either a physical or financial burden on the family. Of course it should be pointed out that some individuals enjoy the sick role and its forced dependency. However, most patients prefer the wellness role and become angry at themselves for being ill, injured, disabled, or unable to cope with their emotional problems. Nurses frequently hear patients say, "My family would be better off without me," "I have been such a burden to my wife," or "I hope my husband remarries when I die." In such instances, the patient internalizes anger and hostility toward the self. The patient may be fearful of exhibiting anger to the staff on whom one depends for care. The internalization of anger may be the result of guilt feelings; the patient may feel guilty for temporarily abandoning a spouse and responsibilities. In addition to internal anxieties, the patient may not be able to cope with external restrictions imposed by the illness and he or she may struggle for independence. Such patients find that becoming dependent upon the hospital staff or family is too threatening.

Internal anxieties may evolve as the patient continues a self-perception as the harmful agent. As a result, the patient uses denial to cope with the anxieties. Physically ill or injured patients, such as those with arthritis, burns, acute myocardial infarction, congestive heart failure, renal failure, CVA, or cancer, are on the verge of being overwhelmed by the threats of their respective illnesses. The anxieties force them to retreat into denial. The schizophrenic patient usually does not perceive himself to be the harmful agent. Rather, the schizophrenic perceives others as the agents of harm. As with patients who are physically ill, the emotional problem creates internal anxieties. He or she may also choose to deny until an overwhelming crisis occurs and denial is no longer possible.

Illness and disability serve to frustrate the individual. One is no longer able to be the principal provider for the family. Besides the restriction of the illness, the role changes that might be necessary serve to bruise an already ailing self-concept. According to Hays, "A blow to the self-view occurs when a person suddenly sees himself more fully, when he grasps the meaning of some dissociated or selectively unattended aspects of experience that are threatening his self-respect."[15] Forced dependency makes the individual, particularly the aged, see oneself as less significant and as a detriment to existing family members. Behaviorally, such an individual may fail to eat, communicate, or follow a doctor's orders. These behaviors demonstrate a lowered self-concept. The patient may unconsciously feel that he or she has minimal social value, so that there is no reason to take care of oneself.

The aged patient may feel that no one really cares or wants to understand, and that there is no help within either the self-system or the interpersonal system. The patient whose body or mind is ill may experience an overwhelming sense of disappointment in himself. As a result, the patient turns the energies inward. It is too threatening to turn them overtly outward; instead, the patient disguises anger. The patient may become negative: "What difference does it make how I feel?" The adult or aged patient may not choose to strike out verbally but may refuse to follow the doctor's orders, showing passive resistance. There are also those patients who can directly express their anger, whether appropriately or inappropriately.

Anger and Hostility Directly Expressed: Externalization

If the patient cannot force the threat away, he or she may express anger overtly toward people in the environment. Nurses, doctors, or even family members can become scapegoats of the patient's anger. In this instance, the child, adult, or aged individual experiences dysfunctional anger. Bowlby states that, "Dysfunctional anger occurs whenever a person, child or adult, becomes so intensely and/or persistently angry with his partner that the bond between them is weakened, instead of strengthened, and the partner is alienated."[16] The external expression of

[15]Hays, *op. cit.*, p. 111.
[16]John Bowlby, *Separation Anxiety and Anger*, Volume II, (New York: Basic Books, 1973), pp. 248–249.

anger and hostility follows a pattern similar to the internal expression of these behavioral responses; first, one perceives a threat; then, one locates an agent of harm.

Perceived Threat

Because society disapproves of outright behavioral expression of anger, the patient may channel anger through demanding or uncooperative behavior. Sometimes these behaviors are perceived as normal or commendable. They represent the patient's attempt to sustain a sense of dignity in an institutional, impersonal setting. Before a person expresses anger directly, he or she must perceive a threat. According to Lazarus, "Anger does not occur unless there is threat. The full reaction of anger and attack with all its motor, affective, and physiological concomitants, requires the presence of threat appraisal. The reaction is then regarded as a process of coping with threat."[17] For the child, adult, or aged patient, the perceived threat may revolve around an unfulfilled or obstructed goal. Depending on the significance of the goal to each age group, the behavioral reaction may be slight or extreme.

The child   An obstructed goal can vary in degree of significance for the young child. Only the child can perceive and evaluate the goal's value. For example, a child might react with anger if unable to watch a particular television program, play with friends, or purchase a new toy. The child might place greater value in a particular television program than playing with friends. These obstructed goals are a part of daily life, and the child eventually becomes familiar with them. Less familiar are the obstructed goals due to illness or injury. The child's goal is to run, play, and ride a skate board; however, a fractured leg temporarily obstructs the goal. Likewise, the child with anemia or leukemia may have similar goals and the energy level does not permit active mobility. The difference between both children is that the latter child's goal may be prematurely obstructed.

Children communicate their anger in a variety of ways. The child's behavioral action may include a variety of responses such as sarcasm, temper tantrum, rudeness, or screaming. These behavioral responses represent both covert and overt manifestations of anger. Initially, the child expresses anger overtly through biting, yelling, spitting, destroying a toy, or striking out at anyone in the environment. These are behaviors frequently seen by the nurse when the child is placed in a threatening clinical situation. The child may be afraid of intrusive procedures or

[17]Richard Lazarus, *Psychological Stress and the Coping Process*, (New York: McGraw Hill, 1966), p. 298.

diagnostic studies. Even a temporary separation from the mothering figure brings about the commonest means of his expression of anger, crying.

The ultimate overt expression of anger is the anger turned inward; the temper tantrum. We have all witnessed the temper tantrum of a child in which he beats himself, rolls around on the floor, and holds his breath. The latter response usually upsets both parents. Of course, this is what the child's anger attempted to accomplish. Fortunately, overt expression of anger such as a temper tantrum is not a usual occurrence for the hospitalized child. Whenever the nurse identifies overt behavior such as spitting, destroying objects, or hitting another child, he or she must assess the behavior's meaning and origin. Only then can the nurse help the child to find other alternative ways of expressing anger or hostility.

The older child has a tendency to manifest anger in less overt ways. The obvious difference between younger and older children is that anger changes from active to passive expression. The older child's behavioral response is that of sarcasm, rudeness, self-centeredness, and negativism. Instead of striking out, the older child chooses not to do anything, thus using active or passive resistance. Passive anger is a difficult behavior for the nurse to break through, especially when expressed by an adolescent. The adolescent is caught between two worlds, one he or she wants and the one he or she is in. The world the adolescent wants contains independence from parental authority. However, insecurity makes the adolescent want to remain in the current world where he or she can be cared for. The hospitalized adolescent is also caught in this dilemma, attempting to show growing independence through sarcasm or negativism. The adolescent's behavior may make it difficult for the nurse to become close and offer security. As a result the tough externalization of covert anger threatens the subtle need for security through dependence.

The adult   Adults, like children, also externalize anger or hostility when a goal is obstructed. The adult's behavioral response can also take the covert form of sarcasm, verbal attack, or rudeness. The adult patient's behavior is often caused by fear and the belief that the self or self-image is threatened. Adults experience a degree of anger or hostility when illness leads to forced immobility or hospitalization. The individual reacts to illness initially with anxiety, which eventually develops to some degree of anger. Lazarus has pointed out that, "high degrees of threat will be associated with tremendous anger, and the intensiy of the behavioral and physiological reaction will reflect the degree of threat. A person may be very frightened or only slightly frightened, and the motor and physiological indicators will also reflect this variation in the degree of threat."[18]

18Lazarus, *op. cit.*, p. 300.

Dependency feelings which accompany terminal cancer, severe arthritis, chronic schizophrenia, chronic emphysema, acute myocardial infarction, or any other debilitating illnesses lead to anger or hostility. It may be that illness obstructs certain goals. For example, a young mother with terminal cancer wants to watch her children grow into adulthood. The executive with chronic emphysema experiences the threat of dependency on a volume respirator coupled with visions of a limited future. These individuals realize that their long term goals of future dreams will go unfulfilled. Regardless of the clinical problem, the factors leading to the biological or emotional crisis are adequate enough to cause intense anxiety and hostility. As with children, the adult may express anger in a variety of ways. Therefore, assessment may be difficult for the nurse.

The schizophrenic patient may have spent an entire life acting out hostile feelings on both a passive and active level. As discussed earlier, the individual during childhood may have been forced to repress anger. It is quite possible that this person never learned appropriate and acceptable ways of coping with anger. Unfortunately, repressed anger which accumulates eventually manifests itself on an action level. For the schizophrenic, the feelings of anger are externalized in crisis. The schizophrenic converts excess anxieties and fears into energy, and the energy must be dissipated externally. When he or she internalizes anger, the schizophrenic feels powerless against threats to biological, psychological, and social integrity. Anger projected externally gives the patient a sense of power. This kind of anger has significance, because it "serves a very useful purpose, if it can be felt and expressed freely, because it usually promotes a pleasant, powerful feeling, which is quite the opposite of the feeling of anxiety for which it is substituted. But it also veils the original threat which gave rise to the anxiety."[19]

Regardless of the patient's illness, anger provides a sense of power that enhances the lowered self-respect and motivates the individual to fight the obstacle interfering with goal achievement. The dream of goal achievement is not unique to children or adults. Aged individuals also have goals they desire to achieve.

The aged   The aged patient is not different from other people who choose independence over dependence. The aged patient has spent more time achieving a level of independence. Forced illness necessitating hospitalization renders the patient powerless, the same type of powerlessness experienced as a child. This alone creates anxiety which can lead to anger centered around altered biological integrity. When aged patients encounter the severe threats associated with their incapacitating illness, disabilities, or disfigurement, "they cannot force their feelings or deal

---

[19]Hays, *op. cit.*, p. 110.

with their interpersonal conflicts without endangering their lives. Their rigid avoidance of changes in their emotional state and conflict tends to perpetuate their emotional and interpersonal problems and increase their frustrations, anger and despair with which, in turn, they cannot manage adequately."[20] Certain forced changes are not always anticipated. Take for example the individual who retires after working all his life. Together with his wife, he has saved his money for the sole purpose of taking long-awaited trips. Suddenly a biological crisis occurs. He has a stroke causing aphasia and partial paralysis. It seems that all his future dreams vanish and what remains is his anger. The goal for which he endeavored so hard is now unobtainable.

Agent of Harm Located

In order for the child, adult, or aged individual to express or externalize anger directly, he or she must identify an agent of harm. It must be kept in mind that the anger or hostility expressed may be displaced onto what the patient believes to be the harmful agent. The harmful agent may only symbolize the true threat. Frequently nurses, doctors, spouses, or parents become the displaced objects for the patient's anger or hostility. They become the individual's scapegoat. Regardless of the patient's age, what he or she fears next to the threat of illness is threat of separation. According to Bowlby, "A period of separation and also threats of separation and other forms of rejection, are seen as arousing, in a child or adult, both anxious and angry behavior. Each is directed toward the attachment figure: anxious attachment is to retain maximum accessibility to the attachment figure; anger is both a reproach at what has happened and a deterrant against its happening again."[21] This reaction to the attachment figure whether to the nurse, doctor, spouse, or parent is due to frustration. There are times, in which, the reaction can affect motivation.

The child The child, while growing older, is no longer considered helpless. Therefore, demands are placed upon the child and he or she must now assume limited responsibility. The new responsibility to self and to the environment evokes threats. The threats coming from the environment are simply reactions to something which the child has done. The child has transferred the previous feelings of himself as the harmful agent to someone or something else in the external environment. The child realizes that if he or she does something wrong it brings disapproval

[20]D. Dudley, C. Wermuth, and W. Hauge, "Psychosocial Aspects of Care in the Chronic Obstructive Pulmonary Disease Patient," *Heart and Lung,* 2, May–June 1973, p. 392.

[21]Bowlby, *op. cit.,* p. 253.

from significant others. The child, through angry behavior, is externalizing hostile feelings. This behavior can be expressed nonverbally as defiant looks at the punishing adult. Another approach is projecting the hostility on the other person by behaving as if the adult was bad. Thus, the child can justify anger. Frequently, in hospital settings, the nurse becomes the other person. When confronted with intrusive procedures or diagnostic studies, the child perceives the nurse or doctor as harmful agents. Therefore, the child may try to attack or avoid them.

The parent who leaves a child alone in the new and threatening hospital environment is also perceived as a harmful agent. Behavioral responses to separation vacillate between anger and love. Separation from the attachment figure for prolonged or frequent periods of time creates feelings of anger. However, the child is so pleased when the parents return to the bedside that he or she expresses love rather than the feelings of anger. The same double bind may exist between the child and the nurse, with neither realizing its existence. True feelings may be accidentally discovered in a play session. A doll may symbolize the child's parents and the child might be found verbally scolding the parent substitute for leaving him or her alone. The parent substitute is less threatening than the attachment figure. Therefore, expressed anger will not lead to love denial.

As with the child who internalizes anger, the nurse must assess meaning and origin of the externalized anger. This is particularly true when anger is directed toward either members of the health team or parents. The child's anger takes the form of reproach toward significant others for having been absent when needed. Only after the nurses assesses the significance of the patient's anger can the nurse skillfully intervene with less threatening means of its external expression. Such external expression might be accomplished through doll playing sessions or through the symbolic language of drawing.

The adult and aged   The adult or aged patient who has had unfortunate experiences with authority figures in the past may become suspicious, hostile, quarrelsome, or angry. Members of the health team become the harmful agent. Similar to children, the adult may either attack or avoid the harmful agent. Lazarus has pointed out that, "the location of such an agent does not permit us to tell whether the coping impulse will be attack or avoidance, since both forms of coping require the specification of an object to attack or to avoid. The kind of harmful agent, on the other hand, is crucial. To the extent that the power of the agent to retaliate against attack is great (when the balance of power strongly favors the harmful agent), avoidance and fear will occur. To the extent the harmful agent is comparatively weak against direct attack, attack will more likely be viewed as a viable coping process. It should be pointed out that overcoming the harmful agent does not necessarily eliminate its capacity for harm; otherwise, if it can be easily overwhelmed, there would be no appraisal of threat in the first place."[22]

To the patient, whether in biological or emotional crisis, the doctor and nurse may come to symbolize the illness itself. This behavioral response may help to lessen some of the personal disappointment consequent to having an acute illness, severe disability, serious disfigurement, terminal illness, or emotional crisis. The individual may feel justified in feeling anger or hostility, but may not be able to demonstrate anger overtly toward the staff. The patient may fear that if he or she expresses outward anger toward the nurse or doctor, they may retaliate by not providing proper care. They may symbolize an agent of harm too powerful to overcome, but a family member, one perceived to be comparatively weak as a retaliation, may be next in line to accept the patient's display of anger. The patient may feel safe in verbally attacking a spouse because his or her role is "to love me no matter what I do or say." The adult or aged patient's behavioral response is an attempt to drive the anger-provoking object away. In this case, the object is illness and its obstruction to goal attainment.

The patient may choose to attack the agent of harm, the nurse, because the nurse is the most dominant individual in the patient's environment. The nurse may not be too accepting of these outbursts. The nurse will probably feel he or she has done nothing to warrant such a behavioral response. If the nurse fails to recognize the meaning behind a patient's anger, the nurse may feel hurt. Furthermore, the nurse may become as angry as the patient, only he or she may not overtly or verbally express it. Instead, the nurse may express anger nonverbally through avoidance behavior by reducing the time spent with a patient. If the nurse responds with overt anger, the patient's anger may increase to the point of threatening the biological integrity. The nurse who reacts overtly or covertly to a patient's angry or hostile response may reinforce the patient's displacement of the origin of the problem toward the health team.

NURSING INTERVENTION: ENERGY MOBILIZATION

The nurse must be able to recognize anger or hostility and explain its meaning to the patient regardless of developmental levels. The nurse must be able to identify overt and/or covert signs of angry or hostile

[22]Lazarus, *op. cit.*, p. 300.

behavioral responses. For example, the child, whose need for growth and autonomy are threatened, acts in a mature way when taking a stand for himself. The child is being difficult to others but to the nurse the behavior is necessary for this particular individual.

Adults may react in the same manner. An adult may find that he or she is being subjected to various diagnostic studies and has never been told the results. The patient finally reaches a level of intolerance and refuses to participate in further studies until he or she is respected as a human being and provided with information. As with the child, the nurse perceives the behavior to be appropriate for the clinical situation. On the other hand, a schizophrenic patient who throws an ash tray at another patient is not demonstrating appropriate expression of anger. It is possible that the anger is justified; however, the manner in which it is expressed is not. Therefore, the nurse must help the schizophrenic channel this excess physical energy into verbal externalization of anger toward the other person involved.

What the patient says and does may covertly camouflage real feelings. What he or she says overtly may serve to make the nurse defensive, thus forcing the nurse away from the individual he or she seeks to help. In facilitating a patient's movement toward resolving the loss phase of adaptation, the nurse must remember two significant factors. First, all behavior is meaningful and goal-directed. Second, anxiety converts into energy, which is subsequently expressed as anger. The anger felt by the individual can serve as a motivation.

Nursing responsibilities consist of helping the patient channel internal energies into appropriate external expression of feelings. As previously mentioned, the patient can be given permission to feel and express anger. The nurse helps the patient, regardless of age, find alternative ways of expressing anger. The externalized anger might be expressed on one or two levels. First, the patient may be encouraged to externalize anger on an action level. For the child, this might involve working with clay in an attempt to dissipate excess energies which could be converted into anger. The clay is nonthreatening and makes no demands upon the child. In addition, the patient might become involved in doll-play sessions and through role playing act out fantasies or anger. Likewise, the schizophrenic patient may need to channel excess energies into sports such as those seen in day-night units. These include volleyball, basketball, or baseball. Here the ball becomes the object of the anger rather than a member of the health team or other patients. The above sports involve little physical contact which might lead to aggressive acts if the patient has accumulated anger.

Other adult or aged patients may need to externalize their anger on the second level, the verbal level. Aggressive action level is an unobtainable goal for the critically ill, terminally ill, or even some chronically disabled aged patients. Therefore, failure on an action level might further increase feelings of powerlessness and worthlessness, thus contributing to their frustration. Consequently, the nurse encourages verbal expression of anger and hostile feelings. The nurse intervenes by helping the patient identify angry feelings and the possible reasons why these feelings arise. Talking together can be one constructive way of appropriately channeling energy that might otherwise be converted into anger. When the adult or aged patient finds appropriate channels for direct expression of anger or hostility, he or she no longer needs to feel guilty for having such behavioral reactions to the stress of illness.

Patients who internalize or externalize their anger or hostility are actually directing their feelings toward a perceived threat; illness, disability, disfigurement, or emotional crisis. The clinical problem, whether cystic fibrosis, leukemia, chronic renal failure, eclampsia, or schizophrenia, threatens the patient's sense of biological, psychological, and social integrity. The basic nursing intervention is to recognize the patient's behavioral response. For example, a patient may say, "I am disappointed," "I am frustrated," or "So go ahead, no one is stopping you." Such statements are covert examples of a patient's anger or hostility. Because the patient may be unable to express anger overtly, it is repressed. Repressed anger can seriously aggravate already existing threats to biological integrity. The nurse must acknowledge the patient's behavior. In so doing, she or he communicates concern and willingness to help. The patient may respond by silence or angry outbursts. Regardless of the response, the nurse must be prepared to accept the patient as is and continue to meet his or her needs.

The significant point is that the nurse recognizes that a particular problem exists. The patient may be unable to express problems concerning personal fears known only to him. The once highly independent individual has difficulty accepting loss of control, power, or independence. To be dependent upon others both frustrates and threatens psychological integrity. Take for example a male patient who is dependent upon hemodialysis. His perceived threat is directed toward his machine. His dependency on a hemodialysis machine and his inability to work may make him resent the fact that his wife must assume the financial responsibility. Patients, in general, sometimes react to the stress of illness, disability, disfigurement, or emotional crisis by withdrawing. When this behavior is assessed, the nurse should provide stimuli to help the patient externalize his ideas or feelings. Just as the nurse recognizes the need to give a patient relief from physical pain, he or she should also acknowledge," the need for allowing the patient to ventilate his feelings in order to help him come to grips with the meaning of emotional pain. This assists him to focus on himself as a 'person' rather than a 'victim' who must survive both his crisis and the strange world of a hospital."[23]

After the nurse recognizes the meaning of a patient's behavior, he or she should help the patient understand its meaning. Beyond assessing the meaning behind anger or hostility, the nurse must assess a patient's readiness to look more closely at a threatening situation. The nurse's goal becomes that of reducing threats perceived by the patient. The nurse should reduce the perceived threat and help the patient look realistically at threats of loss. The nurse can help the patient identify alternative ways of coping with the stress of illness and aid in fulfilling goals. The patient realistically needs honest reassurance that he or she is reaching biological or psychological stability. The patient must be assisted in identification of internal strengths and assets. With support and positive reinforcement, the patient may come to realize that not all future goals are unattainable.

Nurses must realize that not all behavior can be changed. The chronic schizophrenic patient may not want to change behavior because it would imply discharge from the protective or secure hospital setting. The aged individual has difficulty changing behavior simply because change is not one of his or her idiosyncrasies. A patient who recently sustained a severe myocardial infarction realizes the consequences of the illness and the imposed medical restriction. Nevertheless, the patient might continue to enjoy heavy smoking, eating, or strenuous work. These decisions become his and his alone.

The nurse can serve as a catalyst or motivator toward meaningful change. The nurse must also remember that a restorative solution to the problem may not exist. In other words, a patient may be so biologically decompensated that he or she will never achieve stability or a level of wellness. The nurse will not be able to help the patient look at role changes or dependency-independency behavior. The nurse's responsibility may be to help the patient accept the terminal aspects of an illness. In doing so the nurse listens to what the patient verbalizes. The nurse must be prepared to accept direct anger and hostility generated by introspection and intervene to constructively channel the patient's externalized energies.

Anxiety converts into energy. An individual can only accumulate a certain amount of potential energy. It must be released sometime and in some direction, and the release may create problems. Overt expressions of anger may create biological problems for the patient. The patient with a

[23]S. P. Davidson, "Nursing Management of Emotional Reactions of Severely Burned Patients During the Acute Phase," *Heart and Lung,* 2, May–June 1973, p. 371.

decompensated pulmonary or cardiac system cannot tolerate prolonged expression of anger. The potential depletion of stored energy may compensate the individual's ability to perform limited functions. The nurse must therefore establish limits for externalized anger or hostility. By setting limits, the nurse reduces guilt feelings resulting from overt anger expression. Rather than feeling a sense of relief, the patient may feel even greater tension. The patient, particularly the schizophrenic patient, might project guilt feelings onto the nurse thinking he or she was responsible for the behavioral response. Therefore, the nurse must assess those clinical situations in which limits must be set and controls established.

All patients need help in recognizing that their energy outbursts are really anger and hostility. The first step toward understanding and mastering this behavior is for the patient to admit anger. Next, the nurse should assist the patient to identify why he or she is angry. Third, the nurse can help identify the target of the anger. It may be threatening for the patient to admit a loss of behavioral control in becoming angry or hostile. The patient may feel guilty or embarrassed. At this point, he or she needs reassurance that being angry or hostile is a normal adaptive response to illness. If the patient's anger or hostility was displaced on the family, he or she will have to explore reasons why such displacement occurred. This is most important, because a family relationship can become badly damaged. A family member may have become defensive and in the process say things that only serve to hurt the patient. It is conceivable that a fatal complication could occur, thus leaving the family member with memories of their last angry encounter. Such behavior leads to overwhelming guilt. Therefore, the family needs help in understanding the patient's needs. The nurse turns both his or her own energies and those of the family toward motivating the child, adult, or aged patient.

The nurse is in a unique position to assist both the patient and the family. The nurse should learn the reasons behind behavioral responses. The nurse assesses behavior, helps the patient to assess its meaning, and motivates the patient to find appropriate ways of channeling energy. The nurse must keep in mind that a patient who is critically, chronically, or terminally ill may not reward the nurse by becoming symptom-free; he or she may continue to complain of discomfort after all the staff has done. These patients, especially the disabled or terminal, may lack warmth and the capacity to relate. Occasionally one finds a patient who relates only on a hostile or angry level. This patient may never move beyond this level because he or she has successfully coped, using such behavioral responses, in the past. The nurse should support and reinforce the patient's positive attributes. Regardless of behavior, the nurse should acknowledge, understand, and try to motivate the patient toward the affirmative.

REFERENCES

Ammon, Louise, "Expressions of Hostility in Early Labor," *Maternal Child Nursing Journal*, 2, Fall 1973, pp. 215–20.

Baker, Joan and Estes, Nada, "Anger in Group Therapy," *Journal of Psychiatric Nursing*, January-February 1966, pp. 50–63.

Brooks, Beatrice, "Agression," *American Journal of Nursing*, 67, December 1967, pp. 2519–22.

Jaeger, Dorothea and Simmons, Leo, *The Aged Ill*, New York; Appleton-Century Crofts, 1970.

Maier, Norman, "Frustration Theory: Restatement and Extension," *The Psychological Review*, 63, November 1956.

Richter, Dorothea, "Anger: A Clinical Problem," *Nursing World*, December 1958, pp. 22–24.

Robinson, Alice, "Anger," *Journal of Practical Nursing*, 2, July 1971.

Schoen, Eugenia, "Clinical Problem: The Demanding Complaining Patient," *Nursing Clinics of North America*, 2, December 1967.

Suggs, Kathryn, "Coping and Adaptive Behavior in the Stroke Syndrome," *Nursing Forum*, 10, 1971.

10
Space and Territoriality

Historically, in hospitals, interest and concern with space has been limited to determining whether a patient had enough closet or drawer space for his or her belongings, or if there was enough storage space for linen, equipment, and sterile supplies. Space, or the growing decrease of space, is a concern to those responsible for urban development. To conserve space in our crowded cities, we have witnessed the rapid development of high rise apartments. The newer high rise apartments are actually cities within cities. Everything an individual might need is contained in one building. This is tremendous for the older individual who is unable to venture away from home territory. However, more active individuals may begin to feel that they no longer have a personal space or territory. In other words, one lacks territorial ownership, as he or she may not even own the apartment. Efficiency of space and territorial conservation, both in the hospital and community, can actually lead to intrusion into the individual's space and territorial bubble.

In our Western culture a, "relationship between physical and social territory is frequently evident; the amount of space a person has is often related to his personal importance or economic status. For example, a large home on a double lot is generally symbolic of high income and status."[1] Therefore, if a patient has a private room in a hospital, this has some financial significance. On the other hand, there are patients who find themselves in a private room because their terminal illness bothers other patients or because they are confused and noisy.

In the midst of unpredicted affluence and technological sophistication, most members of our culture encounter unnecessary and extensive conflict in their day-to-day interaction with the man-made environment. The discipline of environmental design is committed to the resolution of such conflicts, to the realization and maintenance of appropriate, viable man-environment relationships. The design should be environmentally

---

[1]Margaret Pluckhan, "Space: The Silent Language," *Nursing Forum*, 7, 1969, p. 393.

conducive for the patient's well-being. While man-made environments may be monotonous and unstimulating, they may simultaneously be viewed as chaotic and overstimulating.[2] The routines in various hospital units may be monotonous to the patient; however, the environment may be noisy and overstimulating. Current design of hospitals has taken color into consideration as a pleasant stimulation. The colors are soft and relaxing. Curtains and carpets can be added to hospitals in an attempt to provide a pleasant visual stimulation.

TERRITORIALITY, SPACE, AND PRIVACY DEFINED

People who have studied territoriality have attempted to conceptualize its behaviors in two main ways: as a geographic or spatial phenomenon and as a behavioral phenomenon. For the purpose of applying territorial and spatial concepts to patients, it is best to view territoriality primarily as a behavioral system. According to Carpenter, "the drives and incentives or motives, and the sensory-response and learning process are all different aspects of the behavioral systems of territoriality."[3]

Territoriality

McBride believes that territories are fixed geographical areas which are maintained and defended against intrusion by other members of the same species, and are important in mating, feeding and nesting behavior.[4] Stea further states that with man, "territorial behavior reflects the desire to possess and occupy portions of space, and, when necessary, to defend it against intrusion by others. A distinction also needs to be made between territorial units of individuals, territorial clusters, and territorial complexes involving multiple people, as well as stationary and moving territories."[5] Pastalan indicates that, "a territory is a delimited space which an individual or group uses and defends as an exclusive preserve. It involves psychological identification with the place, sym-

[2]Raymond Struder, "The Organization of Spatial Stimuli," *Spatial Behavior of Older People*, (Ann Arbor: University of Michigan, 1970), p. 113.

[3]C. R. Carpenter, "Territoriality: A Review of Concepts and Problems," *Behavior and Evolution*, (New Haven: Yale University Press, 1968), pp. 228–29.

[4]Leon Pastalan, "Territorial Behavior in Humans: An Analysis of the Concept," *Spatial Behavior of Older People*, (Ed: Pastalan and Carson), (Ann Arbor: University of Michigan, 1970), p. 3.

[5]*Ibid*.

bolized by attitude of possessiveness and arrangements of objects in the area."[6] Hall believes that territoriality is, "behavior by which an organism characteristically lays claim to an area and defends it against members of its own species."[7] Hall also maintains that territoriality is a basic behavioral system characteristic of living organisms, including man, which evolves in the same way as anatomic structure evolved. He further believes that every living thing has a boundary which separates it from its external environment. A nonphysical boundary exists outside the physical one. This new boundary is harder to delineate than the first but it is just as real; it is called the organism's boundary.[8]

Functions of territoriality In the animal world, territoriality offers protection from predators, and also exposes to predation the unfit who are too weak to establish and defend a territory. One most important function of territoriality is proper spacing, which protects against overexploitation of that part of the environment on which a species depends for its living. Territoriality is also associated with status. Man exhibits territoriality and has invented many ways of defending what he considers his own land.[9]

Component parts of territoriality For application to various patients, territoriality is best viewed from several perspectives at once. Lyman[10] has suggested a multifocal meaning of territoriality involving four types of territories. The components consist of body territories, interactional territories, home territories, and public territories. Each of Lyman's component parts of territoriality will be examined in terms of their application to patients, regardless of age or clinical setting.

Whatever theory of territoriality is utilized, as we, "stand in line for coffee, in a tow line on the ski slopes, or in the supermarket check out line, we realize that the recognition of territorial rights is one of the most significant attributes of our civilization. We may even become concerned when someone's cigar or cigarette smoke floats into our air."[11] This has significance in determining the compatability of patients who share rooms.

[6]*Ibid.*, p. 4.

[7]Edward Hall, *The Hidden Dimension*, (New York: Doubleday and Company, 1966), p. 7.

[8]Barbara Minckley, "Space and Place in Patient Care," *American Journal of Nursing*, March 1968, p. 511.

[9]Hall, *op. cit.*, pp. 9–10.

[10]Stanford Lyman, "Territoriality: A Neglected Sociological Dimension," *Social Problems*, p. 237.

[11]Pluckhan, *op. cit.*, p. 390.

Space

Though individual territory and personal space are often viewed as being equal, the two can be differentiated in several ways. Personal space is that space that surrounds us at all times. Territory is relatively stationary and usually much larger in area. An individual, whether hospitalized or at home, will, "delineate the boundaries of his territory with a variety of environmental props, both fixed and mobile, so that they are visible to others, while the boundaries of personal space are invisible, though they may sometimes be inferred from self-markers such as facial expressions, body movements, gestures, olfaction, visual contact and voice intonation."[12]

The concept space has been defined as "room to move about in" and "room to put our bodies in." In and of itself it is a nonentity, but in relationship it has the power to convey meaning. It is essentially that nothingness which exists between "self" as the point of departure and some object or person perceived in the world "out there."[13] According to Beck, "Imminent space is inner, subjective space, the space of unconsciousness, of dreams, of fantasy; it includes the spatial styles and orientation of the individual, and the ingrained spatial notation systems of whole cultures. This is the basic space imposed upon us by the anatomy of our bodies. Consequently, it is also the space involved in the image of our body."[14] Each individual has what is referred to as personal space. This is the area immediately surrounding an individual. The area serves as a body-buffer zone in interpersonal transactions.

Space, then, is seen as sensible space; it has significance according to the purpose for which it is sought and the conditions under which it is experienced. Space becomes adequate if it allows for privacy. The determinants of spatial adequacy, both in its isolation and difference dimensions, lie in part in the nature of the space and in part in the individual and the constraints on his activities.[15] Stea says that, "When space is held collectively by men, their behavior regarding it greatly resembles the behavior of animals defending their individual territories. Hostility is

[12]Leon Pastalan, "Spatial Behavior: An Overview," *Spatial Behavior of Older People*, p. 212.

[13]Pluckhan, *op. cit.*, pp. 386–87.

[14]Robert Beck, "Spatial Meaning and the Properties of the Environment," *Environmental Psychology Man and His Physical Setting*, (Ed: Proshansky, Ittelson, and Rivlin), (New York: Holt, Rinehart, and Winston, 1970), p. 136.

[15]J. Sonnefield, "Variable Values in Space and Landscape: An Inquiry into the Nature of Environmental Necessity," *Journal of Social Issues*, 22, 1966, p. 74.

overt and socialized individual patterns of aggression in men are collectively released."[16]

Privacy

According to Pastalan, privacy may constitute a basic form of human territoriality because of its unique human behavioral state. Privacy may be defined as the right of the individual to decide what information about himself should be communicated to others and under what conditions.[17] From this basic definition, Westin elaborates on the relation of the individual to a social group, stating that privacy is the temporary and voluntary withdrawal of an individual by physical or psychological measures.[18]

Functions of privacy The first function of privacy is personal autonomy. A basic human need is autonomy or the desire to avoid manipulation or dominance by other people. Illness thrusts individuals into a dependent role, one in which they must passively submit to the desires of others. Therefore, the individual's sense of autonomy becomes threatened when intrusion into one's privacy occurs. Patients, depending upon the nature of their illness, may be manipulated, intruded upon, or forced to momentarily live with the decisions made by members of the health team. In this respect, their personal sense of autonomy may feel threatened.

The second function of privacy is that of emotional release, the safety-valve effect. This becomes a major problem for those patients in critical care. Patients who experience their own stress and environmental stress need the opportunity for privacy in order to find emotional release. With the door or curtains pulled making the atmosphere private, the patient can tell the nurse what he or she thinks about the care, food, doctor, or illness.

Privacy is always associated with the management of bodily functions. The bathroom is usually the only place in one's home offering privacy from intrusion. Surveillance of such bodily functions by outsiders is practiced with social approval in hospitals. As much as possible, how-

[16]David Stea, "Space, Territory and Human Movements," *Landscape*, Autumn 1965, p. 13.

[17]Leon Pastalan, "Privacy As An Expression of Human Territoriality," *Spatial Behavior of Older People*, p. 89.

[18]Dorothy Bloch, "Privacy," *Behavioral Concepts and Nursing Interventions*, (Philadelphia: Lippincott, 1970), p. 252.

ever, the nurse should make the surveillance without intruding upon the patient.

The third function is self-evaluation. According to Pastalan, "Every individual needs to integrate his experiences, into a meaningful pattern and to exert his individuality on events. To carry on such self-evaluation, privacy is essential. At the intellectual level, individuals need to process the information that is constantly bombarding them, information that cannot be processed while they are still on the go."[19] A further influence of privacy on self-evaluation is its role in the proper timing of the decision to move from private reflections to a more general publication of acts and thoughts.

The last function is limited and protected communication. It provides the individual with the opportunities needed to communicate confidentially with those he or she trusts, such as nurse, physician, spouse, or minister. Withdrawal into privacy also provides psychological distance. The need for privacy can be nonverbally communicated through facial expressions, bodily gestures or body parts, and others. Verbally the patient may change the subject of a conversation.[20]

Degrees of privacy   The four degrees of privacy are solitude, intimacy, anonymity, and reserve. All four apply to patients, regardless of their age or clinical setting. Solitude as a state of privacy occurs when an individual is separated from the group and freed from the observations of other persons. For example, the isolation patient or patient at the end of the hall in a private room both experience solitude. Solitude may be difficult to attain in those more active areas within the hospital, such as critical care, emergency room, or pediatrics. Solitude in and of itself is the most complete state of visual privacy that individuals can achieve.

The second degree of privacy is intimacy, in which the individual is acting as part of a small unit and is allowed to exercise seclusion. Typical units of intimacy are husband and wife, parents and children, extended family, friendship cycle, or work clique. Whether close contact brings released relations or abrasive hostility depends on the personal interaction of the members, but in that intimacy, a basic need for human contact can be met.

Anonymity, the third degree of privacy, occurs when the individual is in a public place but still seeks, and finds, freedom from identification and surveillance. As a state of privacy, anonymity has less application to hospitalized patients. The individual attempts to merge into the environment or landscape. Such is the case when a prestigious individual is quietly admitted into the hospital. Consequently, one can retreat into a private room and maintain a sense of personal anonymity.

[19]Pastalan, "Privacy," p. 91.
[20]*Ibid.*, p. 92.

Reserve, the most subtle state of privacy, is the creation of a psychological barrier against unwanted intrusion. This arises when the individual's need to limit communication about himself is protected by the willing discretion of those surrounding him. The manner in which individuals claim reserve and the extent to which it is respected or disregarded by others is at the heart of securing meaningful privacy.[21]

As the definitions of territoriality, space, and privacy indicate, every living thing has a physical boundary that separates it from its external environment. There is also a nonphysical boundary which exists outside the physical one. This new boundary is harder to delineate than the first but is just as real. No matter how crowded the area in which the patient temporarily lives, he or she tries to maintain a zone or territory around self. No one knows exactly how much space is necessary to any individual. The amount of personal space needed by each individual varies. Spatial need is dependent upon emotional and physical status, cultural background, and position in the community. The significant question is what happens to the child, the schizophrenic, the adult patient in a critical care unit, or those individuals living in overcrowded conditions when their space or territory is threatened or intruded upon.

APPLICATION OF CONCEPTS TO PATIENTS:

Body Territories

According to Lyman, "there are body territories, which include the space encompassed by the human body and the anatomical space of the body. The latter is, at least theoretically, the most private and inviolate of territories belonging to an individual. The rights to view and touch the body are of a sacred nature, subject to great restriction."[22] The infant learns body territories or boundaries through contact with the physical world. Beck states that, "The infant's active exploration of his physical environment—pushing, pulling, grasping, thrusting—endows space with a primitive concrete meaning. But the infant passes through stages of involvement with different kinds of space. At first, the baby is placed on his stomach (facing down), then on his back (facing up). In the crawling stage, the infant lives in the horizontal plane—his line of sight and mode of exploration are highly uniplanar, action occurs toward and away from objects at his own level of height."[23] The infant, by crawling through this horizontal environment, learns things about the body. The

[21]*Ibid.*, p. 90.
[22]Lyman, *op. cit.*, p. 241.
[23]Beck, *op. cit.*, p. 136.

infant becomes aware of the different pleasures or displeasures obtained from feeling various textures on the hands and knees. In addition, as the infant crawls from room to room, he or she increases spatial distance from the security of the mother.

Beck continues to point out that, "Later the child raises his head, and eventually stands up; he enters the space of the vertical plane—up and down become coordinated, right and left gain more freedom. As the child structures space and forms object relations, innumerable spatial connotations develop."[24] The schoolager's spatial experience, both horizontal and vertical, contributes to ego spatial development. Ego space becomes the child's adaptation of observed to objective space, to produce a logical view of sizes, stages, and distances. Later, the adolescent's territorial and spatial development includes social distance. As the adolescent grows emotionally, spatial distance moves further away from significant ones, such as parents, toward peers.

Ego space becomes a problem for the schizophrenic adult patient. He or she sometimes has difficulty differentiating body territory or boundary from the boundaries of those in the surroundings. The realization of the self is intimately associated with the process of making boundaries explicit.[25] DesLauriers believes that, in the development process of delineation and demarcation the first step is to identify the physical limits of the person's body. The corporal ego feeling is the sensation of the whole body, not only of its weight, but also of its size, extension, and sense of fullness. In schizophrenia, the ego breaks down and ceases to exist as a psychological structure when the conditions necessary to its existence are absent. The schizophrenic person does not experience a relationship to an object and cannot relate to reality because he does not experience himself as real, that is, bounded, finite, separate and differentiated from what is not himself.[26]

The schizophrenic patient may have difficulty realizing where his or her body territories end in relationship to those in the immediate environment. The patient may touch another patient or therapist thinking that the part touched was an extension of his or her own body. The behavioral response can indicate that the patient's own self-concept or body image is not clearly defined in the mind. Yet at another time, when the patient's body territories or boundaries are coherent and consistent, touch becomes a spontaneous means of nonverbal communication. The patient who has difficulty identifying one's own body territories needs

[24]*Ibid.*

[25]Hall, *op. cit.*, pp. 10–11.

[26]Austin DesLauriers, "The Psychological Experience of Reality," *Chronic Schizophrenia*, p. 280.

greater space in which to move. According to Hall, when the boundaries of self extend beyond the body, patients refer to anything that happens within their flight distance as taking place inside themselves.

The aged individual's body territory boundary may be limited due to normal physiological changes associated with the aging process. "Being characterized by a decreasingly sensitive sensory apparatus, one might say that their sensory channels are typified by a greater degree of interference, or that the noise level relative to the information level is increased. Either way, their sensory contact with their social and spatial environment is diminished and they must negotiate that environment with reduced information."[27]

The aged individual is aware of body territories or boundaries. The body image, although changing, is well defined in the mind. The exceptions would be those patients experiencing a stroke resulting in neurologic deficit, loss of a limb, or a sensory impairment resulting from glaucoma or cataract. They must now incorporate a loss. The stroke patient sees the affected limb, but touching it does not elicit feelings of ownership; the limb has no feeling. Therefore, the patient feels it does not belong to him or her. Of course, once the crisis stabilizes and physical therapy begins, the patient, through involvement, becomes reattached to the affected body part. Many aged patients, although aware of their body territories, have difficulty with spatial navigation. The sensory-motor feedback system is less accurate and efficient then that of younger patients. Therefore, the body territories need to be defined according to the objects within the immediate physical environment.

It was stated earlier that the right to view and touch the body is of a sacred nature. Yet the patient, regardless of age or severity of illness, relinquishes the privacy of his or her own body. Shortly after admission into the hospital, the patient's body is explored, manipulated, or intruded upon. Granted the adult patient can maintain a degree of control through refusal to sign consents for intrusive procedures but failure to compromise and submit could greatly hinder the patient's progress. Therefore, the patient complies. Intrusion or manipulation is more likely to invoke the critically-ill patient. Nevertheless, intrusion occurs in varying degrees to all patients.

Intrusive procedures or supportive devices connected to the affected body part make the individual more aware of its temporary or permanent loss. Lyman states, "Body space is, however, subject to creative innovation, idiosyncrasy, and destruction. First, the body may be

[27]Alton DeLong, "The Micro-Spatial Structure of the Older Person: Some Implications of Planning the Social and Spatial Environment," *Spatial Behavior of Older People*, (Ed: Pastalan and Carson), p. 83.

marked or marred by scars, cuts, burns, and tattoos. In addition, certain of its parts may be inhibited or removed without its complete loss of function."[28] Therefore, body territories can be altered due to illness or extended through various pieces of equipment which support the affected body part. Intrusion into the individual's body territory can be a threatening experience in and of itself.

Depending upon the severity of the patient's illness, the intrusive procedures happen quickly. The patient has very little, if any, time to recover between tests and examinations. Subjected to numerous and sometimes repetitious procedures, it is not surprising that the child becomes frightened and the adult becomes angry. Normally, "in every individual the readiness to fight is greatest in the middle of his own territory; it is there he has the greatest chance of winning."[29] This possibility explains why some patients become angry about various admitting or diagnostic procedures. Children become angry or combative out of fear. Possibly the adult has the same fears, though unable to openly express them. Eventually, most patients react by quietly submitting to the intrusion, perhaps because, "when a man's territorial defenses are weakened or intruded upon his self assurance tends to grow weaker."[30] Not only does the patient feel intruded upon by procedures, the patient also feels intruded upon by the health team and environmental props. Environmental props associated with hospitals include the IV poles and bottle, respirator, cardioscope, commode, and others.

Interactional Territories

Interactional territories refer to any area where a social gathering may occur. Surrounding any interaction is an invisible boundary, a kind of social membrane.[31] The mother-child interactional territories are close ones. While being breast fed or simply held, the two interactional territories overlap or integrate into one. It is during the close interaction that basic needs of security, love, touch, and food are being fulfilled. Beck points out that, "Meaning is derived from a satisfaction of needs, needs which have spatial qualities. Food-objects, tool-objects, danger-objects, pleasure or love objects acquire special significance for the child. Mother is too close or far away and food is consumed (put inside or spit out.)"[32]

[28]Lyman, *op. cit.,* p. 242.

[29]Mickley, *op. cit.,* p. 511.

[30]Julius Fast, *Body Language,* (New York: M. Evans and Company, Inc., 1970), p. 53.

[31]Erving Goffman, *Behavior in Public Places,* (New York: Free Press of Glencoe, 1963), pp. 151–165.

[32]Beck, *op. cit.,* p. 136.

The child's first interactional territorial experience is with mother. The success of this encounter permeates other relationships, including the relationship to father. The young child makes a claim of boundary maintenance around self through the clustering of "his" or "her" toys. The child does not share them with other children. If someone invades the boundary, thus temporarily disturbing the cluster, the child displays great displeasure at the invasion. Initially, children parallel play with each other, thus protecting and maintaining the safety of their clustered objects. In time, as trust is established, the child learns to share toys and the closed territorial unit becomes an interactional one. The child moves towards social interaction.

The aged individual's interactional territories may not be as mobile as those of younger people. Nevertheless, many aged people maintain social intercourse through group activities. The individual's personal circle of friends becomes constricted due to the death of loved ones. Many aged individuals maintain the desire for social interaction with others and extension of their territories into the territory of others. Social interaction helps to lessen the pains of loneliness. On the other hand, some aged individuals seem to revert back to periods of solitude, in which interactional territories become constricted to self. In other words, his interactional territories constrict.

Lyman's belief is that, "Interactional territories are characteristically mobile and fragile. Participants in a conversation may remain in one place, stroll along, or move periodically or erratically. They may interrupt only to resume it at a later time without permanently breaking the boundary or disintegrating the group."[33] Interactional territories become a problem for schizophrenic patients. Horowitz believes that, "Measurement of personal space, the area immediately surrounding an individual, demonstrates its reality and its function as a body-buffer zone in interpersonal transactions."[34] As discussed earlier, the schizophrenic patient may have difficulty realizing his or her body territories. Therefore, the schizophrenic seems to require more interactional territory or boundaries than the normal individual.

Horowitz and his associates studied both schizophrenic and normal persons, observing their sensitivity to physical closeness. They were concerned with the first distance at which discomfort became conscious enough so that the subject preferred no further closeness. They termed the area defined in this way the body-buffer zone and found that schizophrenics were more sensitive to physical closeness than normals. Thus, they concluded that the schizophrenics have larger body-buffer

[33]Lyman, *op. cit.*, p. 240.

[34]Lt. Mardi Horowitz, "Body-Buffer Zone Exploration of Personal Space," *Archives of General Psychiatry*, 2, 1964, p. 651.

zones.[35] The nurse-therapist who works with schizophrenic patients may observe spatial maneuvers of the patients. The patient moves toward the therapist until both territories overlap and then moves backward, thus separating both territories once again. This phenomenon can be explained dynamically, structurally, and developmentally. Dynamically, this behavior appears to be directly related to a decrease or drastic reduction of narcissistic cathexis of bodily boundaries, which leaves the schizophrenic person psychologically undifferentiated and somewhat boundless. Structurally, the patient may be unable to experience a relationship with an object, namely the therapist. Developmentally, the schizophrenic condition can be described as a dramatic representation of a level of behavior where the various psychological functions are undifferentiated, unintegrated, and lacking goal-directedness and true reality value.[36]

Home Territories

Home territories are areas in which the participants have a relative freedom of behavior and a sense of control over the area. Home territory can also be referred to as a territorial unit. When the individual leaves the territorial unit because of illness, two other behavioral characteristics of space become evident. Stea believes that, "The first is personal space defined as a small circle in physical space, with the individual at its center and a culturally determined radius. The second is the territorial cluster, enclosing those people (or other territorial units) frequently visited and the paths taken to reach them."[37]

The hospital room becomes the patient's new home territory or territorial unit. Some patients, depending upon their biological crisis or social status, may require or request greater space within their territorial unit. We must also keep in mind that the hospital itself is a territorial complex with each specialty unit, general floor, diagnostic, or service department representing a separate cluster. Those individuals whose condition is too critical or disturbed may remain in their territorial unit while representatives from the various diagnostic or service clusters come to their bedside to collect pertinent data. The individual who is able to leave the territorial unit will move into the hospital cluster that corresponds to his or her diagnostic needs. The passage through the various clusters is analogous to moving through the various rooms of a house or home territory. The only difference is that the patient may not feel a personal attachment to each hospital cluster as with the home. If personal

[35]*Ibid.*, pp. 651–56.
[36]DesLauriers, *op. cit.*, p. 280.
[37]Stea, *op. cit.*, p. 14.

security is possible within the hospital, the patient finds it in his or her own territorial unit.

Regardless of the patient's age, the territorial unit is the patient's crib, bed, or room. It must be kept in mind that territorial units are man-made, designed environments. As designed environments, they may not always have the patient's interest in mind. Instead, they are designed for the efficiency of the health team. According to Struder, "Designed environments are systems of energy and matter interposed between humans and ambivalent forces in the impinging macroenvironment."[38]

All patients observe some sense of territoriality, whether learned or instinctive. Furthermore, it becomes important for the individual to maintain an element of control over his or her immediate space. For some patients such control is not always possible or realistic, for example, the critically-ill patient who enters a territorial unit in biological crisis and is unable to lay territorial claim. The critically ill patient is unable to lay territorial claim by hanging up clothes in the closet, finding the bathroom or urinal, pacing off the size of the unit, or placing personal belongings in a night stand. Because of the seriousness of the biological status, the patient enters his or her territorial unit on a stretcher which may be three feet wide. The patient is then moved from the stretcher to the bed by two or three nurses who lift this patient into the new territory. The patient is unable to get a spatial feel for this new territorial home, not even the width of the bed.

Once the patient is lying in bed, the side rails are immediately raised to ensure continual safety. Most patients are connected to a cardioscope so that the cardiac pattern can be evaluated for rate, rhythm, and regularity. The various tubes or wires that are inserted or connected to the patient may further limit mobility in bed, thus making the patient dependent upon one portion of the total spatial claim of four feet. The patient's sense of privacy is temporarily, sometimes permanently, lost. The patient's body, like those of most patients, is poked, percussed, probed, and generally intruded upon in an attempt to assess and diagnose his problem. In addition, various environmental props might become necessary and are placed in the patient's territorial unit. Such environmental props as the arterial line, central venous pressure, oxygen tubing, IV tubing, Foley catheter, nasal-gastic tube, volume respirator, and/or cardioscope support the fact that the patient is sick. Such hospital props serve to restrict the patient's territorial unit. The patient may feel surrounded by a shroud of equipment.

Intrusion by members of the health team or hospital environmental props diminish the patient's sense of privacy. Privacy is important to

[38]Struder, *op. cit.*, p. 102.

most individuals, no matter where they are. The nurse should remember that there are some cultures in which privacy has less significance than in Western culture. Nevertheless, the nurse should assess its meaning to the patient for whom he or she cares. Barton points out that, "Every patient, no matter how sick he is, needs some privacy and a place he can call his own where he may store his personal possessions. After all, man, like other animals, has territorial instincts."[39]

The territorial unit has an orienting effect for the aged patient. Davis believes that the effects of unfamiliar territory are more rapidly induced in the elderly and more profound, leading to temporary states of confusion, anxiety, and disorientation.[40] Familiarity of the territorial unit is achieved by the aged individuals in one of two ways. First, if possible, he or she can ambulate through the environment thus laying territorial claim. If not possible, the nurse can verbally claim the territory for the patient by explaining where personal belongings are located within the territorial home. Second, the aged patient achieves familiarity within the environment by placing personal environmental props. It is not unusual for the nurse to find environmental props such as glasses, purse, pictures, favorite pillow, sweater, tissues, address book, and even a piece of toast wrapped up from breakfast, in the patient's bed. Each prop has a certain space within the total territory of the bed and room. We who are determined to be professionally neat nurses have a tendency to remove these props in order to straighten the bed or simply to get them out of our way. If we do this, then the older patient may find himself bounded by a spatial world that works against the establishment of personal and social identity.

Another territorial characteristic of the aged patient is the tendency to collect many small objects, more so than with other patients. The nurse may find the night stand, like the bed, cluttered with various objects or props. "The pattern of cluttering is very important in the organization of space for the elderly, and at the risk of sounding ludicrous must be one of the critical elements for achieving an ordered space. A cluttered spatial environment satisfies, not too surprisingly, most of the structure-points so far uncovered that the elderly use in environmental transaction, providing for: heightened peripheral visual stimulation, increased tactile involvement, greater kinesthetic awareness, and a sense of closeness so important in interpersonal transactions—by reducing the distance between objects to little more than an arm's length."[41] Therefore, instead of

[39]R. Barton, "The Patient's Personal Territory," *Hospital and Community Psychiatry*, 17, 1966, p. 336.

[40]Robert Davis, "Psychologic Aspects of Geriatric Nursing," *American Journal of Nursing*, 68, April 1968, p. 802.

[41]DeLong, *op. cit.*, p. 86.

straightening out the night stand and putting objects away, the nurse could be much more therapeutic with the elderly by simply leaving the stand cluttered.

To cope with the environment within their territorial unit, the aged patient appears to depend upon quite different sensory information than do other patients. For example, the aged appear to pay more attention to information channeled through the peripheral receptors of the eye, which magnify movement. Therefore, since many aged have impaired vision, they have difficulty visually assessing the span of their territory. When possible, the boundaries of territory should remain reasonably constant. The territory is in every sense of the word an extension of the organism, which is marked by visible and invisible territorial markers. It is important to note that once the aged patient's territorial unit is established, changes within it may not be easily tolerated. Lorenz discovered in his studies that innate behavior mechanisms can be thrown completely out of balance by small, apparently insignificant changes in environmental conditions.[42] Adjustment and adaptability to change are greatly reduced in later years.

Most hospitalized patients have a territorial unit or space of their own even if it is shared between two (semiprivate) to four (ward) other patients. The psychiatric patient is the exception, having to share a territorial unit with between ten and thirty other patients. Needless to say, the patient sharing space with one other patient may have a greater sense of ownership than the patient who must share a space with ten to thirty patients. The latter really does not feel a sense of personal ownership to the territory in which he or she finds their physical being. According to Colman, "It is striking how often the hospitalized mental patient and the prisoner do not have a home of their own. If it is true that these people with least potential for social adaptation are in most need of territorial strengths, then not having a home is a circular dilemma. They have lost (or never had) the skills to build one, yet its absence deprives them of the supporting structures they need."[43]

Like the critical-care patient, the psychiatric patient needs a space or territorial unit of his or her own. Such space should not be shared by other patients. However, the design of many psychiatric facilities or units is geared to economize space rather than to facilitate the inhabitant's sense of identity. It has been stated that, "To deprive a person of a space of his own is, in a very real way, to deprive him of part of his identity."[44] Space

[42]Konrad Lorenz, *On Aggression*, (New York: Harcourt Brace and World Inc, 1966), p. 46.

[43]Arthur Colman, "Territoriality In Man: A Comparison of Behavior in Home and Hospital," *American Journal of Orthopsychiatry*, 38, April 1968, p. 467.

[44]DeLong, *op. cit.*, p. 83.

and privacy provide the patient with a feeling of autonomy and individuality.

Public Territories

Public territories have limited application to the hospitalized patient. Public territories are those areas within the hospital cluster that might not be used by the patient, but rather the family. Such areas are the family waiting room, coffee shop and/or cafeteria. Besides these areas, the family also has access to the patient's territorial unit. Children under the age of fourteen are the exception. They may not have access to the territorial unit in which a mother, father, sister, brother, or grandparent is hospitalized. According to Lyman, "Public territories are those areas such as parks, roads, etc. where the individual has freedom of access, but not necessarily of action, by virtue of his claim to citizenship. These territories are officially open to all, but certain images and expectations of appropriate behavior and of the categories of individuals who are normally perceived as using these territories modify freedom."[45]

USE OF PROXEMICS IN NURSING INTERVENTIONS

The nurse has a primary responsibility for early detection of territorial deprivation and territorial disorientation, so that he or she may either prevent its occurrence by manipulating environmental stimuli, or help the patient to adapt better to the new environment. The relationship between space and a feeling of freedom has potential therapeutic significance. "Spatial changes give a tone to communication, accent it, and at times even override the spoken word. The flow and shift of distance between people as they interact with each other is part and parcel of the communication process."[46] A less dramatic approach, "is the nurse's everyday use of space as a message system to convey her attitudes and intentions to the patient. For example, support may be given to a patient who is feeling isolated and estranged by moving closer. On the other hand, the patient's personal space must be respected and no unwanted intrusion made."[47] A willingness to be somewhat close spatially conveys

---

[45]Lyman, *op. cit.*, p. 237.

[46]Edward Hall, *The Silent Language*, (New York: Doubleday and Company, 1959), p. 160.

[47]Mardi Horowitz, "Human Spatial Behavior," *American Journal of Psychotherapy*, 19, 1965, p. 27.

the message of a desire to be close in other human-to-human transactions. Such a desire or message may serve to quiet the restless and agitated patient as well as to support one who seems to be withdrawn.

Man's sense of space has a bearing on the ability to relate to other people, to sense them as being close or far away. The anthropologist, Edward Hall, has coined the term proxemics and identified four distance zones commonly used by people; intimate, personal, social, and public.[48] Little points out that, "For a given individual each of the zones (intimate, casual-personal and social) has quite stable boundaries although they may fluctuate depending upon the immediate situation. In a subway during the rush hour, for example, one's zone of intimacy extends to his outer clothing, no further. Personal space may thus be considered as a series of fluctuating concentric globes of space, each defining a region for certain types of interaction."[49] The nurse working with patients can specifically use all but public distances.

Intimate Distance

At intimate distance, the presence of the other person is unmistakable and may at times be overwhelming because of the greatly stepped up sensory inputs. Sight, olfaction, heat from the other person's body, sound, and feel of breath all combine to signal unmistakable involvement with another body.

There is a close and far phase of intimate distance and the nurse who provides direct patient care moves between them. Because the nurse does technical procedures, involving touch, to the patient, he or she has territorially entered into an intimate distance, close phase. Children, particularly infants, require their nurse to use the intimate distance zone. The hospitalized child frequently needs to be held, fed, and diapered. The nurse may spend most of the time intervening in the intimate distance zone.

Use of the intimate distance may be threatening to the schizophrenic patient. Even though the nurse-therapist does not bodily touch the patient, physical presence may nevertheless be viewed as intrusive. Therefore, touch might be misconstrued as an attack. Consequently, the nurse may use only the personal and/or social distance. Of course there are occasions, when appropriate, that the nurse-therapist will need to touch the patient. Such touch intervention is in the context of support.

The nurse has become accustomed to forcing his or her presence on the adult patient at those times which best suit the nurse's schedule. For

[48]Pluckhan, *op. cit.*, p. 393.

[49]Kenneth Little, "Personal Space," *Journal of Experimental Social Psychology*, 1, 1965, p. 238.

example, it is traditional to bathe a patient in the morning. The patient, however, may normally take a bath in the evening. Therefore, the nurse needs to be flexible and together with the patient decide upon a time that meets the patient's needs, not the nurse's. Also, the patient may have had a difficult or sleepless night with many intrusions into the territorial unit. Consequently, the patient wants to sleep rather than be further intruded upon with a bath. The nurse may choose to give the patient a relaxing backrub to help reduce tension so that he or she might sleep.

The close phase of intimate distance involves touch and manipulation of the patient's skin. This can be reassuring and pleasurable to some patients. Again, the bath is a good example. If the nurse is unhurried in approach, he or she can use this time to talk with the patient, get to know the patient as a person and not do the bath just as a task but attempt to evoke relaxation. Touching the burned patient's skin might not be viewed as pleasurable, but associated with pain.

If the nurse makes frequent intrusions upon the patient's intimate territory, he or she may react with hostility or anger. The patient, regardless of age, is cognizant of the nurse's intrusive behavior. It is significant for the nurse to keep in mind that at intimate distance, the presence of the other is unmistakable. When the nurse starts an IV, takes blood pressure, or inserts a Foley catheter, he or she has territorially entered into an intimate distance-close phase. Since the readiness to fight is the greatest in the middle of a person's own territory, the patient must be verbally prepared before the nurse enters into the intimate-close phase territory in order to prevent aggressive behavior from the patient. The nurse must also assess the appropriateness of frequent intrusions upon that territory. Rather than intruding into the patient's territory uninvited, it is wise for the nurse to ask permission to enter.

Intimate distance is most effective when applied to the aged patient. According to DeLong, "Intimate-personal transactions among the elderly are characterized by very high levels of sensory involvement. The inner boundary is at a point inside the skin, and the outer boundary falls at the distance of an extended forearm. Body orientation is generally at right angles or greater, with a side-to-side orientation not at all uncommon."[50]

Because the aged patient's sensory process may be limited, the nurse should intervene by moving into the patient's intimate territory. Through intimate distance, the patient is able to see, hear, and touch the nurse. This becomes important to the aged patient who is hard of hearing, has poor vision, or has difficulty ambulating. As with the adult, the intimate zone involves touch. It seems that the aged patient, more than other patients, relies heavily on tactile involvement; the nurse should use touch, and then the nurse and the patient's territories overlap. Because

[50]DeLong, *op. cit.*, p. 72.

touch has significance to both people involved, it may not be seen as intrusive. Important ways of using touch are: (1) ambulating the patient with arms around him or her, (2) combing the hair, (3) shaving the patient, (4) putting lotion on the feet, or (5) simply holding one's hand.

In addition, the intimate distance-far-phase is also useful when working with aged patients. This distance zone is approximately 6 to 16 inches. At this distance the aged patient is able to see, touch, and hear the nurse. This is imperative for the aged patient who has loss of hearing or loss of vision. The aged patient is able to touch the nurse and know the voice is connected to a body. Also, the close phase offers the aged patient a feeling of security and protection against harmful stimuli. This may well serve to meet needs for belonging, for closeness to a human being who has become significant. Of course, this is true of all patients regardless of age, but it seems most appropriate to those individuals like the aged with sensory loss. At the close phase, the nurse is able to touch the patient in an effort to convey warmth, caring, and understanding.

All patients need time to adjust to their new home territory or territorial unit. During the initial adjustment phase, the nurse may intervene verbally to orient the patient to spatial and territorial surroundings. If the patient appears to be relatively stable after admission, the nurse talks to the patient. The nurse attempts to give the patient an opportunity to recover psychologically before proceeding with any intrusive procedures. When possible, the nurse may include the patient's family in the orientation process. By orienting the family and patient simultaneously, the nurse saves time; time that could be better spent with the patient. In addition, family inclusion gives the nurse a chance to assess the family relationships, what further teaching may be needed, and their level of anxiety. The family has a much more positive feeling toward the hospital cluster, and more specifically the territorial unit, if they are initially included and told of the staff's expectations of them. While the family and patient are together, the nurse may spend time taking a brief nursing history. While obtaining the nursing history, he or she can take the time to explain some of the unit's routines, and together with them decide how the patient can fit into that routine.

Personal Distance

Personal distance is the distance consistently separating the members of noncontact species. It might be thought of as a small protective sphere or bubble that an organism maintains between itself and others.

Personal distance-close phase is a distance of 1½-2½ feet. At this distance, one can hold or grasp the other person. Where people stand in relationship to each other signals their relationship, or how they feel toward each other, or both. For example, the nurse working in isolation may choose to stand in the doorway and talk to a patient rather than putting on a gown in order to move into personal close distance. By standing in the doorway, the nurse has nonverbally communicated that he or she does not have the time or interest to enter into the patient's territory.

It is at the personal-close distance that the patient can reach environmental props located on the nightstand. However, if the patient's condition is serious, as indicated by the presence in the critical care unit, he or she is not allowed to reach the night stand, which is territorially his or hers, because this activity increases the demands on an already compromised biological system. Environmental props should be arranged on top of the night stand for all patients. In this respect the patient can see pictures of family, glasses, cards, or flowers. Infants can have mobiles hung over their cribs. Children can place their favorite stuffed animal or blanket nearby if not in bed. The various environmental props may be the individual's only reminder of home. Nurses should encourage the family to bring environmental props from the patient's children or grandchildren. Patients who have children or grandchildren enjoy receiving drawings which can be taped to the wall. This reassures the patient that he or she is not being forgotten.

The nurse can give the patient's spouse something from the hospital for the children or grandchildren so that communication between the two continues. In addition, the nurse must remember to keep the patient's nightstand close by rather than pushed out of reach in an unobservable corner. If the patient cannot reach the night stand due to the seriousness of illness, he or she may request that environmental props be placed in bed.

It is at the personal-close distance that the nurse can sit beside the patient and talk. If either patient or nurse choose to touch the other, it can be accomplished. By sitting within the patient's personal territory, the nurse is communicating an interest or desire to be there. This is of particular significance to the schizophrenic patient. According to Howells, "communication among individuals tends to be maximized between individuals positioned opposite to one another."[51]

Personal distance, far phase, (3-3½ feet) is possibly the best territorial zone for communication with the schizophrenic patient. Hall states that with personal distance, far phase, subjects of personal interest and involvement can be discussed.[52] It is within the zone of 3-3½ feet that the nurse can lean toward a patient, thus intruding in the patient's territory.

[51]Lloyd Howells, "Seating Arrangements and Leadership Emergence," *Journal of Abnormal and Social Psychology*, January-June 1962, p. 148.

[52]Hall, *The Silent Language*, p. 113.

Leaning as an intrusion, "acts as an external force on the patient, brings his awareness to the boundaries that must be transgressed in order for the experience to be meaningful to him."[53]

Initially, while in emotional crisis, the schizophrenic patient is sometimes unable to differentiate body boundaries from those of the nurse-therapist. Therefore, safe and appropriate intrusion makes the schizophrenic more aware of his or her own body-buffer zone. Des-Lauriers believes that in the early part of contact with the therapist, the patient's identity is defined by the physical boundaries of the body so that separation and differentiation from the therapist is basically a matter of relationship in space. In this context, to be oriented in space means to relate to the therapist as a separated and differentiated physical object outside of one's own boundaries, and experienced as such whenever these cathected boundaries are transgressed.[54]

The nurse uses personal-close phase to help an aged patient ambulate around the bed or in the bathroom. Younger patients may not need such close assistance while ambulating. The aged patient who no longer needs the bedpan and can be assisted to the bathroom is able to lay territorial claim to the bathroom. This is also a good time for the nurse to increase a patient's perception of the territory by showing where his or her clothes are hung and by allowing the patient to examine the nightstand. As the aged individual increases immediate territorial adaption to the area around the bed and the room, the chances of territorial disorientation are decreased.

Social Distance

The social distance, close-far phase, is a distance of 4-12 feet. This is the distance completely out of the patient's territorial unit. In critical care units it may be the space between the patient's bed and the nurse's station. There may be a glass barrier or screen separating the nurse's station from the patient. They can still see each other but are unable to hear what is being said. When there is a lull in the pace, the nurse may want to retreat into the heart of his or her personal territory; the nurse's station. The distance between both patient and nurse becomes social far phase. By remaining in the nurse's station, the nurse is able to peek into some patient's personal territory. The patient may view visual surveillance as a type of intrusion; however, the patient prefers it over constant physical intrusion.

At social close phase, the nurse should remember to knock before

---

[53]DesLauriers, op. cit., p. 297.
[54]Ibid.

entering. If the patient asks for curtains to be pulled to be left alone, the nurse should treat that territory like he or she would the patient's home. Before opening the curtains, the nurse should seek permission to enter.

In conclusion, the concepts territoriality, space, and privacy are gaining more recognition in patient care. The nurse must intervene to decrease or control technological over-stimulation and territorial deprivation, and to promote territorial adaptation as soon as possible. A skillful nurse brings together two territorial boundaries; the nurse's and the patient's. Patients frequently voice complaints about intrusion into their personal territory, either by equipment or hospital staff. Even though territoriality is instinctive, the nurse should relinquish claim of the territorial cluster to the patient. Because the nurse works daily in the territorial cluster, he or she may feel possessive about the total territory including the space in which the patient is located. The nurse may temporarily forget to knock on the patient's door or announce herself outside the curtains before entering into the patient's territory. The patient needs to feel that the bed or territorial unit is his or hers. In this respect the patient feels an inner strength.

REFERENCES

Allekian, Constance, "Intrusions of Territory and Personal Space," *Nursing Research*, 22, May–June 1973, pp. 236–41.

Alpern, Mathew, *Sensory Processes*, Brooks-Cole, 1967.

Altman, I. and Lett, "The Ecology of Interpersonal Relationships: A Classification System and Conceptual Model," *Social and Psychological Factors in Stress*, New York: Holt, Rinehart and Winston, 1970.

Ardrey, Robert, *The Territorial Imperative*, New York: Dell, 1969.

Engebretson, Darold, "Human Territorial Behavior: The Role of Interaction Distance in Therapeutic Interventions," *American Journal of Orthopsychiatry*, 43, January 1973, pp. 108–16.

Felipe, N.J., "Invasion of Personal Space," *Social Problems*, 14, 1966, pp. 206–14.

Goffman, Erving, *The Presentation of Self in Everyday Life*, New York: Doubleday, 1959.

Hall, Edward, "A System for the Notation of Proxemic Behavior," *American Anthropologist*, 65, 1963, pp. 1003–27.

———, *The Silent Language*, New York: Doubleday, 1959.

Hildreth, Arthur, "Body-Buffer Zone and Violence: A Reassessment and Confirmation," *American Journal of Psychiatry,* 127, June 1977, pp. 1641–45.

Kinzel, A. F., "Body-Buffer Zone in Violent Persons," *American Journal of Psychiatry,* 127, 1970, pp. 59–64.

Leigh, Hoyle, "A Psychological Comparison of Patients in Open and Closed Coronary Care Units," *Journal of Psychosomatic Research,* 16, 1972, pp. 449–57.

Levine, Myra, "Knock Before Entering Personal Space Bubbles," *Chart,* 65, February–March 1968, pp. 58–62.

Lorenz, K., *On Aggression,* New York: Bantam Books, 1967.

Proshansky, Hana, *Environmental Psychology: Man and His Physical Setting,* New York: Holt, Rinehart and Winston, 1970.

Roberts, Sharon, "Territoriality: Space and the Aged Patient in Intensive Care Unit," *Psychosocial Nursing Care of the Aged,* (Ed: Burnside), New York: McGraw-Hill, 1973.

———, "Territoriality: Space and the Schizophrenic Patient," *Perspectives in Psychiatric Care,* 7, 1969.

Sommer, Robert, *Personal Space,* Englewood Cliffs, N.J.: Prentice-Hall, 1969.

11
Loneliness

Loneliness is a subject which has gained increasing recognition over the past several years. Long before professional groups began studying loneliness and its application to infants, prisoners, isolated adults, or the aged, the poets and novelists were aware of it. Their essays or poems reflected personal experiences with loneliness. Today people find themselves living within a highly transitory, mobile, and changing society. People are moving toward and away from each other with great rapidity. Therefore, relationships have a tendency to be only temporary. Consequently, people feel the void of lost friendship. To guard against the void feeling and the loneliness that results, people shy away from involvement beyond the superficial level. In the process of avoiding the thing they fear, these become even more lonely.

Individuals, regardless of age or social position, experience loneliness at some point in their life. Loneliness knows no age limit as it affects the very young and the very old. Feelings of loneliness seem to be more acute during hospitalization. Even though the hospitalized patient is surrounded by many stimuli, he or she can still experience the overwhelming feeling of loneliness. The nurse realizes that, ". . . the patient is the most important person in the hospital. He is, therefore, the center of much attention from all kinds of people. In spite of this he is probably the loneliest person in the hospital. People come and go, but few really encounter him as a person."[1]

In one way or another, loneliness becomes the experience of us all. By accident, or by intent, circumstances are so arranged for many of us that we are not aware of our own loneliness. According to Lopata, "One of the characteristics of loneliness is its infusion in all three time dimensions, the past, present, and future. People often feel lonely for a person, object, event, interaction, scene, or mood which had been experienced in

---

[1]Kathryn Hurlburt, "The Loneliness of Suffering," *Canadian Nurse*, 61, April 1965, p. 299.

the past."[2] There are circumstances in which loneliness occurs when we have no control. The loss of a loved one or separation due to hospitalization are such experiences. In each instance, contact is severed or temporarily removed from the significant others in our daily life. It may be at this time that we realize the importance contact has been or is with the significant other in our environment.

According to Hoskisson, "It is only when we are aware that we require contact with another human being or an environment, that we are aware of loneliness. Sometimes loneliness is apparent and sometimes not, so that we can well be alone without this need and in the limited sense we are not lonely, although all of us from the cradle to the grave need human contact."[3] Once the individual becomes aware of the absence of contact, one may choose to deny or avoid loneliness. The individual may choose not to be aware of being lonely out of the necessity to avoid it. "In other words, in a certain sense, loneliness has a value: it coerces us into consorting and communicating. It makes social life, culture and human institutions possible."[4]

Even though the individual is permanently or temporarily severed from contact or human relationships, the ". . . solitary state gives the individual the opportunity to draw upon untouched capacities and resources and to realize himself in an entirely unique manner. It can be a new experience. It may be an experience of exquisite pain, deep fear and terror, an utterly terrible experience, yet it brings into awareness new dimensions of self, new beauty, new power for human compassion, and a reverence for the precious nature of each breathing moment."[5] The individual may learn new things about the self which can help in coping with future experiences of loneliness.

DEFINITIONS AND FUNCTIONS OF LONELINESS

Before focusing entirely upon the concept loneliness, it would be of value to examine what Peplau believes to be the difference between lonesomeness, aloneness, and finally loneliness. Patients, regardless of their age or clinical problem, will experience all three at different times during their hospitalization. Therefore, the nurse should be aware of their existence.

[2]Helena Lopata, "Loneliness: Forms and Components," *Social Problems*, 17, Fall 1969, p. 250.

[3]J.B. Hoskisson, *Loneliness*, (New York: Citadel, 1965), p. 26.

[4]*Ibid.*, p. 11.

[5]Clark Moustakas, *Loneliness*, (Englewood Cliffs, N.J.: Prentice-Hall, 1961), p. 7.

Lonesomeness

The feeling of lonesomeness is not an unusual experience. It happens to each one of us at various times in our lives. Lonesomeness, "implies being without the company of others but recognizing a wish to be with others."[6] An individual can experience lonesomeness when separated from contact with others. Likewise, one may be surrounded by family, staff, and other patients yet continue to feel lonesome. The individual acknowledges the need to feel close to other people and frequently is able to express this feeling. He or she may assume responsibility for reversing the feeling by requesting more patient-family or nurse-patient contacts. If mobility is possible, the patient may extend to others on a social level. Social encounters with other patients may even have a therapeutic effect on both people. They may share their concerns and possibly even their feelings of lonesomeness.

Aloneness

Aloneness, "implies being without company. It may signify a singular position, such as being alone in making certain kinds of decisions which affect living."[7] There are individuals in life who chose to be alone. The creative individual who paints, writes, invents, or discovers retreats from the presence of others. To this individual, being alone gives time to contemplate and ideate. In this respect it is possible to be alone without being lonesome. The individual can choose to be alone in order to accomplish a goal.

On the other hand, a patient, not by choice, may experience aloneness. The patient feels aloneness when making decisions that have a future effect upon himself and the family. The child must receive an injection or experience surgery alone. Parents cannot substitute themselves in place of the child. The patient who signs a preoperative consent for bilateral nephrectomy knows that he or she alone must make the final decision. Other people have a role in the decision; however, it is the patient who experiences the event alone. Possibly this is the rationale behind telling a patient of impending surgery several days in advance. The consent is usually given to the patient to sign the day or evening before the event. This gives the patient time, in the aloneness, to think through the decision. The patient may not want to be alone in the decision; however, physiologically the body has given no other choice.

[6]Hildegard Peplau, "Loneliness," *American Journal of Nursing*, 55, December 1955, p. 1476.

[7]*Ibid.*

Loneliness

According to Hoskisson, "Loneliness is the conscious experience of separation from something or someone desired, required or needed. It is not solitariness, for there the separation is not felt, nor is it lack of physical or social contact, for as we all know the presence of people does not assuage it. So there must be experienced a need, a desire for contact, and an inability to make it."[8] Lopata points out that, "A person may feel lonely when no one else is present, when a particular other is absent, when interaction patterns treat him differently than he desires, or when aspects of the situation make him feel alienated from those with whom he could develop different relations."[9] Sullivan stated that man is a gregarious animal with a need for contact with others; when this need is unfulfilled, it is expressed in loneliness. When action is taken to avoid or relieve tension or loneliness, there is enhancement of self-esteem.[10]

Peplau believes that loneliness is not a chosen state. Often the lonely person is not aware of the reason why he or she does certain things when experiencing loneliness. Loneliness can then be defined as an unnoticed inability to do anything while alone. Often loneliness is not felt; instead the person has a feeling of unexplained dread, of desperation, or of extreme restlessness.[11] According to Francel, "Loneliness is in essence the inability to love, combined with a negation of being; or to describe it otherwise, the lonely person has the terrifying experience of being unable to conceptualize himself as real or having existence. This is both a cognitive and affective unconscious dynamism; it is out of the person's awareness."[12] The loneliness and fear of all patients, regardless of age, becomes our fear and concern. When we begin to encounter the patient's fear and loneliness, we also begin to encounter our own. Not every individual desires this kind of encounter. Rather, it is an encounter that is avoided as much as possible.

Functions of loneliness Loneliness involves a unique substance "of self," a dimension of human life which taps the full resources of the individual. It calls for strength, endurance and sustenance, enabling a person to reach previously unknown depths and to realize a certain

[8]Hoskisson, *op. cit.*, p. 37.

[9]Lopata, *op. cit.*, p. 250.

[10]Harry Sullivan, *Interpersonal Theory of Psychiatry*, (New York: Norton, 1953).

[11]Peplau, *op. cit.*, p. 1476.

[12]Claire Francel, "Loneliness," *Some Clinical Approaches to Psychiatric Nursing*, (New York: Macmillan, 1963), p. 178.

nakedness of inner life."[13] It is interesting to note that, ". . . the individual in being lonely, if let be, will realize himself in loneliness and create a bond or sense of fundamental relatedness with others. Loneliness rather than separating the individual or causing a break or division of self, has the function of expanding the individual's wholeness, perceptiveness, sensitivity, and humanity. It serves to enhance the individual's realization of humanity. In loneliness the individual is definitely alone, cut off from human companionship."[14]

Moustakas believes that there is, "a power in loneliness, a purity, self-immersion, and depth which is unlike any other experience. Being lonely is such a total, direct, vivid existence, so deeply felt, so startlingly different, that there is no room for any other perception, feeling or awareness. Loneliness is an organic experience which points to nothing else, is for no other purpose and results in nothing but the realization of itself."[15] The experience of loneliness serves the function of helping the individual look within. As we look toward self it is believed we commune with self. "He discovers life, who he is, what he really wants, the meaning of his existence, the true nature of his relation with others."[16] As the individual reaches completion of the loneliness experience, he or she realizes its purpose. Again, this function or purpose is that the person has grown, matured, and reached out for others in a deeper and more vital sense.

Just as loneliness can have long-term positive functions, it can also have some negative effects. Loneliness can become unbearably immobilizing. It is the potential immobilizing side effect of loneliness that should concern the nurse. As Moustakas has pointed out, loneliness as it applies to all individuals can be examined in two ways. First, there is the loneliness of self-alienation and self-rejection which is not loneliness at all but a vague and disturbing anxiety. This aspect of loneliness is referred to as loneliness anxiety. Second, there is existential loneliness which inevitably is a part of human experience.

THE INDIVIDUAL'S EXPERIENCE WITH LONELINESS

Loneliness as a condition of existence can lead to new awareness and insight into oneself. It has the potential of creating new images and ideas regarding the being of an individual. As a concept, "existential loneliness

[13]Moustakas, *op. cit.*, p. 8.
[14]*Ibid.*, p. 47.
[15]*Ibid.*, p. 8.
[16]*Ibid.*, p. 102.

is an intrinsic and organic reality of human life in which there is both pain and triumphant creation emerging out of long periods of desolation. In existential loneliness man is fully aware of himself as an isolated and solitary individual while in loneliness anxiety man is separated from himself as a feeling and knowing person."[17] Existential loneliness is also referred to as the real experience of the individual. Loneliness anxiety is more diffuse and many times is experienced by all patients after the initial crisis. Needless to say, the patient can simultaneously experience both types of loneliness. The difference lies in the intensity of the experience. Existential loneliness is the real experience of the here and now whereas loneliness anxiety involves more attention toward fear of aloneness or fear of future implications.

Existential Loneliness: Real Experience

Wolfe believes that existential loneliness is an essential condition of creativity, that out of the depths of grief, despair, and the shattering feeling of total impotency springs the urge to create new forms and images and to discover unique ways of being aware and expressing experience.[18] Moustakas states that, "fear, evasion, denial, and the accompanying attempts to escape the experience, will afflict and separate him from his own resources so that there is no development, no creative emergence, no growth in awareness, perceptiveness, sensitivity."[19] Therefore, the loneliness experience can isolate or separate the patient from his or her own experience.

Freida Fromm-Reichmann describes the real experience of loneliness as, ". . . such that one cannot communicate with people who are in the grip of it. Once they emerge from it, they do not wish—or they are unable—to talk about their loneliness or about any topic which is psychologically connected with it . . ."[20] The real experience or existential loneliness involves two major components, namely, the threat of illness and the loneliness of both psychological and physiological pain.

Sullivan has explained the developmental process of the phenomena called loneliness. He believes that the components of loneliness begin in infancy and continue through each developmental period. Sullivan refers to these components, "as being related to the need for tenderness in infants, the need for expressive play in children, the need for peers in the juvenile era, and the need for a more intimate kind of

[17]*Ibid.*, p. 24.
[18]*Ibid.*, p. 33.
[19]*Ibid.*, p. 35.
[20]Marita DeThomaso, "Touch Power," *Perspectives in Psychiatric Care*, 9, 1971, p. 131.

relationship in preadolescence. He believes that lonely people lack the kind of experience that they should have in these development stages."[21]

The threat of illness   Illness, with its threat to biological integrity, is a real experience; real in the sense that the threat involves potential loss of a part, whole, or life itself. The real experience of illness causes existential loneliness. Illness may be either an old or new experience to the patient. In either instance, the illness with its threats creates loneliness. It involves separation and isolation from the secure and the familiar. This is a particular problem for the very young patient.

Hospitalization removes the child from familiar and secure surroundings. The child is placed in a new environment with new experiences. According to Spenner, "He is surrounded by strange people and equipment. The child does not choose to be hospitalized, yet he can do nothing to change the situation. He is often forced into a state of increased dependency and made to feel small, powerless, and insecure. He is subjected to numerous threats to body integrity, such as injections, surgery, and/or diagnostic procedures."[22]

The child, unlike adult patients, may have little or no previous experience with illness. Any prior experience might be associated with usual childhood illnesses none of which required hospitalization and each of which was accompanied by attention from a mothering figure. Hospitalization was a subject foreign to the child's thinking. The child may associate it with a school friend who, due to a fractured leg, was hospitalized. In addition, a child's only contact with health professionals may be annual visits to the dentist or pediatrician for routine examinations. Therefore, to become ill and subsequently removed from one's own home, bed, friends, dog, toys, and parents can be devastating and have long term effects upon the child.

Hospitalization, whether sudden or planned, creates feelings of abandonment within the child. Moustakas believes that, "For years medical people have known that hospitalization may do a child more harm than good—not only in contributing to his sense of abandonment, but in the development of terrifying fears, anxiety, and traumas which survive long after the physical defect has been rectified."[23] The real experience of illness requiring strange pieces of equipment or intrusive procedures facilitate loneliness anxiety. To the small child syringes, needles, bottles, tubes, thermometers, and wires all seem to take greater than normal proportions. Each, in varying degrees, communicates threats that seem

[21]Sullivan, *op. cit.*, pp. 260–62.

[22]Dorothy Spenner, "A Preschool Child Copes with Hospitalization," *Maternal Child Nursing Journal*, Spring 1974, p. 41.

[23]Moustakas, *op. cit.*, p. 36.

to remind the child of his or her illness, smallness, and helplessness. The child seems to have little control over the environment. Crying may be the only defense in a seemingly defenseless environment. For children, the threat of illness, including the potential of surgical intervention, revolves around the fear of abandonment and fear of strange invading procedures.

Illness may or may not be a new experience to the adult patient. Take for example the individual who receives an antibiotic for a cold and develops a drug reaction leading to eventual acute renal failure. Another example is the adult male who, while driving to work, sustains an acute myocardial infarction. Each individual never anticipated that illness and its threat of loss would come at this point in life. Illness was something that only happened to the very old or disabled, not to someone in the early forties.

Other adult patients may not have been so fortunate throughout their lives. Illness and its recurrence may be a continued threat facilitating feelings of loneliness especially when hospitalization becomes necessary. According to Stockwell, "When a person is hospitalized, he becomes more acutely aware of his human separateness. The disease, the trauma, is happening to him, and no one else can experience this for him. There is no escape from his body capsule. In the hospital, the opportunity for relating is minimal. He is surrounded by strangers who relate to him in the most intimate way, yet with an aura of detachment. Loneliness becomes overwhelming. Physical stress leaves him helpless, as bodily functions are out of control. Lonely and helpless, to whom can he turn."[24] Physical illness creates one type of existential loneliness whereas psychological illness creates another.

The schizophrenic patient may not realize he or she is lonely. Others may be aware of it but try to deny its existence. "It may be experienced not primarily as loneliness but as depression or anxiety; and vice-versa, patients may speak of loneliness when they really may be experiencing something else such as emptiness or dependency needs."[25] Furthermore, Burton points out that, "The need to be more than what mundane life offers is the characteristic need of the schizophrenic patient. What in life for others is a meaningful form of existence becomes for the schizophrenic person the absurd, with no reconciliation possible."[26] Loneliness and alienation is central to the schizophrenic's psychological illness. It has been said that the loneliness preceeds schizophrenia rather than follows

---

[24]Martha Stockwell, "The Third Hand: A Theory of Support," *Journal of Psychiatric Nursing,* 8, May-June 1970.

[25]Jack Rubins, "On the Psychopathology of Loneliness," *American Journal of Psychoanalysis,* 24, 1964, p. 153.

[26]Arthur Burton, "On the Nature of Loneliness," *American Journal of Psychoanalysis,* 21, 1961, p. 36.

it. Loneliness is what forces the individual into the complex state of schizophrenia. The illness thrusts the schizophrenic into contact with others equally as lonely.

The threat of illness makes the aged individual more vulnerable. In contrast to the young and middle aged, the aged patient is known to be liable to loss of physical integrity, attachments, and/or activities. Illness serves to immobilize the patient further, isolating him. Chronic illness may keep the patient immobilized or restricted to one's own home or a convalescent home. Acute illness necessitates hospitalization. Many aged patients no longer have significant others; therefore, the real experience of illness is a lonely one. Furthermore, the aged patient's energy depletion and sensory loss contributes to physical immobility. When these factors, together with illness, make the individual lonely, he or she has a tendency to exaggerate a physical illness. Naturally, the aged patient expects to have some discomfort. However, if left alone without social or physical contact, physical ills will consume all attention.

The threat of both physical and psychological illness can lead to existential loneliness in each developmental stage. Its threats include the most significant threat, to life itself. The potential threat to life and/or physical loss can be a lonely one to the individual. Illness does not only imply a physical event; it also becomes a psychological event. The illness and threat of loss or disfigurement creates both psychological and physiological pain. Both types of pain are real experiences to the individual and therefore create feelings of loneliness.

The psychological pain   Psychological pain occurs when the individual must maintain a separateness from others. The separateness of existential loneliness involves three components. These components are separateness from contact with significant members of his or her life, separateness from the body, and separateness from his or her values and ideas. Children are especially vulnerable to the first component.

The temporary abandonment that leads to feelings of loneliness in the child is hospitalization. To be hospitalized alone implies separateness from significant others, particularly the mothering figure. In her place are strangers, rules and regulations, routines, and frightening pieces of equipment. According to Moustakas, "The cold marble floors; the impersonal rules and regulations; the extreme bleak whiteness everywhere; the desensitized atmosphere; the neat, empty categorial arrangement of food and beds, external to the individual child and his personal preferences; the constant checks and routines; the frequent medication and shots which he does not comprehend; the disrespect for the integrity of his wishes and interests; the absence of genuine human warmth; and, the presence of surface voices, surface smiles, and superficial words and meetings; all enter into the loneliness of hospital life."[27] The health team cannot fully comprehend the terror experienced by a child who feels alone in the hospital environment.

The psychological pain the child experiences cannot be measured beyond his or her tears. As discussed earlier, illness alone is a threatening experience. However, to be left alone with one's illness without familiar supportive assistance is even more threatening to the child. The child needs parents ". . . in every painful experience to help him bear the loneliness of living with strangers who often apparently care more about x-rays, charts, and shots, and temperatures, and tests, than they do about him. There is no one, absolutely no one, who can comfort the child, and give him the strength to face his ordeal except his mother or father or some person to whom he is significantly related."[28] Even when the mothering figure is present, the child can still experience loneliness. This is because there are hospital experiences that the child must inevitably face alone. The child alone must experience the various diagnostic tests, intrusive procedures, or surgery. Therefore, there are times when the child will realize loneliness as an individual. "This is the inevitable loneliness of human existence. But when the child is abandoned, his terror lives inside. He will always remember the lonely, isolated hours of abandonment."[29]

The child requires a mothering figure present with each new and significant experience. Eventually, as the experience becomes less threatening and/or painful, the child reaches a readiness point whereby he or she is able to be alone. Therefore with supportive assistance from the health team and significant others, the child's psychological pain will not be of overwhelming intensity.

The adult patient, like the child, who discovers he or she has a disease, illness, or surgical need finds one isolated or separated from fellowmen. The patient is now different and the difference may only be in the label temporarily worn; "patient." Once the individual receives the label of "patient", he or she is automatically separated from others; family, friends, or colleagues. This person has a distinction all his or her own. To the patient, this distinction represents failure not success. The patient is then placed in a protective community with other people who have the same label. As the diagnosis is confirmed, the patient is given a further more specific distinction. This person is now a schizophrenic, cardiac, renal, or pulmonary patient. With the above distinction, the patient is removed from the larger patient community to a more specific

---

[27]Moustakas, *op. cit.*, pp. 35–36.

[28]*Ibid.*, p. 37.

[29]*Ibid.*, p. 38.

community such as a psychiatric or critical care unit. Hopefully, "The experience of separation or isolation is not unhealthy any more than any condition of human existence is unhealthy. Ultimately each man is alone but when the individual maintains a truthful self-identity, such isolation is strengthening and induces deeper sensitivities and awareness. In contrast, self-alienation and estrangement drive one to avoid separation."[30] The nurse helps a patient maintain self-identity by personalizing his or her care.

When a person is hospitalized, that person becomes more acutely aware of human separateness. The disease, the trauma, the anxiety, or the depression is happening to him. No one else can experience this for him. There is no escape from the body. The schizophrenic's anxieties and fears create loneliness through social isolation. The social isolation further contributes to the psychological pain of existential loneliness. As a defense, social isolation allows the individual to avoid contacts. The schizophrenic fears that self-esteem will further decline because of potential rejection by others. For the general hospitalized patient, the environment creates feelings of separateness and isolation. Not only is the adult patient separated from significant others, but also from his or her own body.

Many times patients feel that the health team is more interested in their diseased organ, fantasies, wires, or tubes than in them as a whole. The individual can feel separated from either the physical or psychological being. Physically, the patient feels removed from the body as though watching it undergo various diagnostic tests, procedures, or treatments. Such separation is most threatening to the schizophrenic patient. The disassociation and disharmony between the mind and body involves confusion over boundaries. He or she fails to realize where the body ends and external objects begin. Fantasies and hallucinations contribute to a state of separateness. The individual experiences loneliness in either instance. The loneliness may be even greater if the patient feels that the body or mind is a place for research or the application of new treatments.

As with the adult, the aged individual also experiences psychological pain of loneliness. It is quite possible that the aged individual has previously experienced separateness from significant others and the body. Unlike younger patients, the aged patient may have lost close friends, parents, or a spouse. Furthermore, his or her physical being may have required hospitalization throughout the years. What is specific to this patient is the separateness from familiar environment, values, and ideas. For the aged patient, unfamiliarity with the environment creates loneliness. Whether hospitalized or at home, physical immobility contributes to social isolation.

[30]*Ibid.*, p. 34.

As a human being, the aged individual experiences psychological pain when he or she no longer feels valued. The value and ideas regarding health care and its delivery may be totally different from those of the nurse or physician. The patient feels compelled to compromise values and ideas to those planning and guiding personal care. The patient has difficulty assimilating all the events and changes within the environment. "Social forces also contribute to the psychic impoverishment and depersonalization of the aged person. Part of this is due to the inability of the aged person to assimilate, with any degree of comfort, the impact of fast moving events to which he is exposed."[31] Existential loneliness can be psychologically destructive to the individual if the ability to cope is reduced. The patient feels hopeless and helpless.

The physiological pain   There are three ways in which all patients, regardless of the developmental stage, respond to physical pain. The individual may choose to ignore the pain, realistically react to the pain, or overreact to the pain. In the first instance the patient may avoid or ignore its existence. The child learns that pain is associated with intrusive treatments, injections, therefore, denying its existence.

Older patients feel that the pain will limit or immobilize, thus reducing the ability to interact with the environment. The patient feels that submitting to the pain will limit the ability to participate in activities with family or friends. Essentially, the patient avoids the loneliness he or she assumes the pain will create. Most patients realistically react to their physical pain. They see their pain as real and tangible. The patient can only inform others when it occurs and hope that the medication will relieve it.

Last, there are those patients who overreact to their pain. The same type of pain ignored or reacted to by one patient may be intolerable to another, to the point of overreaction. The child may overreact to gain the sympathy of a mothering figure. The adult may overreact to gain the nurse's attention and therefore decrease loneliness. The more, "pain the patient experiences, the more he becomes preoccupied with the avoidance of further pain. His defenses become phobically organized in that all of his fears may become focused on the needle or the pill or some treatment procedure. One or another of these factors is perceived as the source of all discomfort; it is therefore regarded as something that must be avoided, regardless of the consequences insofar as the illness itself is concerned."[32]

Regardless of its origin, physiological or psychological pain can be

[31]David Tannenbaum, "Loneliness in the Aged," *Mental Hygiene,* 51, January 1967, p. 94.

[32]Sydney Smith, "The Psychology of Illness," *Nursing Forum,* 3, 1964, p. 41.

unbearable. According to Burnside, "If the alleviation of pain is one goal, then one may need to integrate the aloneness or loneliness that may be concurrent with the pain."[33]

Loneliness Anxiety: Fear of Aloneness

Loneliness anxiety results from a fundamental breach between what one is and what one pretends to be, a basic alienation between man and man and between man and his surroundings. Moustakas believes that "Loneliness anxiety is a widespread condition in contemporary society. The individual no longer has an intimate sense of relatedness to the food he eats, the clothing he wears, the shelter which houses him. He no longer participates directly in the creation and production of the vital needs of his family and community. He no longer fashions with his own hands or from the desires of his heart. He has been sharply cut off from primary groups and from family and kinship ties. He lives in an impersonal urban or suburban community where he meets others not as real persons but according to prescribed rules of conduct and prescribed modes of behavior."[34]

In its clinical application, loneliness anxiety implies fear of aloneness. The patient realizes that he or she alone must experience the unknown. This involves fear of aloneness in the hospital environment and in the vagueness of the new or altered future. The patient alone must go through the admission rituals. Second, he or she alone must integrate the necessary changes of the future into being.

As with existential loneliness, loneliness anxiety involves two major component parts; fear of aloneness in the environment and fear of aloneness in the future. Each fear may not be communicated by the patient thus pushing the patient further into the loneliness and aloneness feared. In the patient's mind he or she is in the process of becoming an emotional or physical cripple. "In his aloneness, man reaches out to others to make some contact. He may do this by direct means such as relating to another person or group or by indirect means such as creative expression through art or writing. Either method is a means to the same end. It is man's effort to overcome his separateness."[35]

Fear of aloneness in the environment   The fear of aloneness in the environment begins the minute a patient arrives in the hospital. Fear of

[33]Irene Burnside, "Loneliness in Old Age," *Mental Hygiene*, 55, July 1971, p. 395.

[34]Moustakas, *op. cit.*, p. 25.

[35]Clark Eloise, "Aspects of Loneliness: Toward a Framework of Intervention," *Developing Behavioral Concepts in Nursing*, (Ed: Loretta Zderad and Helen Belcher , Atlanta: Southern Regional Education Board, 1968), p. 33.

aloneness applies to all developmental stages. Even though there are people within the environment with whom the patient interacts, the interaction may have little significance. This is particularly true for the hospitalized child. As with existential loneliness, the child experiences a separateness with significant people in his or her life. What remains are strangers. The strangers make the child realize aloneness in a foreign and sometimes technical world. Needless to say, the child feels less than whole. It is the mothering figure who initially provides the whole. Fortunately wholes are dynamic and as the child develops the whole grows. Therefore, other significant people, in time, can assume the mothering role. This is possible when the child feels a sense of relatedness to members of the health team. According to Rubins, "The feeling of healthy relatedness as well as separateness of the self from others, of the self as an independent entity, depends on many factors. Among these are the infant's tactile-visual-auditory contacts as well as his emotional relationships with parent figures."[36]

Regardless of the potential for relatedness, the child must face certain experiences alone. While experiencing aloneness the child tries to find explanations for what is happening internally and externally. The personal feelings of helplessness, smallness, and separateness cause the child to feel lonely. Fear of aloneness forces the child to validate the meanings of observations and experiences with others.

Because of diffuse internal feelings, the process of loneliness anxiety may not be overtly manifested or communicated by the adult patient. Coupled with loneliness, will be a feeling of aloneness. The patient alone is the one experiencing the pain which brought him or her to the hospital. Others can ask questions about the pain or prescribe an analgesic, but the patient alone endures the frustration of pain. He or she alone must experience the continual poking and probing of the admitting physician who attempts to gather data. The liver and abdomen are palpated; the chest is percussed; the eyes, ears and nose examined; and the cardiac status assessed. The patient alone must experience the initial diagnostic procedures necessary to confirm the data obtained from the doctor's poking and probing. He or she alone is subjected to the intrusion of various needles and tubes, must lie under the X-ray machine, breathe rhythmically into a volume respirator, or remain motionless as an EKG machine records a cardiac rhythm. The patient alone must be told what all the poking, probing, and intrusive tests show and hear the frightening diagnosis and experience the potential threat to his or her life. All of these experiences occur in a strange environment. The "painful experience of loneliness denotes the sensation of feeling alone and at the same time having the awareness that one needs a connection with his fellowman. Loneliness is not only a factual acknowledgment of being by oneself, but

[36]Rubins, *op. cit.*, p. 159.

it indicates an urgent desire to re-enter human contact."[37] The patient can fill the voidness or loneliness felt for human contact. The patient re-enters human awareness by becoming acquainted with the nurse.

The schizophrenic patient fears aloneness while simultaneously fearing closeness. Frieda Fromm-Reichman believes that the schizophrenic's, ". . . fear of closeness involves the arousal of anxiety that all social closeness, however desirable, might be followed by subsequent rejection. Because of his weak self, the schizophrenic fears that social closeness can endanger and even destroy the boundaries between his own identity and that of the other person."[38] While experiencing loneliness, the schizophrenic, ". . . seeks companionship even though intensely anxious in the performance. When, because of deprivation of companionship, one does integrate a situation in spite of more or less intense anxiety, one often shows, in the situation, evidence of a serious defect of personal orientation."[39]

The aged individual is often fearful of communicating feelings of aloneness and loneliness. These feelings are threatening and the patient wonders whether or not communicating them will resolve the conflict. Tannenbaum points out that, "Talking with another aged person who faces a similar situation is frequently not constructive either, since what he is actually seeking is difference—a different orientation to his feeling and doing. Voicing his impressions to a younger person may seem equally fruitless since he may feel that it is unlikely that a young person could possibly understand his feelings."[40] The aged individual needs to communicate with the nurse. In this respect they no longer remain strangers. Furthermore, the fear of aloneness in the environment diminishes.

Fear of aloneness in the future   More important than the patient's fear of aloneness within the environment is the fear of aloneness in the future. It not only involves the individual's future but the future of his or her family. The child's future might involve frequent trips to the hospital for additional diagnostic studies, emergency treatments, or surgery. With each additional hospitalization, the child brings new fears and anxieties. In the interim between hospitalization, the child has matured into a new stage of development. Consequently, the child must deal with different fears and expectations. As Spencer said, "He is a child with unique needs

[37]DeThomaso, *op. cit.*, p. 114.

[38]Freida Fromm-Reichman, *Psychoanalysis and Psychotherapy*, (Chicago: University of Chicago Press, 1959), pp. 210–12.

[39]*Ibid.*

[40]David Tannenbaum, "Loneliness in the Aged," *Mental Hygiene*, 51, January 1967, p. 97.

and talents, who comes to the hospital with his own ways of coping with life and with the stresses and crises that characterize the course of growing up."[41] The child's future may then require that he or she learn ways of adapting to physical limitations or disabilities. Supportive help from the parents, health team, and friends makes the future brighter.

The adult patient fears the transitional aloneness of moving from the sick to well role, with its changes. The patient may actually fear the aloneness of these changes. Initially, the patient may not realize that the changes are not made totally alone, having support from family and health team. This realization comes later during the hospitalization. However, in the beginning the patient alone must be the one to accept these changes and incorporate them into a new life style.

The transition path toward change is lonely. The changes may mean one cannot be as active as before, travel as extensively as before, or return to a previous job. Only the patient can know the meaning change has for him. The family can assist in the transition; however, the patient alone must make the decision to accept or reject change. Within the lonely process of either accepting or rejecting change, the patient goes through the psychological pain of mourning. As stated earlier, the anxious patient goes through the process of becoming an emotional or physiological cripple. The patient may not realize that the changes which take place will not render him a cripple. The patient needs to communicate fears to the nurse so together they can verify their validity.

Ironically, the patient may reject help from others—the same others with whom he or she wanted to have a sense of relatedness. Smith stated that, "the individual faces in his illness the trial of unfamiliar states of dependency and passivity which may prove frightening and arouse considerable resistance to the acceptance of help."[42] Once the patient communicates fears he or she no longer experiences aloneness.

Within the developmental process, the aged patient is the most vulnerable in terms of future implications. The aged patient lives in a social world that is changing at a faster pace than can be comprehended. The various changes cause the aged individual to feel he or she no longer has a significant place or role. Illness added to normal physical changes associated with aging further limit contributions. It is understandable that many aged people experience loneliness in their present and future worlds. Moustakas believes that, "There is no longer a place for old age, no feeling of organic belonging, no reverence or respect or regard for the wisdom and talent of the ancient. Our elder citizens so often have feelings of uselessness, so often experience life as utterly futile. Old age is fertile soil for loneliness and the fear of a lonely old age far outweighs the fear of

---

[41]Spenner, *op. cit.*, p. 41.

[42]Smith, *op. cit.*, p. 39.

death in the thinking of many people."[43] The aged individual needs to feel significant within the future. As with all patients, the aged patient needs to communicate fears with the nurse. In this respect the aged patient realizes that someone else in the immediate environment is aware of his or her internal thinking.

The patient, regardless of developmental stage or reason for being hospitalized, seeks to eliminate feelings of both existential loneliness and loneliness anxiety. The nurse realizes that the patient's own desire for relatedness becomes the vehicle through which he or she may guide the patient out of this loneliness.

NURSING IMPLICATIONS

In nursing situations, the nurse does ". . . not deal directly with the patient's loneliness but rather with his defenses against experiencing the pain of loneliness—the plausible structure he has erected to cover up the problem and hide it from himself and from others."[44] The patient who feels alone and isolated from others may feel threatened by the potential loss of boundaries. In other words, the patient fears the loss in the ability to discriminate between the subjective self and the objective surrounding world. The nurse helps the patient maintain a sense of boundary. The concept of boundaries will be discussed relevant to both types of loneliness.

Existential Loneliness: Real Experience

The nurse assists the patient in overcoming existential loneliness by minimizing the threat of illness and minimizing both psychological and physiological pain. Each component part of existential loneliness or the real experience will be discussed in terms of its boundaries.

Minimize threat of illness   Boundaries of illness become manifested as the patient shares in detail those events which led to hospitalization. The patient goes into great detail in relaying the minute-by-minute activities prior to the crisis. Such behavior applies to all patients, regardless of age. Children may share in detail those events leading to their accident. For example, the child discusses how he or she sustained a broken leg when struck by a car. Other children may share a detailed account of an

---

[43]Moustakas, *op. cit.*, p. 26.
[44]Peplau, *op. cit.*, p. 1476.

event prior to their surgery. Such events include the number of turns right or left before the stretcher reached the elevator and ultimately the operating room. The details become the child's means of coping with anxieties and fears. The nurse who realizes their significance to the patient will listen attentively. Initially, the details may seem rather tedious and boring to the nurse; however, their expression minimizes the patient's loneliness. The patient has shared concerns and thoughts with someone else.

Basically, for the adult and aged patient the details have two functions. First, they give the patient an opportunity to work through the guilt feelings for having become ill. Guilt evoked by one's illness can be a very lonely experience. The patient may make statements such as, "The business is dependent upon me," "my wife really depends on me," "my husband has never had to manage the house and children alone," or "my children are too busy to bother with me." All these statements imply feelings of guilt. The nurse intervenes to minimize the individual's guilt feelings by allowing the patient to share what specifically causes guilty feelings. Second, the nurse helps the patient identify strengths of the family members remaining at home and the business associates assuming the work load. Finally, the nurse can encourage the patient to share feelings of guilt with the family. The patient may need direct reassurances from those people for whom he or she feels the guilt.

The second function of sharing the details is the patient's way of seeking support and clarification. In other words, by sharing details the patient is indirectly asking if he or she could have precipitated the problem. By sharing the precrisis events, the experience remains real but need not be a lonely one. The patient, in sharing activities which led to the biological crisis, is also asking the question "will it happen again?" The patient wants to know the boundaries of the current illness. All patients, regardless of their reason for being hospitalized, hope that the boundaries will not extend to permanent loss of function, whole, or life itself. The mere thought of such a possibility can make the patient lonely.

The nurse's goal is to move the patient toward developing expanding boundaries of illness rather than constricting ones. The nurse teaches the patient the positive stages of healing and therapy. For example, the cardiac patient is taught physiological boundaries in terms of scar tissue. The nurse teaches the patient the stages of healing, time spent with each stage, and levels of activities possible in each stage. The psychiatric patient is taught alternative ways of coping with anxieties and fears. The ability to understand problems and develop new resources for coping will determine the time boundary of the emotional illness. Likewise, patients with physical dysfunction are also given a possible time boundary in which their illness will reach some level of stability. This includes the teaching process and its various stages. The child needs to know how long the leg will be in traction or in a cast. The nurse provides the patient with the realistic but positive boundaries. Consequently, the real experience of crisis diminishes and the new experience of restoration begins. Besides minimizing loneliness by helping a patient to realistically look at boundaries of an illness, the nurse also minimizes both psychological and physiological pain.

Minimize psychological pain   The three components of psychological pain are separateness from contact with significant people in one's life, separateness from the body, and separateness from values and ideas. The nurse attempts to minimize psychological pain by fostering relatedness in these three areas.

The nurse realizes that patients, regardless of age, feel more secure knowing that significant members of their life are nearby. Sullivan refers to, "The human need for contact and tenderness in order for one to be equipped to negotiate the stages of development satisfactorily. With a deprivation of human relatedness, a person must defend himself against total annihilation of self through a substitutive production of fantasies which cannot be shared by others."[45]

Relatedness occurs on two levels. First of all, there is physical relatedness. Physical relatedness exists between the patient and nurse, family, or other patients. Nurses foster relatedness between children through various play activities involving two or more other patients. The psychiatric patient can attain a sense of relatedness through group therapy. The patient discovers other individuals with similar problems or needs. Other hospitalized adult patients attain physical relatedness not necessarily through other patients but rather through frequent visits by significant members of their family or social community. Physical closeness with significant people, whether the nurse, family, or other patients, diminishes the individual's feelings of loneliness. The need for such physical closeness may be paramount in the initial stage of illness. Children and the critically ill realize the need for closeness. Therefore, it seems only reasonable that family members be permitted to remain quietly at the patient's bedside.

Nurses also facilitate physical relatedness through the intervention of touch. Naturally the nurse must assess those patients who would view touch as threatening and/or painful. The schizophrenic patient with an identity problem or the very agitated paranoid patient may react negatively to touch. Likewise, the burn or severely disabled arthritic

[45]Cited in Madeline Guptan, "An Interruption in Loneliness: The Use of Concrete Objects in the Promotion of Human Relatedness," *Journal of Psychiatric Care*, 9, July-August 1971, p. 23.

patient may view touch as painful. For most patients touch represents momentary release from loneliness. DeThomaso believes that, "The need for intimacy and physical as well as interpersonal closeness, develops throughout life, but the greatest need is experienced in preadolescence. Since touch is a form of contact, it is not surprising that touch and loneliness form some sort of dyad in human experience."[46] Older patients particularly enjoy touch.

It was mentioned earlier that relatedness occurs on two levels, the first being physical relatedness. Second, it occurs as relatedness to one's illness, injury, or disfigurement. In order to facilitate such relatedness, the nurse includes the patient's family in the teaching. The nurse, together with other members of the health team, explains to both individuals what the illness, injury, or disfigurement implies, the treatment plan and nursing care. Again nurses can use play activities in teaching smaller children. Dolls can be substituted for the patient. Dressings can be placed on the doll and the child encouraged to help the nurse change these dressings. A variety of creative approaches can be used to lessen the child's fears and hopefully enhance a sense of relatedness to an affected body part.

Needless to say, the nurse must assess a patient's readiness to learn and comprehension of teaching input. Any teaching plan must be initiated, when realistic, early in the patient's hospitalization. If not accomplished early then the patient, family, or spouse may not attain a sense of relatedness to the illness. The nurse's goal, regardless of the patient's age, is to facilitate relatedness through knowledge. Together the patient, family, or spouse can share the experience, thus minimizing each individual's feelings of loneliness.

The second way in which the nurse minimizes psychological pain is by facilitating the patient's sense of relatedness to the boundaries of his or her own body. The nurse helps the patient feel a part of the diagnostic and therapeutic regime that is happening to the body. When the nurse attaches various wires or tubes to the body, he or she also attaches meaning to them. If pieces of equipment are attached or treatment procedures are done without explanation, the patient will not achieve a sense of relatedness to them. Meaningful explanations help the patient to feel less an object in a strange environment.

The last way in which the nurse minimizes psychological pain is through the ability to foster a sense of relatedness to values and ideas. Both of these may have been temporarily threatened by the crisis. Again, the patient becomes aware of boundaries in terms of limits or restrictions. Boundaries or limits become those activities which the patient can do and those activities which must be temporarily postponed. The word "can" is

---

[46]DeThomasa, *op. cit.*, p. 113.

stressed rather than "can not." The words "can not" signify a loss and loss precipitates feelings of loneliness. In most instances, the patient will return to a relatively stable level of wellness and will not need to make major changes. Together the nurse and patient discuss limits that the current crisis has dictated.

Minimize physiological pain   The nurse assesses when a patient is experiencing pain and intervenes to alleviate it. The nurse realizes that a patient may complain of pain in the foot, chest, finger, hand, leg, or as Peplau said, "any other organ that could be called into service to indicate the pain of loneliness."[47] As discussed previously, patients may react in one of three ways to pain; ignore it, realistically react to it, or overreact to it. Regardless of the reason, pain to the patient is a real experience. Therefore, it cannot be ignored. The nurse must assess the meaning pain has to both types of patient—the one who chooses to ignore it and the one who chooses to overreact to it. The degree of intensity is not the important factor. The important element is how the individual reacts.

The nurse may discover that the patient who overreacts to pain is seeking attention. Therefore, the nurse intervenes to provide the patient with the necessary attention. This is accomplished through purposeful communication with the patient. Through communication the nurse attempts to move the patient out of isolation and existential loneliness. "Persons who are in a state of deep isolation and loneliness can communicate and be communicated with only in the most concrete terms; one cannot break through their isolation with abstraction."[48] Keeping this in mind the nurse begins on the patient's level and moves accordingly. Usually the patient is left with the boundaries of his or her thoughts. The mind is left to focus on any physiological pain feelings. Therefore, it is imperative that the nurse spend 10-15 minutes giving the patient full attention. A consistent time each day will be the key that unlocks the door of loneliness and minimizes physiological pain.

Loneliness Anxiety: Fear of Aloneness

In helping the patient cope with loneliness anxiety, the nurse has two goals. First, the nurse intervenes to foster the patient's relatedness to the environment. Second, the nurse fosters the patient's relatedness to the future. Both goals involve the establishment of boundaries.

[47]Peplau, *op. cit.*, p. 1479.
[48]Guptan, *op. cit.*, p. 23.

Foster relatedness to the environment   The nurse fosters environmental relatedness by helping the patient to establish boundaries of location. In regard to boundary of location, the patient needs to know the proximity of the bed to the family room, nurse's station, or other departments. In addition, the patient needs to know the relationship of personal objects within the environment. Personal objects such as toys, pictures, flowers, radios, or cards help to reduce feelings of loneliness. These objects are especially important for the small child and the aged patient. Personal objects may represent their security and identity. Aged patients need more relational elements in their environment. Unfortunately, what is often seen is isolation. The patient is isolated from activities due to fear of injury. Such protection forces the patient to disengage rather than engage with the environment.

Patients also need to know their boundary of location in relationship to other patients. A patient may need to have territorial boundaries defined. This would include the relationship of the bed, night stand, bedside table and chair to others. Once the patient knows physical relationships or boundaries to objects within the environment, he or she feels a sense of territorial relatedness and ownership. The nurse must realize that the patient's bed becomes the only reference point. Everything else either revolves around or away from the bed. Therefore, in orienting the patient, the nurse should define the boundaries of location in relationship to the bed. The patient then becomes oriented to the dimension of physical boundaries whether they be curtains, objects, walls, or rooms. After the patient and/or nurse have established appropriate boundaries of location, the nurse then helps the patient to establish boundaries of the future.

Foster relatedness to the future   In order to foster a sense of relatedness to the future, the patient must believe that a future exists. The nurse continually reassures the patient that a future does exist. The future is significant to all patients. However, the past is equally meaningful to the aged patient. To realize being in the future, one must have the memories and reassurances of a past. Together the nurse and patient relive the past through reminiscing activities. This can be accomplished on a one-to-one or group level. The health team helps each patient derive meaning from the future. If the patient feels that his or her life will not have meaning, that patient succumbs to regressive behavior or dependency. The nurse intervenes to help the patient focus on the positive aspects of the future. The patient soon realizes that the boundaries of the future are not limited. With realistic guidance from the health team, the patient realizes the loss is not as overwhelming as anticipated. The patient no longer fears aloneness in his or her own future. Instead, the patient has a sense of relatedness to it and a sense of significance in it.

In conclusion, the nurse assists the patient in formulating boundaries of illness, location, and future by helping the patient maintain a sense of relatedness to others through meaningful contact. Finally, the nurse fosters meaningful communication utilizing a variety of therapeutic techniques. All of these factors lead the child, adult, or aged patient out of a world of isolation and loneliness.

REFERENCES

Barry, Maurice, "Depression, Shame, Loneliness and the Psychiatrist's Position," *American Journal of Psychotherapy*, 16, 1962.

Berblinger, Klaus, "A Psychiatrist Looks at Loneliness," *Psychosomatics*, 9, March-April 1968, pp. 96–102.

Bowman, Claude, "Loneliness and Social Change," *American Journal of Psychiatry*, 112, September 1955, pp. 194–98.

Buhler, C., "Loneliness in Maturity," *Journal of Humanistic Psychology*, 1, Fall 1969.

Ferrcira, Antonio, "Loneliness and Psychopathology," *The American Journal of Psychoanalysis*, 22, 1962.

Fromm-Reichmann, Frieda, "Loneliness," *Psychiatry*, 22, 1959.

Greer, Ina May, "Roots of Loneliness," *Pastoral Psychology*, 4, 1953.

Knight, Theresa, "Loneliness: A Clinical Nursing Problem," *Interpersonal Relations*, (Ed: Maloney, Elizabeth), Iowa: Brown, 1966.

Mark, Frank, "A Project for Nursing Homes to Combat Loneliness, Anxiety, Boredom," *Nursing Homes*, April 1973.

Mercer, Lianne, "Touch: Comfort or Threat?" *Perspectives in Psychiatric Care*, 4, 1966, pp. 20–25.

Mintz, Elizabeth, "Touch and the Psychoanalytic Tradition," *The Psychoanalytic Review*, 56, 1969, pp. 365–76.

Munnicks, J., "Loneliness, Isolation and Social Relations in Old Age," *Vita Humana*, 7, 1964, pp. 228–38.

Norris, Catherine, "The Work of Getting Well," *American Journal of Nursing*, October 1969, pp. 2118–21.

Riesman, Davis, *The Lonely Crowd*, New Haven: Yale University Press, 1950.

Steig, William, *The Lonely Ones*, New York: Duel Sloan and Pearce, 1942.

Tournier, Paul, *Escape From Loneliness*, Philadelphia: Westminister Press, 1962.

Von Witzleben, Henry, "On Loneliness," *Psychiatry*, 21, February 1958 pp. 37–43.

Weigert, Edith, "Loneliness and Trust—Basic Factors of Human Existence," *Psychiatry*, 23, 1960.

12
Body Image

The concept, body image, has found application in many diverse disciplines and levels of thinking. It has potential usefulness over a wide range of disciplines. Historically, one finds the concept referred to in studies of psychiatric problems, neurological problems, hypnotic phenomena, drug effects, psychotherapy results, and psychosomatic illness. Each expert handles the concept in a segmented fashion according to his or her own specialty. Consequently, the concept has not been examined or applied in a holistic way in literature. Body image is an exciting concept because it provides a way of thinking about one's body and how, through the body, one relates to the environment. "This internal mental representation of one's body is elaborated out of all the interoceptive stimuli that reach the cerebral cortex and all the experiences in which an individual perceives his body as a meaningful part of his subjective world."[1]

Nurses are becoming increasingly more aware of the body image concept. They realize that any individual, no matter what the level of wellness or illness, cherishes and guards his or her wholeness. Our culture is based upon wholeness. Beauty and the achievement of beauty is represented by a total body. Television commercials foster this image. Rarely is the deformed represented through mass media. An exception would be televised telethons for various debilitating illnesses such as cerebral palsy, muscular dystrophy, or arthritis. It is interesting that, "Despite evidence on social, vocational, and intellectual competency, the deformed are exposed to a kind of stereotyping which is socially disadvantageous. Pervasive as these attitudes are, there is a reality basis for the high concern manifested by patients with physical deformities."[2] Whether or not the individual can identify with various commercials, he

---

[1]W.A. Cantrell, and S.H. Frazier, "Psychiatry for the General Practitioner," In Arieti, S. (Ed) *American Handbook of Psychiatry*, 3, (New York: Basic Books, 1966).

[2]L.C. Kolb, "Disturbances of the Body-Image," *American Handbook of Psychiatry*, 1 (New York: Basic Books, 1959), p. 83.

or she is still a whole being. The individual's, "wholeness must depend not only on the private resources of his own body but equally on the interaction in which he unceasingly is engaged with his environment."[3]

The human body image develops through sensory messages from the inner surface of the body and from the outer surface in contact with the environment. This implies a degree of exchange between man and the environment. One has a feeling of self-contained independence which enables one to move through the environment without restrictions. However, injury, illness, or disfigurement sets limitations or restrictions on a sense of freedom. A person may no longer feel a sense of uniqueness. Alterations in body image may lead to disturbances because of possible limitations. In addition, disturbances of body image can occur when the individual fails to accept the body as it is and to adapt to it. The individual experiences a conflict between the way the body is now perceived and how he or she actually mentally visualizes the body.

BODY IMAGE DEFINED

A person's body, as perceived or evaluated, plays a significant role in determining security and sense of self-esteem. The body concept includes all of the perception and knowledge concerning one's own body appearance, boundaries, limits, and inner structure. Therefore, body image becomes the image that an individual holds in the mind of his or her own body. The image then becomes the way the body appears to self. The individual perceives himself to be tall, short, thin, or fat. The image may be fifty pounds lighter than that perceived by others. "Body image forms an integral part of an individual's conception of his personality, his worth, and his relations with other people."[4]

According to Schilder, "Body image is a gestalt or a unified pattern for organizing sensory input. Although body image has a physiologic basis, it is composed of physical, psychologic, and social experiences. Thus, body image not only includes an individual's personal and psychologic investment in his body and its parts, but also has a sociologic meaning for both the individual and society."[5] Fisher believes the term refers to the body as a psychological experience, and focuses on the individual's feelings and attitudes towards his own body. It is concerned with the individual's subjective experience with his body and the manner

[3]Myra Levine, "Pursuit of Wholeness," *American Journal of Nursing,* January 1969, p. 98.

[4]E.V. Olson, "Immobility: Effects of Psychosocial Equilibrium," *American Journal of Nursing,* April 1967, p. 794.

[5]Paul Schilder, *The Image and Appearance of the Human Body,* (New York: International Universities Press, 1950).

in which he has organized these experiences. The assumption is that as each individual develops, he has the difficult task of meaningfully organizing the sensations from his body—which is one of the most important and complex phenomena in his total perceptual field.[6]

Body image involves a number of things. It represents a unity between temporal, environmental, and interpersonal factors. The term also implies an interpersonal experience of the individual's feelings and attitudes toward one's body and the way one organizes these experiences. For example, a lady who weighs 230 pounds decides to diet and lose weight. With supervised dieting, she loses approximately 90 pounds. Even though she has lost considerable weight necessitating a new image, including smaller dress size, the lady's concept of herself remains that of obese. Other people may perceive her new image as slender; however, her own visual image remains unchanged. She has not assimilated her new image into her being. Another individual may feel inferior or unattractive because of a large nose. It is interesting that body orifices or protuberances are significant in orienting one to his own body as well as to the environment and bodies of others. The individual may compare his nose to those of others with less protruding ones. His comparison leads him to alter the size of his nose. Even with a new nose, the individual discovers that his feelings still exist. These feelings regarding his image have been internalized over a span of many years. Consequently, it takes time to change the concept he holds of his self and body image. Much of the editing of the experiences that go into making and modifying the body image is not conscious, and no one can describe his or her own total body image. According to Kolb, "The body image must be considered as a psychologic entity deriving from past experiences and current sensations. It is built up through the years from physiologic, psychologic, and social components organized by the central nervous system, which serves as an integrative agent."[7]

Body image is a part of self-concept. How well a person likes the self, his or her concept, is related to the definiteness of body image. The definiteness of an individual's body implies how well defined or structured it has become from early childhood to present. Of course, the child's perception of body image can be related to personality variables in the child and how adults reacted to the child. Definiteness of body image also comes through body boundaries. Body boundaries become a vehicle or aid in maneuvering about in the external world. Knowledge of the limits of one's body boundaries is essential for judging whether or not a given space can be moved into without actually testing the situation. In

[6]Seymour Fisher, *Body Image and Personality*, (New York: Dover Publications, 1968), p. 10.

[7]Kolb, *op. cit.*, pp. 749–69.

order to reinforce body boundaries, the individual must move through the environment and use the boundaries. The individual who is immobilized through illness or injury cannot use the body-image boundaries. According to Arnhoff, "Body-image boundaries, therefore, will deteriorate due to disuse, and judgements about these boundaries will become inaccurate."[8]

Each individual moves around a mental image of one's own appearance. This image may or may not be consistent with actual body structure. The body image, as an entity, derives itself from past and current experiences. It is usually described as evolving gradually in the course of a learning process in which the individual experiences the body in manifold situations and also notes the reactions of others to it. The individual may or may not be conscious about the image projected. By and large a person's body, as one perceives and evaluates it, plays an important role in determining security and sense of self-esteem.

Schonfield summarizes body image definitions by referring to it as a complicated constellation of elements, both conscious and unconscious, which represent the following: (1) the actual subjective perception of the body; (2) the internalized psychological factors arising out of the individual's personal-emotional experiences, as well as the distortions of the body concept expressed as somatic delusions; (3) the sociological factors, namely how the parents and society react to the individual's interpretations of their reactions; and, (4) the ideal body image formulated by the individual's attitudes toward his body derived from identification with the bodies of other persons.[9]

NORMAL DEVELOPMENT OF BODY IMAGE

Through the course of an individual's growth and development one builds an image of his or her own body. The image that emerges is determined by both interpersonal and intrapersonal experiences. These experiences are the result of tactile, kinesthetic, and visual perceptions. Intrapersonal experiences are integrated into the individual's being or self over time. The integration facilitates development of a personal frame of reference from which body change is registered. Both development and maintenance of an image of self are dependent upon perceptual feedback between the individual and the environment. An understanding of nor-

---

[8]Franklyn Arnhoff, "Body Image Deterioration in Paraplegia," *Journal of Nervous and Mental Diseases*, 137, July 1963, p. 88.

[9]W.A. Schonfield, "Body Image in Adolescents—A Psychological Concept for the Pediatrician," *Pediatrics*, 31, May 1963, pp. 845–55.

mal body image development from childhood through old age is imperative in understanding an individual's reaction to alteration of an image.
Normal development of body image will be examined as it pertains to the
child, adolescent, adult, and aged.

Childhood

The child, while moving through the environment, integrates experiences from it, masters it, and responds to it. In the process of doing so
the child is continually resynthesizing body image and self-concept. Body
image and self-concept are developed during the childhood years (see
table). Consequently, the body image of the child is like clay. It is capable
of being molded and reshaped according to adjustments and reorganizations that need to be made—all of which eventually change body boundaries. The definiteness of the child's body boundaries is determined by
how well structured the child perceives the body image to be. Such
definiteness of the child's image is fundamental to his or her identity.
Blaesing believes that, "The child's concept of his body image or the
degree of definiteness of his body boundaries is expressed in the way the
child interacts with his environment, and can be identified in his values,
attitudes, and feelings about himself."[10] The child's body image emerges
as a result of changes occurring in the developmental stages of infant,
toddler, and schoolage years.

The infant   The infant does not have a physical body image. The
infant's image occurs on a feeling level. The infant experiences comfort,
hunger, satisfaction, pleasure, displeasure, and pain. In addition, the
infant differentiates his or her body from other objects through motor or
kinesthetic sensations. A crucial factor in the development of body image
is stimulation. An environment deprived of tactile stimulation can impair
the infant's ego development. In addition, the level of anxiety may
actually increase because the infant does not experience security from
tactile sensation.

Initially, the infant's body image is centered around the mouth. It is
here that he or she experiences the greatest degree of pleasure. Changes
occur during the infant's first year that enable differentiation of the body
image from the external world. He or she becomes aware that the body is
separate from all others, including mother. The infant's initial experience
of his or her own body and its separateness becomes the foundation for
other life experiences. The initial experience is dependent upon how well
the infant is cared for. An infant who has been well taken care of and

[10]Sandra Blaesing, and Joyce Brockhaus, "The Development of Body Image in the
Child," *Nursing Clinics of North America* 7, December 1972, p. 597.

STAGES OF BODY IMAGE DEVELOPMENT DURING CHILDHOOD

INFANT	TODDLER (1–3)	PRESCHOOLER (3–6)	SCHOOLAGER (6–12)
Unable to differentiate body from other objects in the environment (e.g. hand vs rattle)	Able to differentiate between self and the environment	Interested in one's own identity "I"	Sense of industry vs inferiority period
Attitude toward own body: bites fingers, hand, or toes	Due to increase in physical growth, toddler experiences modification in body image	Identifies with parental model	Learns how to interact socially with peers
Develops trust relationship which contributes to further development of positive self-concept	More aware of significant others	Increase growth of language, intellectual and motor skills	Increase development of sex role identification
	Developing a sense of autonomy	Beginning sexual curiosity	Further development of intellectual skills by testing them against peers
	Learning mastery over environment through development of: basic motor skills language skills bladder-bowel mastery		Increasing concern with how others see one's body
			Growing knowledge about the body and how it works

271

whose needs were met will experience a sense of trust. A sense of trust enables the infant to develop a positive self-concept. On the other hand, the infant whose needs are not met by significant others in the environment will experience mistrust. The infant who develops a sense of trust is ready for the next stage of development.

Toddler   The toddler, because of growing and sometimes active involvement with the environment, is capable of greater differentiation between self and the environment. The toddler is continually modifying body image. Modification takes place because size is changing. In addition, the toddler experiences greater motor skills which enable him to explore the environment. It is during the toddler stage of childhood that mastery of the body is a principle task. The toddler learns who he or she is in relationship to the environment which signifies the world. Furthermore, it is a time when one begins to learn how to manipulate the environment and control one's own body. The toddler who is unable to master both the body and the environment may experience feelings of helplessness, inadequacy, and guilt.

Parental figures are those people who facilitate the toddler's mastery of body and environment. The parents are the most significant people in his or her world. Blaesing has said that, "Their approval or disapproval of the toddler's behavior and physical features is conveyed verbally as well as nonverbally. The attitudes of parents impart an indelible impression on the child's concept of himself, his body, and its functions. The child's valuation or devaluation of his own body reflects the value ascribed to it by those who take care of him."[11]

Preschooler   The preschool stage revolves around the child's discovery of what kind of person he or she is to become. The "I" aspect of the child's personality becomes stronger and the body image is more clearly formed in his or her own mind. Sex role identification and differentiation between sexes is an important developmental component of this stage. Boys learn from their fathers desirable idiosyncrasies of boys; independence, muscular build, and interest in athletics. Girls learn from their mothers those stereotypic attributes of girls such as gentleness, feminine appearance, and interest in less aggressive activities.

Schoolager   The school age child's body image focuses on further differentiation or identification of sex roles, how to interact with peers, and development of learning skills. This is a time when psychosocial problems may become evident. If the child is emotionally disturbed he or she may be less tolerant of the physical self. The child's intolerance may

[11]*Ibid.*, p. 599.

take the form of disruptive behavior in the classroom. The child's physical self may be normal. However, emotionally the child is unable to accept the physical self and may become preoccupied with some aspect of appearance. "The child's concept of his body image is a primary indicator of his degree of personality organization and ego strength. The way a child organizes his experiences during the various developmental phases determines his body concept and his degree of body boundary definiteness."[12]

Adolescent Physical growth leads to change in body image. Growth is a major characteristic of the adolescent period. It is during this time that growth occurs rapidly. The physical changes that result from growth become evident not only to the adolescent but to others as well. Because of the rapidity of changes, the adolescent cannot deny them. As a result, he or she is compelled to change the body image. The adolescent perceives the body in two ways. First, the adolescent perceives the body according to its appearance. Second, he or she perceives the body according to its usefulness to the adolescent. If the body permits one to accomplish goals then it has use or purpose. On the other hand, if the body is perceived as limited in its usefulness then one feels handicapped. Both perceptions make the adolescent, more so than the child, aware of body image. The adolescent is very much aware and concerned with his appearance.

The adolescent years are filled with an almost sudden interest in clothes, hair, and complexion. During preadolescent days, a boy might wear the same pair of pants to school for one week. The adolescent boy, on the other hand, must have a different pair of pants for each day of the week. Parents sometimes have difficulty keeping up with the various changes. Just when the parent thinks he or she understands one's own adolescent, he again changes and assumes a new image. It is during this rapid period of growth that the adolescent becomes more aware of certain parts of his or her body. Furthermore, it is a time when the adolescent is sensitive about those body parts that are changing. The changes that occur bring about two consequences. "First, a subsequent change in body image is called for in the adolescent himself, and second, others will respond to his bodily changes and thus communicate their values about the body to him. The adolescent uses these to evaluate himself."[13]

Adolescence is a phase of high ideals. It is a time of peer comparison and contrast. One teenage girl's larger than average bust size becomes the envy of less endowed girls. Likewise, the deepening voice and facial hair

[12]*Ibid.*, p. 606.

[13]Mary Dempsey, "The Development of Body Image in the Adolescent," *Nursing Clinics of North America* 7, December 1972, p. 615.

of one boy may become the focus of attention or envy of other boys. Both adolescents may become sensitive about their physical changes and new images. Sensitivity can lead to an accurate body image or a distorted view of one's self. The girl with a large bust may be perceived as being sexy. Her own image may be quite the opposite. On the other hand, she might assume a sexy appearance and build her image according to the perception of others rather than how she feels herself. The adolescent girl then develops a distorted perception of her body or a part of it. The same would apply to the adolescent boy who becomes preoccupied with his masculine voice or facial hairs. Both may attribute undue significance to the new changes.

Adolescents unhappy with their body image may distort it in an attempt to bring it up to his or her ideal. Those unable to achieve their ideal may discredit their bodies. The adolescent may feel inferior in comparison to peers. In time and with parental support, the adolescent adjusts ideals to more realistically encompass one's own body image. According to Dempsey, "Most adolescents revise their ideals and their fantasies about their body when they clash with reality. They become reconciled to any physical limitations; they eventually accept the image of the adult body."[14]

Adulthood

The developmental stage of young adulthood continues to be a time characterized by growth and change. Those biological growth changes of adolescence are completed. The body image is a result of having experienced the physical, social, and psychological changes associated with adolesence. The difference in adulthood is that people differ in their experience of body boundaries. Fisher believes that, "Some perceive the boundaries as definite, well articulated, and clearly separated from their environs. For others, the boundaries are vaguely defined and represent only a hazy contour. The more definite and clearly articulated an individual's body image boundaries, the greater is his tendency to show high reactivity in boundary regions such as the skin and muscle, and low reactivity in interior sectors, for example, the heart."[15]

Throughout the years the adult has developed certain feelings about the body and its parts. One's feelings are dependent upon the function a particular body part serves. In other words, the body part is perceived as either a functional tool or central to the body image. For example, an

---

[14]*Ibid.*

[15]S. Fisher, "Sex Differences In Body Perception," *Psychological Monographs*, 78, 1964, pp. 1–22.

individual's eyes can be seen as a tool for seeing. They permit one to move through the environment with an element of ease. To another individual, the eyes may represent a central part of facial feature. Such an individual may say that "people are attracted to him because of his blue eyes." To him the need for glasses threatens a youthful image and sense of attractiveness. He may have difficulty integrating the change in self-image. However, if the eyes were viewed as a tool used for mobility or reading, one is better able to integrate or assimilate the new change.

Men and women vary in their body boundaries. The variation is in the definiteness of body boundaries. For example, women seem to have a more definite sense of body boundaries than men. Women are more likely to perceive alterations in the face region, perhaps because of the social significance attributed to the female face. In addition, the face is most consistently used to register expressive emotion, and women are more skilled at this; it is socially acceptable. Therefore, women are more confident and less anxious about the function of the face and more aware of the facial changes.[16] The female devotes more attention to the body than does the male; she arrives more quickly at a realistic concept of her body. The role of the woman is more explicitly identified with her body and its functions; a woman more nearly equates self with body. Man's role and status has typically been defined in terms of his achievement rather than in terms of body attributes. This body awareness in the female involves boundary regions while for the male it reflects experience pertaining to digestive aspects, that is, the gastrointestinal tract.[17]

In general, an adult's body image and self-concept are the results of social evolution. In our society, a normal appearing body image is favored. Therefore, an individual's self-image can influence how constructive or expansive his or her world becomes and one's success in it. An adult's self-image becomes a dynamic interrelationship between three vital components: self-concept, identity, and personality. Usually an individual who feels positive about the body image projects a positive attitude. He or she soon discovers that people are attracted to one's positive personality and self-confidence.

The middle years of life, between the ages of 45 and 65, continue to represent changes, particularly in the growth cycle. The middle aged individual experiences physical and psychological changes. He or she notices that certain parts of the body seem to age at different rates than others. The once slim individual may notice a gradual increase of his or her weight. This is particularly true for the menopausal woman. Men may notice a thinning of the hairline and decrease in physical strength. Both realize a loss in their once youthful images. Associated with the loss is a

[16]*Ibid.*
[17]*Ibid.*

realization that their bodies may no longer be strong and healthy. Furthermore, the once boundless energy seems dissipated into accomplishing less strenuous goals. Of course, those adults who have physically maintained their bodies through proper diet and activity may not experience physical strength or energy loss.

Those who see middle age as loss of physical power evolving into an image of oldness might attempt to alter their appearance. Such alteration usually involves imitating youth in their dress and style of living. Murray believes that, "What the person does with his appearance is based on maturity and image of self as well as on social and advertising pressures. To blindly imitate youth denies the mature person's own past and experience, valid in its own right. The excitement of the middle years lies in using the experience, insights, values, and realism acquired during the years of living. Honesty about perceiving the body outwardly makes for an inward security."[18]

Aged   The aging process brings about a marked change in the self-concept. Psychologically, the aged individual goes through depression and disengagement. He or she becomes disengaged through loss of leadership roles and occupation. In addition, "the later years of life bring physical and social, and therefore mental and emotional changes. Two critical events that affect self-concept are retirement and eventual loss of the spouse, as well as loss of other close family and friends. The decline of physical powers, although possibly intruding into one's self-concept as early as the forties or fifties, will be more strongly felt in the late sixties and thereafter. This heightens fears of incapacitation and the nothingness of death."[19]

Physical changes in body image can lead to dependency on supportive devices such as dentures, hearing aid, glasses, cane, walker, pacemaker, or wheelchair. Other physical changes include a slowing gait, wrinkles, loss of hair, postural changes, reduction in sensory-motor function, and loss of strength. Regardless of physical changes in body image, the aged individual may seem young. To some people retirement is not the end but rather the beginning of a new life. As a result, retirement does not represent a rocking chair or a life of nothingness. Many aged people have maintained interest in activities other than those related to work or family. Involvement in their environment and the people therein becomes increasingly more significant to them. This is why the aged individual responds to the emotional climate of the environment.

[18] Ruth Murray, "Body Image Development in Adulthood," *Nursing Clinics of North America 7*, December 1972, p. 623.

[19] A.M. Rose, and W.A. Peterson, *Older People and Their Social World*, (Philadelphia: F.A. Davis, 1965).

The emotional climate takes the form of support, interest, and encouragement. It is through the warm relationship of others that the aged person develops a realistic body image.

A normal body image and self-concept are the result of learning, maturation, one's perception and others' perception of self. Each of the above are carefully interwoven throughout one's life time. An individual's body image, no matter what the age, can change for reasons other than through normal growth and developmental processes. These reasons may be the result of disease, illness, injury, surgery, or even pregnancy. The alterations in body image that result are capable of creating a crisis.

ALTERATIONS IN BODY IMAGE

Alterations in body image can be as minor as a bruise or as major as disfigurement or surgical loss. Even something as insignificant as a bruise or small cut draws the individual's full attention to the affected body part. The altered body part may not seem as attractive as before the change, no matter how subtle the change is. Of course, the more significant the change the more threatened is the individual. Patients who experience major alteration, such as in pregnancy, illness, injury, or surgery, are in fact experiencing a crisis. As a result of the changes, the patient's image must go through a reorganization process. According to Murray, "This person is encountering a situation which is stressful to the degree that the usual pattern of responses, behavior, and coping mechanisms is inadequate to handle the present feelings resulting from this event."[20]

The patient experiencing alteration in body image will go through four phases, each of which are attempts to reintegrate the new image. The success of one's passage through each phase is dependent upon perception of the actual alteration, the physiological status of the individual, one's age, the nature of the illness, the duration of disability, and previous coping abilities. Alteration in body image of any patient, regardless of age or sex, will be examined according to Lee's four phases.[21] The four phases, through which each individual must move after an illness, injury, disease, disfigurement, or surgical loss, are impact, retreat, acknowledgment, and reconstruction. The patient's perception of the body contains the preinjury or preillness image. The patient is forced to alter the concept of the body. The change, no matter how minor or major, must be assimilated into one's being.

[20]Ruth Murray, "Principles of Nursing Intervention for the Adult Patient with Body Image Changes," *Nursing Clinics of North America*, December, 1972, pp. 697–98.

[21]Jane Lee, "Emotional Reactions to Trauma," *NCNA*, December 1970, p. 583.

Impact

Adaptation to alteration in the body's function and structure depends upon the nature of the threat, its significance to the patient, previous and current coping ability, the response from significant others, and the assistance available to the patient and family as changes occur. The impact phase has different significance to the child, adolescent, adult, or aged patient. The difference is in its degree and meaning. The child may not fully realize the impact of an altered image. This is because his or her image is always changing, consequently, the new change can be incorporated. The adult or aged patient, on the other hand, may fully realize the impact of the altered image.

Alterations in body image can occur slowly, such as a gradual increase in weight, arthritis, pregnancy, or quickly, as with injury, acute illness, disfigurement, or emergency surgical alterations. One patient may have experienced prior warning resulting in an eventual alteration in body image. In this respect the change can be acknowledged over time. Other patients, through sudden alteration, are thrust into a new experience for which they have had no previous warning. The effect it has on the individual, regardless of age, will depend on the degree of alteration, the duration of time involved in the change, and the meaning the altered part has for the individual. Each of the above effects has different implications for the child, adolescent, adult, or aged patient as they go through the impact phase.

Children are hospitalized for various reasons—some are more biologically serious than others. Nevertheless, to each child the experience or reason is threatening. This is especially true for the child experiencing a first hospitalization or separation from the family. Hospitalization may result from a diagnostic evaluation, elective surgery, or an emergency. Most health problems require that the child undergo some diagnostic and/or treatment procedures, each of which seems mysterious and frightening. Many of the procedures are of an intrusive nature. The small needle of a syringe suddenly appears twice as large. With most diagnostic procedures, the child initially does not realize any threat to body image or integrity. The first realization comes when he or she sees a bandage. Bandages are not threatening to the child because they are less immobilizing and more familiar. The threatening part is what the bandage covers.

Diagnostic procedures may have less mysterious connotations than surgery. Most children have experienced some diagnostic procedures, whether blood studies or X rays. Surgery, on the other hand, may be a new experience. Likewise, an emergency situation such as an accident, fracture, appendicitis, or respiratory problem necessitating immediate hospitalization can also be a new experience. Surgery and emergency situations can be more difficult to cope with because they contribute to gross stress reaction.

Hospitalization for elective surgery or an emergency causes a stress reaction. The child can be prepared for possible body image changes that might occur as a result of surgical alteration or loss. An emergency, on the other hand, offers no prior warning that a change in image is imminent; for example, the life-threatening emergency of burns or an automobile accident. "The multiple facets associated with the child's reactions would include the nature of the traumatic event and associated circumstances which may involve his guilt, his age and stage of development, the quality and quantity of family upheaval, which would be dependent upon its preexisting status, and lastly, the care provided him in the hospital."[22] Again, the child's realization of the impact comes when he or she sees the dressing, cast, traction, burned skin, or feels the pain.

Unlike the familiarity of small bandages, dressings, casts, traction, or pain are more immobilizing and threatening to the child. Each draws the child's attention to the altered body part. In addition their immobilizing effect, may seriously define his body boundary and his location in space.[23] Furthermore, surgical loss or paralysis due to injury, contractures, and disfigurement are constant reminders of the event and the altered body image. Other than the dressings, casts, tractions, or pain, the child may not fully realize the impact of the altered body image.

Unlike the child, the adolescent is more aware of body boundaries and body changes. As a result, alterations in the adolescent's body image can be more traumatic. The adolescent has greater ego involvement with the altered part than the child. After all, he or she and the altered part have been together for a longer period of time.

One alteration of body image unrealted to injury, loss, or trauma is adolescent obesity. It represents a change, and depending upon the duration of obesity, it represents a crisis. As discussed earlier the adolescent is very concerned and preoccupied with appearance. The attention to appearance continues until attention can be directed to objects outside the self. Of course, obesity is also a major problem of adulthood. Nevertheless, it seems to have particular significance to the adolescent. The obese adolescent has difficulty identifying with the slim actress, actor, rock singer, politician, or friend who represents a fantasized idol. According to Stunkard, "Several factors predispose an obese person to the

[22]Milton Fujita, "The Impact of Illness or Surgery on the Body Image of the Child," *Nursing Clinics of North America*, 7, December 1972, p. 634.

[23]Irene Riddle, "Nursing Intervention to Promote Body Image Integrity in Children," *Nursing Clinics of North America*, 7, December 1972, p. 655.

development of a disturbed body image: age of onset of obesity, presence of emotional disturbances, and negative evaluations of obesity by others during formative years. Persons becoming obese in the adolescent period are more likely to have body image disturbances than those with onset in childhood or adult life. Emotional disturbances are frequent in persons whose obesity is of juvenile onset and the body image disturbance is the dominant feature of the emotional disorder."[24] Body image disturbance in the obese adolescent can revolve around feelings of depersonalization. The depersonalization takes the form of distorted thoughts and perceptions about the body. He or she may perceive the body to be smaller or larger than it is in reality.

Altered body image may have its greatest impact on the adult. Alteration can result from injury, loss, or disfigurement. Loss includes such problems as myocardial infarction, nephrectomy, hysterectomy, mastectomy, amputation of an extremity, radical excisions of face and neck, colostomy, or ileostomy. The adult has spent many years developing the body image and self-concept. Furthermore, it has become a foundation point for his or her identity. Therefore, any changes to its structure and appearance is perceived as a threat. The degree or severity of the threat may be related to the individual's ability to adapt. How an individual adapts can depend upon previous alteration in body image, body part altered, and the meaning the affected part has to the individual. A certain body part may have tremendous significance to the patient. "If these organs become diseased or have to be removed, the threat is greater than if an organ unimportant to the person is affected. The degree to which this loss of bodily control creates loss of customary control of self, physical environment, time, and contacts with others is very closely related to the degree of threat felt."[25]

It is understandable that an individual undergoing body changes can experience feelings of frustration, despair, or anger. The nurse assesses whether or not the behaviors are adaptive or maladaptive. In other words, the patient who continues to despair or be angry for a prolonged period of time may be thought of as maladapting. Futhermore, the surgical dressings, tubes, drains, or wires make the patient all the more cognizant of loss or disfigurement.

"To lose or be threatened with the loss of a complex, coordinated, and controlled functional activity which has been achieved and integrated into the personal system is to lose or be threatened with the loss of

[24]A. Stunkard, and M. Mendelson, "Obesity and the Body Image: Characteristics of Disturbances in the Body Image of Some Obese Persons," *American Journal Psychiatry,* 123: 1967, pp. 1296–1300. Copyright 1967, the American Psychiatric Association. Reprinted by permission.

[25]Ruth Murray and Judith Zentner, *Nursing Assessment and Health Promotion Through the Life Span* (Englewood Cliffs, N.J.: Prentice-Hall, 1975), p. 229.

self. Psychologically, the loss, or threat of loss, of self is equivalent to loss of life. Emotional responses serve as warning signals of the extent of danger, and we immediately mobilize energies for self-protection and self-preservation."[26] The loss and resulting change threatens the patient's sense of identity or self-esteem. Our culture places emphasis on a perfect or whole body. Therefore, any alteration in one's image implies failure.

As discussed earlier, certain body parts assume more significance than others. The breasts, uterus, face, and heart have particular implications. The patient who experiences a myocardial infarction becomes preoccupied with an internal body organ; the heart. According to Smith, "If there is failure of the heart, then there is also failure of life. The damaged part is still there, and it is functioning; it is pumping. However, the ability to rely on that heart is no longer present to the extent that it was before the myocardial infarction occurred."[27]

The loss or altered body part, whether internal (invisible) or external (visible), has special significance to the adult patient. External alterations, because the changes are obvious, create a more difficult adjustment, the exception being pregnancy. Adjustments to a disfigured body arouse feelings of threat. The individual may desire to abandon the body because he or she feels a loss in the body's ability to attain perfection. During impact phase, the adult patient focuses attention on the body part which is injured or lost.

The aged patient is threatened by the most debilitating of all changes in body image. Chronic illness, a stroke, or amputated limb due to peripheral vascular insufficiency may confine the aged individual. Body boundaries are dependent upon the individual's ability to move through the environment. Loss of a limb, paralysis of a limb, or debilitating illness threatens mobility. "When the middle-aged person is on bedrest or limited in mobility because of his illness, normal outlets for aggression displacement are not available. He feels restricted with a narrowed life space. Dependency-independency conflicts are reactivated when the patient is completely cared for by a person in the nurturing role, an experience especially threatening to the man in America."[28] Movement is essential for the individual's sense of well-being. However, the qualities of movement, action, or function are not enough. The aged individual must be able to control them. Illness or injury signals a loss of control.

Arnhoff points out that, "Numerous sensory experiences contribute in integrating one's body image into a highly organized arrangement. As

[26]Reva Rubin, "Body Image and Self Esteem," *Nursing Outlook*, June 1968, p. 22.

[27]Catherine Smith, "Body Image Changes After Myocardial Infarction," *Nursing Clinics of North America*, 7, December 1972, p. 664.

[28]Murray and Zentner, *op. cit.*, p. 274.

the number of environmental and body organ influences are cut down due to organic brain damage, as is seen in the person with a stroke and confinement to bed or wheelchair, the person loses his orientation to his body sphere."[29] The aged patient's body may not serve its normal function of contact with the environment. The wheelchair becomes a barrier between the body and the external world. "Hence, body image boundaries are no longer subject to the contact with the environment that provides the feedback necessary for adequate current evaluation of the body's status."[30] In addition, the patient's judgment regarding body boundaries becomes inaccurate. As a result, the patient may fall or injure oneself thinking he or she can do more than is biologically realistic. Arnhoff indicates that, "chronic illness necessitating confinement to bed, hemiplegia, paraplegia and various other disabilities which result in restricted environmental interaction have been shown often to result in personality disruption of some magnitude."[31]

Most patients in the impact phase manifest behaviors of despair, discouragement, and passive acceptance. Their energies turn inward in an attempt to cope with changes in their body image. Suddenly the nurse assesses that their anger and hostility is misdirected toward the health team and/or family. The patient realizes the impact of the altered body image, whether it be disfigurement due to burns, paralysis, amputation of breast or leg, or chronic debilitating illness. The resulting behavior is a projection onto others of the guilt and shame they feel for themselves. Each might feel a sense of failure in his or her own body. In time, the patient, regardless of the age or alteration, does expand beyond self and into one's environment. He or she moves into the retreat phase.

Retreat

It is during the retreat phase that the patient becomes aware of the injury, illness, loss, or disfigurement. The impact phase permitted the patient to dissociate the body from the event. However, as the shock and threat of death subsides, the reality of the problem becomes apparent. With this sudden realization comes a new array of feelings. The immediate reaction is to run. However, the immobilization created by the injury or illness does not permit one to do so. Instead, he or she can only emotionally retreat from the problem that must inevitably be faced. When one looks at one's self, he or she perceives someone else's body, not his or her own. This is especially true for the stroke patient who touches the

---

[29]Arnhoff, *op. cit.*, p. 88.
[30]*Ibid.*, p. 88.
[31]*Ibid.*, p. 88.

altered body part and feels nothing but a sense of numbness. The normal body image processes have been interrupted. The retreat phase gives the patient an opportunity to mourn the loss.

For the child, the retreat phase is a time of self-awareness and return of behavioral controls. The child who is immobilized due to severe injury such as burns or trauma resulting in multiple fractures is unable to discharge emotional energy through motor activity. Instead, the child may be forced to focus attention on the altered body part—burns, dressings, traction, or casts. The child who is unable to channel energy into motor activity may retreat into a verbal display of energy. Such a display takes the form of regressive behavior. Regressive behavior can be manifested by the child's defiance or stubbornness. The burned child hopes to avoid painful therapy and gain supportive attention through regressive behavior.

Altered body image for the adolescent has many dimensions. Unlike the child and adult, the altered body part affects both the adolescent and his or her peers. The peer group becomes a mirror through which the adolescent sees the self. Adolescence is a time of preoccupation with the self and is characterized by self-consciousness. Self-consciousness becomes magnified when a permanent damage to body part or loss of function occurs. The obese adolescent who feels self-conscious may hide behind loose-fitting clothes. Other adolescents deny their obesity by wearing tight-fitting clothes. Both behavioral responses serve to draw attention to the adolescent. Initially, the adolescent retreats into denial. However, as time progresses, the adolescent begins to reintegrate the body image. Reintegration and reorganization of body image is imperative because, "when an individual fails to reorganize his body image over a period of time following distortions or changes in his body, he has not made the appropriate psychologic adaptation. Such maladaptive states often occur in individuals for whom the integrity of the preillness or preaccident body image was overvalued in maintaining self-esteem."[23]

As mentioned earlier, the adult has greater ego involvement with the altered body part. In addition, the meaning of the body defect to the individual is highly important. To the female patient, loss of her breast or uterus implies, according to society, loss of feminity and attractiveness. To the male patient, loss has similar implications. Loss of body function through myocardial infarction or loss of part due to amputation implies more than the part; it also involves loss of his masculinity and integrity. The male patient experiences more than physical loss, he also expereinces social loss. Kolb says, "Depending upon the individual, the loss may have any meaning such as heroic sacrifice or a deserved punishment, a realization of helplessness and vulnerability, a conviction of loathsome-

---

[32]Kolb, *op. cit.*, p. 764.

ness, a despicable mutilation to be hidden or accepted, or a rejection of the part with defiance toward society and social customs."[33]

Like the adolescent, the adult also retreats into denial. According to Mosey, "Denial of the loss is common, the denial often spreading to surrounding body parts. With limited ability to master the environment, the individual frequently develops a negative attitude towards his total body or the specific impaired part."[34] The loss of a body part or function threatens the individual with loss of self. "Since the self molds experience to avoid conflict with the image, the patient may deny that it is he to whom this even has happened."[35] The latter event can happen with patients who experience internal organ loss or alteration, such as the patient with a myocardial infarction or hysterectomy. The alteration is not visible to others or even himself; therefore, its occurrence can be denied. Denial of myocardial infarction is reinforced by society's attitude toward the individual. He or she is looked upon as being less productive regardless of physical capabilities.

Denial is difficult for the individual whose altered body part is visible to oneself, it not others. Such an alteration would be mastectomy, colostomy, amputation, or other disfigurement due to injuries. As a result, "Acute disturbances of body image may occur following surgical or traumatic dismemberment when the basic body image persists in spite of the visible or apparent loss of a body part."[36]

The aged individual fears becoming disabled or being an invalid. Both situations would make the aged patient dependent upon others for help. Such fears force the aged patient to retreat into regressive behavior. Regressive behavior, while temporary, is the patient's way of adjusting. Murray states that, "The increasing powerlessness and loss of authority status thus lessens the respect from others."[37] The most difficult alterations in body image for the aged are those resulting from amputations and strokes. With other debilitating illnesses such as arthritis and emphysema, the individual has learned to compensate for them throughout the years. However, amputation or strokes occur without warning. The aged patient must learn new ways to move through the environment. Both losses arouse feelings within the aged patient. The loss can symbolize the imminent approach of death. "Reactions felt by the patient with a stroke may also be felt by one with an amputation, that is, there

[33]*Ibid.*, p. 765.

[34]Anne Mosey, "Treatment of Pathological Distortion of Body Image," *The American Journal of Occupational Therapy,* 23, September-October 1969, p. 414.

[35]Florence Brown, "Knowledge of Body Image and Nursing Care of the Patient with Limb Amputation," *Journal Psychiatric Nursing,* 2, 1964, pp. 397–409.

[36]Joan Luckmann and Karen Sorensen, "Disturbances of body Image," *Medical-Surgical Nursing: A Psychophysiologic Approach,* (Philadelphia: Saunders, 1974), p. 83.

[37]Murray, *op. cit.,* p. 626.

may be feelings of guilt and shame, worthlessness, loss of wholeness, and vulnerability."[38]

Each of the above patients reacts differently to altered body image. The child and aged individual retreat into regressive behavior. On the other hand, the adolescent and adult retreat into denial. Both behavioral responses are temporary. The retreat phase allows the individual, regardless of age or problem, to reorganize body image in an attempt to acknowledge the loss.

Acknowledgment

The patient, regardless of age, has suffered an alteration in body image, the result being a change in physical appearance. The reality of such a change must be faced if the patient is to continue daily existence. The phase of adjustment is to help the patient acknowledge the alteration, which is equated with loss of body image. The acknowledgment phase brings about a period of mourning the loss. The patient must acknowledge a loss regardless of the degree involved. The patient realizes that he or she no longer can hide or retreat.

Depending upon the degree of altered body image (that is, extensive burns or multiple fractures), the acknowledgment phase is a time when the child begins to recognize strengths. Prior to this the child saw only losses. Hopefully, the biological crisis stabilizes so that the child can increase his or her motor function. Such an increase can serve as an encouragement to the child of improvement. Furthermore, motor activity helps channel excess energy that during the retreat phase was expressed as behavioral responses. Mobility becomes important for the hospitalized child. It permits the child to move through the environment and become involved with other children. In this respect socialization can take place. Children with similar body-image changes can share their experiences. Such sharing can help the child acknowledge a loss.

Like the child, the adolescent acknowledges changes that have occurred in body image. During this time, the adolescent takes in bits and pieces of information regarding the change. He or she also may become involved with those in the environment. To the adolescent, the external world, composed of the health team and fellow patients, is becoming more significant. How these people, including the family, react to the adolescent's altered image sometimes determines his or her own acknowledgment and eventual acceptance. With both the child and adolescent the goal is to increase use of their bodies for environmental contact. Arnhoff believes that, "By alleviating or preventing deterioration in the

[38]Beverly Leonard, "Body Image Changes in Chronic Illness," *Nursing Clinics of North America*, 7, December 1972, pp. 693–94.

body image through increased and continued use of the body for environmental contact, personality deterioration and dysfunction may be minimized."[39]

For the adult and aged patient, acknowledgment can imply that both experience a loss of their individuality and uniqueness. Permanent disabilities force the patient to lose not only his or her uniqueness but also social freedom. It is during the acknowledgment phase that the patient discusses the details or events which led to hospitalization. The patient then will discuss the altered body part in an attempt to integrate the precipitating event with the eventual alteration. This is particularly true for amputees and stroke patients. According to Ullman, "As a result of an alteration in the way the patient perceives his extremity, he is led to certain misinterpretations of his experience. He is, however, capable of correcting these misinterpretations, so that they remain at a transitory, subjective level and are generally never mentioned unless a specific inquiry is made."[40]

As adult or aged patients are forced to use the altered part, they must acknowledge it as part of their whole body. Supportive devices such as protheses, canes, walkers, or wheelchair are objects which are either attached to the body or actually participate in the body's movement. These devices help the patient extend body boundaries through movement within the environment. As with the child and adolescent, movement serves to encourage the adult or aged patients. It helps them focus on their strengths rather than losses. Once the patient has acknowledged his or her altered body part, that patient is ready to move into the rebuilding or reconstruction phase.

Reconstruction

In the pathophysiologic process that causes loss of function or part, or disfigurement, ". . . the discrete interactions may be disrupted because the individual organs or systems are incapable of performing their required interacting role. But even in the presence of disease, the organism responds wholly to the environmental interaction in which it is involved, and a considerable element of nursing care is devoted to restoring the symmetry of response—symmetry that is essential to the well-being of the organism."[41] Reconstruction occurs in varying degrees. Reconstruction does not imply perfection. Regardless of the degree of reconstruction, the individual is encouraged to try new approaches to

[39]Arnhoff, *op. cit.*, p. 91.

[40]Montague Ullman, "Disorders of Body Image After Stroke," *American Journal of Nursing*, 64, October 1964, p. 89.

[41]Levine, *op. cit.*, p. 98.

life. During the retreat and acknowledgment phase the patient mourned a loss. Now, during the reconstruction phase, he or she tries to adapt to changes in body image.

The child in the reconstruction phase, ". . . develops the capacity to represent visually relationships, fears, wishes, threats, and injuries as part of the self, or as something affecting the self . . . the child can conceive or imagine the workings of his body as well as desired or feared happenings to his body."[42] A significant part of the reconstruction phase concerns how others view the child's body image. The child's family must remain patient through the seemingly long period of hospitalization. The impatient family and health team can interfere with the child's ability to reintegrate an adequate body image. The child may be caught in a double bind. He or she struggles to maintain an individualized self-image while simultaneously wanting to maintain dependence on others. Consequently, "the body image of the hospitalized child is influenced by the attitude of others around him, his stage of development, and the illness event. The quality of the child's relationship with significant others is crucial in reintegration of his body image."[43]

The alteration in body image and the restitution measures to restore self-esteem are viewed as a significant indication of an adolescent's reaction to illness and hospitalization. Interaction with a peer group is an essential part of body image reconstruction. The adolescent with an altered image needs to become involved in activities so he or she can use this experience to compare his or her body with others. Peer involvement in the hospital will prepare the adolescent for post-hospitalization social encounters.

The goal for all patients experiencing an altered body image is to help achieve the highest level of reconstruction possible. The cardiac patient reorganizes a style of living in which to incorporate a new image. The change is a physically visible one. Except for congestive heart failure and edema, the individual looks the same as before the event. There may be little or no limitation in physical activity. Consequently, one feels a more positive attitude toward living than during the impact and retreat phases. The patient feels as if given a second chance. He or she may pay more attention to the new image in terms of activity, rest, and diet, and have a new appreciation for the family.

The aged patient reconstructs the altered image and life similar to the adult patient. The aged patient is also dependent upon the family for understanding and support. Depending upon the age of the patient, friends may be few. Therefore, primary strength comes through existing

[42]Richard Kaufman, "Body Image Changes in Physically Ill Teen-Agers," *Journal American Academy of Child Psychology,* 11, January 1972, p. 157.

[43]Fujita, *op. cit.,* p. 648.

family members. The nurse helps the family work through their feelings about the alteration. As with the patient, the nurse assesses the meaning of the change with the family.

NURSE SUPPORT OF ALTERED IMAGE

The nurse attempts to support the patient while moving through the various phases involved in the altered body image. Within each phase of the adaptation process, the nurse assesses the individual in relationship to the altered body part, intervenes to help the patient cope with the threat of change, and evaluates the effectiveness of the intervention. Regardless of the patient's age, the nurse assesses the significance of the altered body part, previous attitude toward illness and the affected part, previous experiences with hospitalization, the significance of other's perception or reactions to the change, and current knowledge of the severity of the illness or disfigurement. The nurse and other members within the health team help the patient accept and adapt to changes in body image. Each supportive member does this through sensitivity to the patient's needs and anxieties expressed in each adaptative phase.

Initially, the nurse is submerged in the responsibility of admitting the patient into the hospital. These responsibilities include life-saving treatments and procedures. During the initial impact phase the patient is exposed to numerous intrusive procedures. The procedures may be necessary; however, they threaten the patient's sense of wholeness. "Intrusive procedures, such as enemas, catheterizations, injections, diagnostic procedures involving intubation or scoping, and surgery which may realistically be mutilating, also symbolically increase anxiety, feelings of vulnerability and a sense of altered self."[44] The nurse must realize that the interventions may create psychological stress. Therefore, the nurse must not give all his or her energies to the physical aspects of illness.

The nurse should intervene on all levels, thus assisting the patient physically and psychologically to cope with the impact of alteration. In doing so, the nurse assesses the patient's definition of his or her own crisis. As previously mentioned, the nurse learns the patient's perception of what happened and what will happen to him. This will help the nurse and health team anticipate potential behavioral responses. The patient who expresses guilt over an altered image may later despair. Further- more, the patient who projects the crisis as originating outside of self may later express anger or hostility. Denial follows anger or hostility. The

[44]Murray, *op. cit.*, pp. 699–700.

patient may refuse to participate in his or her care. The child might throw a temper tantrum or cry. The adolescent may avoid treatments. The patient who refuses to participate in his or her care may not want to look at the disfigurement. To the patient, the refusal behavior is rational. Likewise, the nurse should realize that the patient's behavior is normal for the situation. During behavioral outbursts, the patient needs the nurse's continued support and acceptance. The patient, particularly the younger patient, is sensitive to the reaction of others. Therefore, the nurse's attitude can hinder or facilitate how the patient eventually accepts the altered image.

As the nurse more fully understands the meaning of a patient's behavior, he or she can channel internal energies of despair into involvement in progress. In order to encourage involvement, the nurse intervenes to protect the patient from premature disclosure of the disfigurement. For example, a female patient may not want to view the site of her amputated breast. The nurse realizes that there exists a readiness point, at which time the patient will ask to view the surgical site. Premature disclosure of the site may threaten the patient from any involvement in her own care. The nurse also realizes that in time, as the patient mourns a loss, he or she will independently share the disfigurement with others.

The nursing goal of involvement is to encourage the patient to care for his or her body. To love one's body is to want to take care of it. This becomes difficult for the patient with a visible alteration or disfigurement. Nevertheless, involvement in care teaches the patient to care for the altered body part. Involvement for children includes touching the dressing, bandage, or painful part. In addition, the nurse can encourage the child to look under the dressing at the time it is being changed. Frequent inspection of the altered body part can help to reduce a distorted conception of the image. The same intervention applies to the adult patient with an amputated or paralyzed limb. It is difficult for the patient to identify with either. The patient with an amputated limb can hold the stump while the nurse changes the dressings. In time, the patient learns to assess tissue healing. Likewise, the stroke patient can be taught to become involved with a paralyzed limb. Such involvement takes the form of exercising to maintain the muscle tone and prevent unnecessary contractures.

The nurse and other members of the health team cannot encourage patient involvement if they themselves are not involved. Involvement allows the nurse to be educated by the patient. The patient's needs involve inclusion, affection, and control. Such knowledge helps the nurse look at the patient in light of the altered body part. The nurse needs to know how the patient saw "self" in the past and how he or she sees "self" in the present. Furthermore, the nurse working with patients who experienced alteration of body image is helped if he or she recognizes that body image attack involves, "problems of altered appearance, discomfort, dependence, stigma, social isolation, action and movement limitations, vocational threat, deformity and loss of control."[45]

Another way in which the nurse helps the patient build or reconstruct body image is through encouragement of movement and activities. Movement brings the individual in contact with the environment. Such contact increases sensory stimulation. Patients who are immobilized due to their illness or treatments are unable to physically move through their environment. Movement through the environment gives both sensory and peripheral feedback necessary for body boundary organization. The nurse intervenes to maintain and strengthen the patient's existing physical mobility. In addition, the nurse facilitates visual contact with the environment. This is accomplished through use of mirrors, special glasses, or moving the patient's bed.

Children can use mirrors in order to obtain visual feedback regarding people and objects in the environment. Besides mirrors, the child's physical position can be changed so that the child is able to maintain visual interaction with the environment. Curtains and doors should remain open in an attempt not to isolate the child. Whenever realistic, the nurse can move the child's bed or crib to the unit dayroom. In this respect, the child can maintain social contact. Contact with the environment, whether through visual or physical interaction, facilitates a sense of body or self-boundary.

The adult patient immobilized by tractions, casts or neurological injury can also benefit by the use of mirrors. Mirrors can be attached to the bed. This provides continual visual feedback. Neurological patients who must remain flat in bed require special prism glasses. As soon as biologically possible, the patient should be transferred from the bed to a chair or wheelchair. Again, the nursing goal is to increase the patient's perceptual feedback. According to Kolb, "Body image also helps with the localization on the body surface of incoming sensory impulses and makes possible the performance of motor activitation through the constant relationship of the body to other objects."[46]

Activities are helpful in maintaing tactile and kinesthetic feedback. All patients, regardless of their age, need diversional activities. For the child, diversional or play activities are particularly important. Riddle points out that, "Diversion has a special role in preventing body image distortion, but a child cannot afford to abandon himself for long in any activity while besieged with body integrity fears. As he is helped to

[45]Catherine Norris, "The Professional Nurse and Body Image," In Carlson, C. (Ed), *Behavioral Concepts and Nursing Interventions*, (Philadelphia: Lippincott, 1970), p. 59.

[46]Kolb, *op. cit.*, p. 752.

manage his fears, he should have ample opportunities to lose himself in the sheer enjoyment of engrossing pursuits."[47]

The adult patient also benefits from diversional activities. An occupational therapist can be consulted for suggestions. Hand crafts, molding clay, or squeezing a ball are a few of the many activities which might be utilized by the patient. In addition, the nurse can play games or cards with a patient. Besides providing tactile and/or kinesthetic feedback, the above activities also encourage social interaction.

The nurse intervenes to facilitate social interaction between the patient and the family, friends, and people in the immediate environment—other patients and members of the health team. To reinforce the patient's realistic acknowledgment of the altered body image, the patient may be encouraged to interact with other people who have positively adapted to the same or similar problem. The nurse intervenes to establish one-to-one interaction or small group sessions. Amputees and stroke patients benefit from the knowledge and experience of other patients who share the same visible alteration in body part. The nurse keeps in mind that the patient with an amputation can be stereotyped as being less competent than before. The same stereotype might also apply to the patient with a stroke or myocardial infarction. These patients fear abandonment; therefore, they seek the sympathy of others by maintaining a helpless appearance. The patient is trying to achieve a sense of control over a threatening environment.

Through group discussions, patients can share their fears and frustrations. Group sessions facilitate the socialization process and acknowledgment of alteration in body part. Likewise, children and adolescents also need a similar socialization process. Both the child and adolescent are more comfortable with a one-to-one interaction. However, since peer evaluation is most significant, peer sessions can be utilized to help the patient cope with the altered image.

The socialization process can take place through play activities, watching television, eating, or simply talking. It becomes a time of preparation for further socialization outside the hospital. The child and adolescent can assess each other's reaction to their altered body part. Furthermore, socialization encourages the individual to think beyond self and focus temporary attention on the one with whom he or she is socializing.

The patient's family also needs support. The alteration in body image becomes their crisis as well as that of the patient. As with the patient, the family goes through a similar adaptative process of despair, depression, anger and hostility. The nurse constantly keeps in mind that when the family undergoes the crisis of a stroke, burns, disfigurement, or mutilating surgery, he or she can expect feelings of resentment to be

---

[47]Riddle, *op. cit.*, p. 657.

displaced onto him or her. The family might feel inadequate and helpless, therefore, anger gives them a feeling of power. Resentment may be the strongest from families with children. If the alteration of body image in the child was the result of a home accident, the family's resentment could be displaced guilt. The members of the family blame themselves for the alteration. It is quite possible that the family might even resent the child. The visible altered body part serves as a constant reminder of their inadequacies. Knowing this, the nurse intervenes to shape the family's attitude toward the damaged body part. The process begins with the onset of the alterations. This is the time in which the ground work is laid for the development of a reorganized or disturbed body image.

The nurse's many interventions ultimately lead the patient to reconstruction. The nurse attempts to help the patient reconstruct the altered body image as early as possible. The patient needs constant realistic encouragement that the illness or injury is progressing in an affirmative direction. A disfigurement, like scars or loss of a limb, may create internal feelings of worthlessness. The nurse must be aware of such feelings and help the patient to feel the significance, even within the crisis. The nurse draws upon the patient's internal and external strengths. The amount of internal strength depends upon the patient's concept of self, body image, and self-esteem prior to the injury. If the patient had a well-defined image, the nurse has a much easier time moving the patient along the health continuum. However, if the patient has a poor body image or self-concept, the task will be difficult.

Most of the actual reconstruction exists between the patient and family. The adaptive changes made to the altered body part depend upon them. Each is aware of the physical, psychological, or social loss. However, each is aware of the gains in terms of new approaches to their future and new strengths.

In conclusion, the nurse initially is a strong quiet being at the patient's bedside. As the patient's nurse, he or she is ready to realistically help the patient through the adaptive phases of illness or injury. While caring for the patient, the nurse gains knowledge about the patient's self and body image concept. On the basis of this knowledge, the nurse assists in planning for the future. The nurse, through goal-directed intervention, positively influences the patient's reorganization of the altered body image into something meaningful and worthwhile.

REFERENCES

Cardone, Samuel, "Psychophysical Studies of Body-Image," *Archives General Psychiatry* 21, October 1969, pp. 464–69.

Cleveland, Sidney, "Group Behavior and Body Image," *Human Relations,* 15, 1962, pp. 77–85.

Corbeil, Madeline, "Nursing Process for a Patient With a Body Image Disturbance," *NCNA,* 6, March 1971, pp. 155–63.

Dixon, J.C., "The Relation Between Perceived Change in Self and in Others," *Journal of General Psychology,* 73, 1965, pp. 137–42.

Dlin, Barney, "Psychologic Adaptation to Pacemaker and Open Heart Surgery," *Archives General Psychiatry,* 19, November 1968, pp. 599–610.

Dorpat, T.L., "Phantom Sensations of Internal Organs," *Comprehensive Psychiatry,* 12, January 1971, pp. 27–35.

Fisher, Seymour, "A Further Appraisal of the Body Boundary Concept," *Journal of Consulting Psychology,* 27, 1963, pp. 62–74.

———, "Body Image Boundaries in the Aged," *Journal of Psychology,* 48, 1959, pp. 315–18.

Gerstmann, Josef, "Psychological and Phenomenological Aspects of Disorders of the Body Image," *Journal of Nervous and Mental Disease,* 126, 1958, pp. 499–512.

Mathis, James, "Obesity—Sin or Savior?" *Psychosomatics,* 6, May-June 1965, pp. 499–72.

Orbach, Charles, "Modification of Perceived Body and of Body Concepts," *Archives General Psychiatry,* 12, February 1965, pp. 126–35.

Rubin, Reva, "Cognitive Style of Pregnancy," *American Journal of Nursing,* March 1970, pp. 502–508.

Ware, K.S., "Body Image Boundaries and Adjustment to Poliomyelitis," *Journal Abnormal Social Psychology,* 55, 1957, pp. 88–93.

Williams, Robert, "Body Image and Physiological Patterns in Patients with Peptic Ulcer and Rheumatoid Arthritis," *Psychosomatic Medicine,* 26, 1964, pp. 701–709.

Zimny, George, "Body Image and Physiological Responses," *Journal of Psychosomatic Research,* 9, 1965, pp. 185–88.

Zion, Leela, "Body Concept As It Relates to Self-Concept," *The Research Quarterly,* 36, pp. 490–95.

Zubek, J.P., "Effects of Prolonged Sensory and Perceptual Deprivation," *British Medical Bulletin,* 20, 1964, pp. 38–42.

Author Index

Subject Index